THE SCIENCE
AND
FINE ARTS OF FASTING

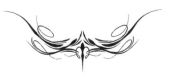

HERBERT M. SHELTON

Martino Publishing
Mansfield Centre, CT
2013

Martino Publishing
P.O. Box 373,
Mansfield Centre, CT 06250 USA

ISBN 978-1-61427-448-3

© *2013 Martino Publishing*

Cover design by T. Matarazzo

Printed in the United States of America On 100% Acid-Free Paper

The
Hygienic System:
Orthotrophy

Fasting

By

HERBERT M. SHELTON

D.P., N.D., D.C., D.N.T., D.N. Sc., D.N. Ph., D.N. Litt., Ph. D., D. Orthp.

PUBLISHED BY

DR. SHELTON'S HEALTH SCHOOL
SAN ANTONIO, TEXAS

First Edition 1934
Third Revised Edition 1950
Fourth Revised Edition 1963

WANT OF APPETITE is not always a morbid symptom, nor even a sign of imperfect digestion. Nature may have found it necessary to muster all the energies of our system for some special purpose, momentarily of paramount importance. Organic changes and repairs, teething, pleuritic eruptions, and the external elimination of bad humors (boils, etc.), are often attended with a temporary suspension of the alimentary process. As a rule, it is always the safest plan to give Nature her own way.

—FELIX L. OSWALD

INDEX

DEDICATION

T O A NEW ERA, *which has just begun to glow in the gold-red light of Eos, the goddess of dawn, while the deluge of medieval susperstitions is fast assauging, and many a submerged truth has reappeared like a bequest of a former and better world, to stand as way-marks on the road to a true Science of Life — its name a prophecy that links its destiny with invisible but strong ties, to the fate of the dainty butterfly: a grovelling grub entombs itself as a chrysalis in a cocoon whence it comes forth a being of celestial beauty, a winged flower of rainbow colors and pure silk, a fitting emblem of the fruition of life's renewed effort to assert its original purity and healthfulness—that no longer considers depravity and wretchedness as the normal condition of man, and happiness as the reward of a self-abhorring suppression of all natural desires; that rejects the blind confidence in the efficacy of an abnormal and myterious remedy, and realizes that the physical laws of creation find an echo in our innate monitor, this book is dedicated by*

—THE AUTHOR

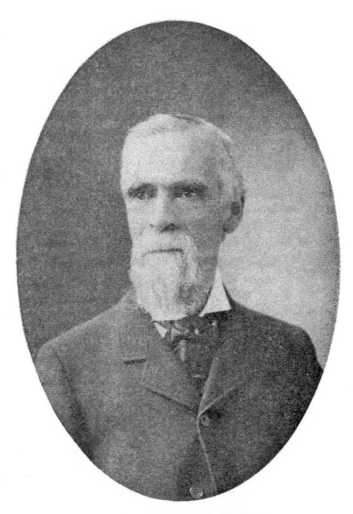

EDWARD HOOKER DEWEY

P URE JOYS never pall; uniformity is uniform happiness if the even tenor of our way is the way of nature. And nature herself will guide our steps if the exigence of abnormal circumstances should require a deviation from the beaten path. Remedial instincts are not confined to the lower animals; man has his full share of them; the self-regulating power of the human system is as wonderful in the variety as in the simplicity of its resources. Have you ever observed the weather-wisdom of the black bind-weed? — how its flowers open in the morning sun and close at the approach of the noontide glare; how its tendrils expand their spirals in a calm, but contract and cling, as with bands, to their support when the storm-wind sweeps the woods? With the same certainty our dietetic instincts respond to the varying demands of our daily life. Without the aid of art, without the assistance of our own experience, they even adapt themselves to the exigencies of our abnormal conditions, and our interference alone often prevents them from counteracting the tendency of dire abuses.

All dietetic needs of our body thus announce themselves in a versatile language of their own, and he who has learned to interpret that language, nor willfully disregards its just appeals, may avoid all digestive disorders — not by fasting if he is hungry, or forcing food upon his protesting stomach, not by convulsing his bowels with nauseous drugs, but by quietly following the guidance of his instincts.

Nature's health laws are simple. The road to health and happiness is not the labyrinthine maze described by our medical mystagogues. In pursuing their dietetic codes one is fairly bewildered by a mass of incongruous precepts and prescriptions, laborious compromises between old and new theories, arbitrary rules, and illogical exceptions, anti-natural restrictions and anti-natural remedies. Their view of the constitution of man suggests the King of Aragon's remark about the cycles and epicycles of the Ptolemaic system: "It strikes me the Creator might have arranged this business in a simpler way."

—FELIX L. OSWALD

Introduction to The Fourth Edition

A few years ago Louella Parsons said in her column, *Movie-Go-Round,* "I found out the reason that Gloria Swanson has been in complete seclusion since she's been in Hollywood. She's been on a water diet for eight days and has taken off 15 pounds. The only nourishment she had was to put carrots and other vegetables in water, let them soak, and drink the juices." I think that she meant that Miss Swanson drank the water in which the vegetables had soaked. This is not, strictly speaking, a fast, as we employ the term in this book, but it is so nearly so that Miss Swanson may be said, for all practical purposes, to have been fasting.

It is significant that no criticism of Miss Swanson was offered. Perhaps this may be taken as evidence of a changed attitude towards fasting and near-fasting. Twenty-five years ago, when the first edition of this book was issued, Miss Swanson would have been the subject of much criticism and ridicule and she would have been warned that if she did not give up such "faddish" practices and eat plenty of "good nourishing food," she would die of anemia, pneumonia or other disease thought to be the result of such practices. Indeed, she might have been warned that if she kept it up her heart would collapse and she would die.

In 1927 I was called to see a woman in New York City who had been suffering for an extended period and who had been under the care of a number of the most expensive specialists and medical professors in the city. She had had a number of fancy and expensive examinations and one exploratory operation and had been the victim of two or more consultations. It was decided that the cause of her condition (she had an accumulation of fluid in her chest) was not known and that nothing could be done except to aspirate the fluid at intervals and trust that nature would right matters. She was made weaker by each aspiration and did not recover from one before she *needed* another.

I advised a fast. She feared that, as she was weak already, she would grow too weak to tolerate another aspiration. I stated that the fast would obviate the need for another aspiration. It was debated by the family and I left with the issue undecided. Three days later I received an excited call from the husband who urged me to meet him at his home at once, stating that his wife had been fasting since I left and that she had done it without his knowledge. I expressed satisfaction with her action, but he was disturbed because her physician, who had just visited her and to whom she had revealed what she was doing, had told him that if she went without food for six days her heart would collapse and she would die. I met the husband at their home and we had another conference. It was decided to go ahead with the fast and let the physician, who had washed his hands of the case, saying he would have nothing more to do with it until she came to her senses and ate, go his own way. She fasted twelve days and greatly improved in health. After an interval of feeding she took another fast of thirteen days with further improvement. There were no more aspirations after she began the first fast and the fluid was rapidly absorbed.

The woman recovered her health, was soon back at her duties, and the physician, who apologized for his hasty action, in association with other men who had been on her case before, took her to Mt. Sinai Hospital for a complete check up and she was said to be fully recovered. The physician said that he had been reading up on similar cases and he had found that in Germany they were using fasting in such cases with good results. Strangely, he was unable to find these German references before I placed her on a fast and was unable to offer her any genuine hope. At any rate, the belief that fasting causes the heart to collapse has been left behind and the fear of fasting that once existed has been weakened.

Although at times there appears to be an awakening interest in fasting in the medical profession, the signs prove to be illusory. The profession never gives up its search for *cures* and these it seeks almost exclusively in the realm of poisons—in the exotic, adventitious and hurtful. The unending search for new and more effective *cures* signifies the lack of valid underlying principles to guide the physician in his care of his patient. Perhaps at no other period of history has there been such a rapid turn-over of *cures* as we have witnessed during the past twenty-five years, yet at no time in all past history has there been such a rapid increase in the incidence of and mortality from disease. With all the failures of all the

—8—

cures of the past twenty-five hundred years, the search still goes on for foreign and adventitious substances with which to *cure* disease and no attention is given to the management of the normal things of life to the end that a means of recovery may be found in these elements of living.

In no other area of human activity has any end ever been pursued with a more obsessed devotion and less appropriate techniques than has been the search for *cures*. This search for *cures* in exotic sources stems from a totally wrong conception of the nature of disease and from a wholly mistaken view of its causes. Few people are willing to admit that their imprudences in living are responsible for their diseases. They think that disease is something independent of their bodies, that it is even an entity with an independent existence that attacks them under circumstances over which they have little or no control. It is to their misfortune, rather than to their misconduct that they owe their sickness. This view relieves them of all responsibility for their condition and makes them unfortunate victims of forces beyond their control. Hence their implicit faith in the power of drugs to *cure* them, that is, to exorcise the attacking germ or virus.

Believing disease to have a separate existence, they are easily led to believe that a drug or a combination of drugs can be given to destroy that existence and, then, of course, they will be well again. This view is not only held but fostered by the medical profession, which finds the view financially profitable. Strangely enough, even those who persist in the old view that disease is a punishment sent by God Himself upon sinful men and women, do not hesitate to stay the hand of God with their drugs and treatments. Whether it is believed that disease is a "dispensation of Divine Providence," the invasion of the body by a demon or an attack upon the body by microbes and viruses, the idea that it can be *cured* by drugs prevails and practices based on this belief are in vogue.

Before the origin of the medical profession there existed, and although at a later period, was carried out co-incidentally with magic and religious procedures, a system of caring for the sick that consisted of adjusting the normal needs of life to the crippled condition of the sick organism. Among the measures employed under this system was that of fasting or abstinence from food. There was also a closely related procedure that consisted in feeding foods in smaller amounts or in feeding only certain easily utilized foods. When Plutarch advised: "Instead of using medicine, rather fast a day," he was undoubtedly advising a return to the pre-Hippocratic practice, that he thought that regulation of the way of life was superior to the drugging plan that had developed after Hippocrates. Celsus, who was not a physician, also advised abstinence from food, referring to the first degree of abstinence, "when the sick man takes nothing," and the second degree, "when he takes nothing but what he ought."

I do not agree with the common assumption that fasting, in the beginning, was a religious activity or that it was entered upon as a disciplining measure. Neither do I agree that, in its origin, it had any *spiritual* significance. A practice that is so well rooted in instinct and that is indulged in by both plants and animals, can hardly have originated in religion. That it has been incorporated into most religions and has long been invested by them with disciplinary, spiritual and sacrificial significance is not denied; it is only denied that it had a religious origin. Dr. M. L. Holbrook, a prominent *Hygienist* of the last century, declared: "Fasting is no cunning trick of priestcraft, but the most powerful and safe of all medicines."

"Everything according to law" is the testimony of scientists. Man becomes possessed of earth's treasures as soon as he learns the laws of their production. The discovery of the law is the first step towards exact knowledge. No laws governing drug *operation* have ever been discovered. Drugging, although today accompanied with extensive experimental work, is still, as it must always remain, an empirical practice. As it is an effort to make use of, in one department of nature, things that normally belong in another, there are and can be no laws governing its operations in this other department. Regulation of the way of life, on the other hand, can and must be based on the laws governing life and the relations of these elements to life. Thus it is that fasting, which we shall demonstrate is a normal part of the ways of life, may be carried out according to ascertainable laws of nature.

Much experimental work has been done with fasting, but most of it has been trivial and the results insignificant. For the most part, these experiments have been carried out on healthy animals and near-healthy human beings and they have been set up for the purposes of finding answers to certain problems in physiology. Often they have been set up in such a way as to fail to give the answers to the problems; often they have been of such short duration that the results were misleading. In almost all instances, the interpretations of results have been unworthy of school children.

In a letter to me dated April 4, 1956, Frederick Hoelzel, long assistant to Dr. Anton Carlson of the Department of Physiology of the University of Chicago, says: "I do not know where you and others, including regular medics, get the idea that Dr. Carlson is a great authority on fasting or has published a great deal on this subject except from the publicity he received in newspapers and popular magazines. He has talked a lot on the subject and has promoted studies by others on the subject, but about all he has done personally was to fast less than 5 full days himself in 1914 and that was for a study of hunger during what he called 'prolonged starvation.'"

Contrary to the implications of this statement, I never regarded Carlson as an authority on fasting. The publicity he received did strongly indicate that he was deeply interested in the subject and that he was carrying on experimental work in fasting. But I was always convinced that most of the work he did and most of the work done by his students and assistants was trivial and led nowhere. Like most research, it was a waste of time, money and human talents. As I shall show later, I regard his conclusions from his studies of "hunger" to be erroneous.

Others have done a little clinical experimenting with fasting and semi-fasting, but they have not differentiated between the fast and the limited diets they have fed, so that their conclusions may not be as conclusive as they seem to think. The *Lancet* (London) April 2, 1958 carried an article entitled "The Influence of Fasting on the Immunological Reactions and Course of Acute Glomerulonephritis." Briefly, the experiment was as follows: A test group fasted for the first sixty hours, except for one hundred ml. per day of unsweetened fruit juice. After sixty hours they were placed on a "semi-starvation diet" of sweet fruits and vegetables yielding not more than one hundred calories, until the Glomerular filtration rate increased and the hypertension edema subsided.

The *Control Group* were treated with bed rest and a light diet, which is one of the currently accepted treatments for this disease. It was found in this experiment that those who "fasted" recovered much more rapidly and completely than those who merely had bed rest and a light diet. But the test group did not have a full fast, nor was the period of abstinence of sufficiently long duration to provide for full results. Such tests may have some value, but they certainly fall far short of what is required to determine the value of the fast.

Another series of clinical experiences that have but limited value are those that have been carried out by Walter Lyon Bloom, M.D., in the Peidmont Hospital, Atlanta, Ga. His employment of the fast has been in cases of obesity, all cases being what he described as healthy subjects. They lost weight, they suffered no inconvenience from hunger, they found fasting easy, but they provided Bloom with no experiences or observations that are of dramatic significance. Bloom did come up with the observation that "our present preoccupation with eating at regular intervals has led to the misconception that fasting is unpleasant." His observations showed it to be otherwise.

Such tests as these may serve to confirm what we have known for a long time about the achievements of the living organism in a period of fasting, but they hardly add anything to our knowledge of the subject. In this instance, in the popular accounts given of Bloom's work, readers were warned not to undertake a fast except under the care of a physician (who would have no knowledge of how to properly conduct a fast) because if they had heart disease or liver or kidney disease or anemia, disaster might result. Had Bloom carried out his studies in the sick he would have known how much benefit patients with these diseases might receive from a properly conducted fast.

My opinion is that the time has arrived when the fast should receive more attention and approval. Slowly the ignorance of the past three centuries is being dispelled and it is becoming more and more apparent that our fathers and grandfathers were wrong in their determination to feed the sick "plenty of good nourishing food." Today the oldest natural resort in sickness is about to be re-recognized and mankind is again to benefit from a measure that should never have been abandoned, whether for drugs or for something else. It does not matter to me what the medical profession elects to do; the public is the important factor in this recognition.

Introduction to The First Edition

In presenting this volume on fasting I am well aware of existing prejudices against the procedure. It has long been the practice to feed the sick and to stuff the weak on the theory that "the sick must eat to keep up their strength." It is very unpleasant to many to see long established customs broken, and long cherished prejudices set at naught, even when a great good is to be achieved.

"Shall we not respect the accumulated wisdom of the three thousand years?," ask the defenders of the regular school and their feeding and drugging practices.

Where, we ask, is the wisdom for us to respect? We see little more than an accumulation of absurdities and barbarities. "The accumulated wisdom of three thousand years!" Look at sick humanity around you; look at the mortality reports; look at generation after generation cut off in the very spring-time of life, and then talk of wisdom or science!

In this volume we offer you real wisdom and true science—we offer you the accumulated wisdom of many thousands of years, wisdom that will still be good when the mass of weakening, poisoning and mischief-inflicting methods of regular medicine are forgotten. A brief history of fasting will help to prove the truth of this.

During the past forty years fasting and its *Hygienic* accompaniments have gained immense popularity and the position to which they are entitled by virtue of their intrinsic worth. The advocates of fasting are constantly increasing in number and the strenuous opposition that fasting has had to face from the medical profession and from laymen alike has merely served to advertise its possibilities and the simplicity and reasonableness of the claims made for it. The benefits that flow from a properly conducted fast are such that we do not hesitate to predict that it is the one procedure in disease that will be universally employed when it is once fully understood.

The literature of fasting is not well known to the average practitioner of whatever school. Few of them have made a study of the subject. Likewise, they have had no experience with fasting and lack confidence in its application. A brief review of the history of fasting will serve, therefore, as a background to the subject and will give confidence to practitioner and patient.

As will be shown later, fasting for the many purposes for which it has been employed, has been in use since before the dawn of history. Indeed, it may be said that it is as old as life. As a procedure in the care of the sick, it fell almost wholly into disuse during the Dark Ages and was revived only a little over a hundred years ago.

Records of fasting are found among almost all peoples in both ancient and modern times. Our encyclopedias tell us that, although the objectives of fasting vary among individuals, the aims of fasting fall, for the most part, into two distinct categories: (1) fasting for reasons of spiritual enlightenment, self-discipline and other religious motives; and (2) fasting for the purpose of achieving political ends. Unfortunately the writers of articles on fasting in the encyclopedias have limited themselves too severely in their studies of fasting; perhaps they have done this for the distinct purpose of suppressing many important truths about fasting. Writers of articles for encyclopedias are not addicted to the commendable habit of telling the truth and they are usually from ten to a hundred years behind the march of knowledge.

The authors of the articles on fasting in the various encyclopedias seem to confine their reading and bibliographies to religious fasting. Although none of the present-day encyclopedias that I have consulted carries the old statement that if a man goes without food for six days his heart will collapse and he will die, they carry statements almost as absurd. For example, the article on *starvation* in the latest edition of the *Encyclopedia Americana* carries the statement that the "preliminary" hunger is accompanied with "severe pain," in the stomach and epigastric region generally, thirst "becomes intense," "the face assumes, meanwhile an anxious, pale expression; * * * the skin is said to become covered with a brown secretion." It speaks of the "decomposition and organic decay of the tissues," as though the fasting person is undergoing a rotting process. "The gait totters, the mind becomes impaired, delirium and convulsions may ensue and death occurs." "From 8 to 10 days is regarded as the usual period during which human life can be supported without food or drink. * * * A case is recorded in which some workmen were dug out alive after fourteen days in confinement in a cold, damp vault; and another is mentioned in which a miner was extricated alive after being shut up in a mine for twenty-three days, during the first ten of which he subsisted on a little dirty water. He died, however, three days after his release."

There is, in this description, and there is much more to it (I have merely repeated the high-lights), of "starvation," no differentiation between fasting and starving, little differentiation between fasting with and fasting without water, and a gross exaggeration of the actual developments, together with the addition of fictional elements that are drawn from the realm of the imagination. The bibliography at the end of this section lists exactly three publications one of these dated 1884-5, one dated 1847 and the other dated 1915. But the most important part of the 1915 publication is entirely ignored.

Physiologists who discuss fasting, or as they prefer to term it, *starvation,* are as prone, as are the writers of articles for the encyclopedias, to rely upon a limited and antiquated bibliography. Howell, for example, in his *Textbook of Physiology,* a standard text, relies largely upon Voit. He gives as a bibliography of "original sources," Virchows's *Archives,* Vol. 131, Supplement 1893; Luciani's *Das Hungern,* 1890, Weber's *Ergebnisse der Physiologie,* Vol. 1, part 1, 1902, and finally Benedict's *A Study of Prolonged Fasting,* Carnegie Institute, No. 203, 1915.

Such deliberate suppression of all the accumulated information about fasting makes it extremely difficult for the student of the subject to learn the truth about fasting. Coupled with this suppression of information is the habitual failure of all standard authors to distinguish between fasting and *starving.* Is this done through ignorance, or is it done with *malice aforethought*; is it done for the deliberate purpose of prejudicing the student against the subject? I leave this for the reader to draw his own conclusions.

Fasting in its modern phase had its beginning with Dr. Jennings in the first quarter of the last century. Jennings may be said to have stumbled upon it by accident at a time when his waning faith in drugs caused him to look for other and more dependable means of caring for the sick.

It is quite common to see Dr. Dewey referred to as the "Father of the Fasting Cure." Dr. Hazzard, on the other hand, declares that "Dr. Tanner is justly entitled to first place among the pioneers of therapeutic fasting." I have no desire to detract one iota from the credit due these worthy men, but I must insist that first place belongs to Dr. Jennings, and wish to point out in this connection that Jennings possessed a fairly accurate idea of nature's "bill-of-fare for the sick," before Dr. Dewey discovered it in Yeo's Physiology.

Dr. Henry S. Tanner was born in England in 1831; died in California in 1919. His first fast was begun in July 17, 1877. Dr. Edward Hooker Dewey was born in Wayland, Pennsylvania in May, 1839; died March 28, 1904. In July, 1877 Dr. Dewey witnessed the first case that fasted to recovery, the stomach rejecting all food, and which set him to thinking about and finally employing fasting. Thus the work of Dewey and Tanner began almost simultaneously. However, Dr. Jennings was employing the fast before either of these men were born and wrote about it while they were both boys. Dr. Trall, Sylvester Graham, Dr. Shew, and others of their co-workers were also advocating and using the fast while Drs. Tanner and Dewey were school boys, although one almost never sees these men's names in the literature of fasting. We find Dr. Jennings using fasting as early as 1822 and Graham advocating fasting in 1832. In his work on *Cholera*, which is his published lectures on the subject, first delivered in New York City in 1832, he recommends fasting for cholera and other febrile conditions. The *Graham Journal* advocated fasting in 1837, its first year.

A writer in the *Graham Journal* for April 18, 1837, writing under the title "The Graham System—what is it?" includes in his item by item description of the system the fact that "abstinence should always be preferred to taking medicine—it is a benefit to lose a meal occasionally."

Another writer who signed himself, *Equilibrist*, writing under the title, "Stuff a Cold and Starve a Fever," in the *Journal* of Sept. 19 of the same year, quotes Dr. Beaumont's *Experiments on Digestion*—"in febrile diathesis, very little or no gastric juice is secreted. Hence, the importance of withholding food from the stomach in febrile complaints. It can afford no nourishment; but is actually a source of irritation to that organ, and, consequently, to the whole system. No solvent can be secreted under these circumstances; and food is as insoluble in the stomach as lead would be under ordinary circumstances," and adds, "In other remarks, if I remember right, the doctor states that food has lain in the stomach of Alexis St. Martin from 6 to 30 or 40 hours, unchanged except by chemical affinities (he is here referring to fermentation and putrefaction. H. M. S.) during some of his ill turns. And yet what multitudes think that when they have a 'bad cold' they must eat or they will certainly be sick! Oh! I must 'stuff a cold and starve a fever,' they will tell you, and go at it in earnest; and not unfrequently in this way bring on a 'fever' that will require weeks to 'starve out.'

"I can testify from my own 'experiments' as well as those of Doctor Beaumont, that any person having a 'bad cold' may find entire relief by abstaining from food, one, two, three, or perhaps five or six meals if the case is a bad one, and that too without taking a particle of medicine."

It is worthy of note that Graham and the Grahamites attempted to form their practices in conformity with what was known in physiology while the medical profession, though studying physiology in college, were then as now, forgetting it as soon as they got into practice and followed the time-honored practice of drugging which bears no normal relation to physiology and violates every physiological principle.

Dr. Oswald, who was a contemporary of Dewey, refers to fasting as "the Graham starvation cure." It is quite probable also that Doctors Page, Oswald, and Walter preceded Dewey and Tanner in the employment of fasting. Dr. Page's book, published in 1883, recounts recoveries while fasting and urges fasting in many cases. Dr. Oswald's *Fasting Hydropathy and Exercise* was published in 1900. These three men were all acquainted with the works of Dr. Jennings and were influenced much by him, frequently quoting him. I feel safe in assuming that they also received much from Trall and Graham. In his *How Nature Cures,* published in 1892, Dr. Densmore definitely ascribes his use of fasting to "studying the writings of Trall, Nichols, Shew and other writers and hygienic physicians" forty years before writing his own book.

Laboratory confirmation of the benefits of fasting is not lacking; but it is not needed. Science is not confined to the laboratory and human observation is often as reliable in the field of practice as in that of experiment. Much experimental work with fasting, both in men and animals, has been done by approved laboratory men. Little attention has been given by these men to the value of fasting in "disease" conditions, but their work is of value to us in a general study of the subject before us.

Dr. A. Guelpa, of Paris, employed short fasts in the treatment of diabetes and other chronic "diseases" and wrote a book on *"Autointoxication and Disintoxication: An account of a new fasting Treatment in Diabetes and other Chronic Diseases."* Dr. Herrick Stern published a book on *"Fasting and Under-Nutrition in the Treatment of Diabetes* (the Allen Treatment); while Drs. Lewis W. Hill and Rene S. Ackman wrote: *"The Starvation Treatment of Diabetes,"* in which they gave an account of the use of fasting in diabetes in the Rockefeller Institute.

In 1915 Frederick M. Allen, A.B., M.D., of the Rockefeller Institute Hospital "discovered" the "starvation treatment" of diabetes. Dr. Dewey successfully employed fasting in diabetes as far back as 1878; while Dr. Hazzard employed fasting in diabetes prior to 1906.

In 1923 *"Fasting and Undernutrition"* by Sergius Morgulis, Professor of Biochemistry in the University of Nebraska College of Medicine, was published. It is a most thorough study of fasting, starvation and undernutrition as far as these subjects have been worked out in the laboratory.

Although Prof. Morgulis has a wide acquaintance with the so-called scientific literature dealing with the subject of *fasting* or *inanition,* he voluntarily cuts himself off from all of the literature of so-called therapeutic fasting, and applies such terms as "enthusiasts," "amateurs" and "faddists" to those whose years of experience with fasting enable them to apply it to the care of human beings in the various states of impaired health. In an extended bibliography he mentions, from the many works on fasting by its exponents, only that of Hereward Carrington. Mr. Carrington's book is one of the best books on the subject which has yet appeared, but it is by no means complete or even up-to-date, having been published in 1908. Morgulis ignores the works of Jennings, Graham, Trall, Densmore, Walter, Dewey, Tanner, Haskell, Macfadden, Sinclair,

Hazzard, Tilden, Eales, Rabagliati, Keith and others who have had widest experience with fasting and who have written extensively upon the subject.

Necessarily, this limits his field very largely to the field of animal experimentation and also limits his knowledge of the effects of fasting in various pathological states. In the book there is no information on the proper conduct of the fast. The hygiene of the fast, crises during the fast, danger signals during the fast, breaking the fast—these and other very practical problems are not considered. Neither does he distinguish between *fasting* and *starving*. The omission of these things from a technical book is inexcusable.

Professor Morgulis' masterly work is full of technical data on the effects of abstinence from food upon the body and its various parts. However, since most of its data is based upon animal experimentation, he having elected to ignore the works on fasting by those who employ it, and since what is true of one species is not always true of another, the conclusions he arrives at in this work may be accepted only in a general way and do not always harmonize with the findings of those who employ fasting in men, and particularly in the care of the sick.

Most of the "scientific" works on inanition have little or no value for us in a study of fasting. This is so for the following reasons:

1. Abstinence from food may mean missing one meal, or it may mean abstinence from food until death results from starvation. In these works little or no effort is made to differentiate the changes that occur during the different stages of inanition.

2. Most of the studies (in man) have been in famine victims and these are not cases of fasting, nor do these people suffer only from lack of food. There is often exposure, there is always fear and worry, there are also the effects of one-sided diets. Findings in death in famines are classed as due to inanition and are not differentiated from fasting changes.

3. In total inanition no water is taken and many of the scientific experiments withhold water as well as food from the animals. The results of such experiments cannot be used to determine the results of fasting.

4. Inanition studies are all mixed up with pathologies of all kinds that occasion more or less inanition. Many of the studies of starvation in humans have been complicated with other conditions that account for much of the findings.

5. Studies of fasting changes are so mixed up with starvation changes and changes due to dietary deficiencies and there is so little discrimination between the three types of changes, that these books become very misleading.

6. None of the experimenters has ever observed properly conducted fasts of the sick under favorable conditions, hence they know almost nothing of its value under such conditions.

7. There is another source of confusion in these books. I refer to the frequent use of pathological terms to describe what is not pathological at all. The word "degeneration" is often used when no real degeneration is evident. Or, shall we say that there is a form of *degeneration* that may be properly designated physiological to distinguish it from another form that is distinctly pathological. For example, muscular "atrophy" that follows cessation of muscular work is not pathological. Decrease in size of a part from lack of food with no actual pathological changes in the tissues and no real perversion of its function is not degeneration, though commonly referred to as such in these books.

The same criticism may be made of *Inanition* and *Malnutrition*, by C. M. Jackson, M.S., M.D., LL.D., 1925. In a bibliography covering 108 pages, I was unable to locate the name of any man, other than Carrington, who is in a position to speak with authority on fasting. Jackson's is a very valuable book, crammed with technical data and detailed experimental results, but lacking in any reference to the hygienic value of the fast.

Much valuable work has been done by laboratory experimenters, but it is obviously lacking in certain important particulars. For example, Morgulis points out that fasting decreases sugar tolerance in dogs, but in no other animal. Indeed, he records that fasting is distinctly beneficial in diabetes in man. He records an experiment performed on fasting rats and pigeons in which the rats gave one result and the pigeons an exactly opposite result. In some species fasting diminishes the *reaction* to certain drugs, in other species it increases this *reaction.*

In certain animals, such as the frog, some of the senses are diminished; while in man the senses are remarkably improved. So distinctive is this sign that we regard it as evidence that our patient is fasting. Sight, taste, hearing, smell and touch are all acutened. Hearing and smell often become so acute that the faster is annoyed by noises and odors that are ordinarily unheard and unsmelled by him. Blindness, catarrhal deafness, sensory paralysis and loss of the senses of taste and smell have all been known to yield to the kindly influences of the fast. The cleansing of the system occasioned by fasting quickly revivifies the mental and sensory powers.

While fasting frequently produces temporary sterility in men, it has no such effect in salmon and seals. The gonads of salmon actually undergo a great increase in size while fasting, while both they and male seals fast during their entire mating season. It is only right that I add that it is denied by some that salmon actually fast during this season.

Prof. C. M. Child, of the University of Chicago, experimenting with worms, found that if a worm is fasted for a long time it does not die, but merely grows smaller and smaller, living on its own tissues for months. Then, after it has been reduced to a minimum size, if it is fed it begins to grow and starts life anew, as young as ever it was. While we know that fasting renews the human body, we also know that it will not renew it to the extent that it does the body of the worm. Man is not a worm, nor a dog, nor a pigeon, nor a rat. In a broad general sense, all animals are fundamentally alike; but there are specific differences, both in structure and function and in instinct and *reaction* as well as in individual needs, and for this reason it is always dangerous to reason from worm or dog to man.

This, however, does not hinder us from studying the similarities and differences existing between man and the sub-orders and making whatever use of these studies we may. It may be said that there is one particular in which all animals, including man, are alike; namely, their ability to go without food for prolonged periods and to profit by this.

For the most part the regular profession has either ignored or else denounced fasting. Fasting is a fad or it is quackery. They do not study it, do not employ it and do not endorse it. On the contrary, they declare that "the sick must eat to keep up their strength."

It is gratifying to see that a change is under way. Just recently (1933) a meeting of famous medical consultants from different parts of the British Isles, was held at Bridge of Allen, Stirlingshire, Scotland. The conference was presided over by Sir Wm. Wilcox. Among other notable physicians present were Sir Humphrey Rolleston, the King's Physician, Lord Horder, Physician to the Prince of Wales, Sir James Purvess-Stewart, Sir Henry Lunn, and Sir Ashley Mackintosh.

These men urged the value of fasting in "disease." Sir William Wilson said "the medical profession had been neglectful of the study of dietetics and fasting." Sir Henry Lunn, noted that there were several institutions (nature cure places) in England employing fasting and urged that *fasting is not a matter for "unqualified"* practitioners. Only a short time prior to this Sir Henry had said in the *Daily Mail* (London) that the "unqualified practitioners" were the ones who were *curing* their patients and added, "I am convinced that the result will be that heterodoxy, now claimed as their own possession by various unqualified healers, will become the medical orthodoxy and commonplace of the next generation."

The conference, instead of offering a little praise where it was long overdue, prepared, as Sir Henry had predicted, to steal the thunder of the "Natural Healers," branding these latter as "unqualified."

In 1927 Lord Horder (then Sir Thomas) declared: "I think there is value in the *occasional* missing of a meal, or in the substitution of a meal, *** but the elaborate and prolonged process of actual fasting which requires for its proper carrying out a complete or partial cessation from active work has never seemed to me to promise any benefits."

What caused this eminent medical man to change his mind? Only one thing could have forced him to join the conference in endorsing prolonged fasting—namely: the steady stream of recoveries in "incurable" cases which the British *Nature Curists* and *Natural Hygienists* continue to effect. Are these *Natural Hygienists* unqualified? Dr. Lief addresses the following questions to Lord Horder in the July, 1933 issue of *Health for All*:

"Which of these two is better *qualified* to use fasting as a method of therapy: (1) the practitioner who has studied over many years the special technique of curative fasting, who has administered fasting treatment in very many cases, and so is fully conversant with how to deal with the various crises and reactions that very frequently appear in fasting cases, or (2) the medical doctor, whose profession, as a body, has done nothing for years but condemn fasting, without investigation, and whose present interest in the treatment has only arisen as a result of the remarkable successes and the ensuing popularity of the so-called unqualified man?"

Certainly the study of Materia Medica and years spent in administering drugs cannot qualify one to conduct fasts. No intelligent person can investigate the subject of fasting without endorsing it and without being struck by the marvelous results it produces. But this same intelligence should lead him to fast under the care of one who fully understands fasting in all its details.

I will conclude this introduction with an endorsement of fasting by a physician of the highest standing, who, twenty years after he made the statement below, still endorses and employs fasting. In 1922 Major Reginald F. E. Austin, M.D., R.A.M.C., M.R.C.S., L.R.C.P., British Army Medical Service, wrote "some sixteen years experience of the treatment of the sick and ailing with the aid of fasting has convinced me that many of the so-called complications and sequelæ of disease are largely the result of forcing nourishment into an organism that is telling one as plainly as it can: 'For heaven's sake keep food way from me until my appetite returns. In the meantime, I will live on my own tissues.'"

Definition of Fasting

CHAPTER I

Nutrition may be conveniently divided into two phases—positive and negative—corresponding to periods of eating and periods of abstaining from food. Negative nutrition has received the terms fasting, inanition, starvation. Fasting and starving are separate phenomena, well demarked from each other. Inanition covers both these processes.

Fast is derived from the Anglo-Saxon word, *faest*, which means "firm" or "fixed." The practice of going without food at certain times was called fasting, from the Anglo-Saxon, fasten, to hold oneself from food. Like most English words, the word fasting has more than one meaning. Thus, the dictionary defines fasting as "abstinence from food, partial or total, or from proscribed kinds of foods." In most religious fasts abstinence from proscribed foods is all that is meant. We may define it thus: *Fasting—is abstention, entirely or in part, and for longer or shorter periods of time, from food and drink or from food alone.*

A misuse of the term fasting, is quite common. I refer to the use of the word fasting when a particular diet is referred to. We read and hear of fruit fasts, water fasts, milk fasts, etc., when talking of a fruit diet, a milk diet, etc. A fruit fast is abstinence from fruit; a milk fast is abstinence from milk; a water fast is abstinence from water.

The dictionary defines a *diet* as a "regulated course of eating and drinking, a specially prescribed regime. The daily fare, victuals, allowance of food; rations." To "diet" is "to regulate or restrict the food and drink according to a regime; to eat carefully or sparingly. To take food; to eat."

Fasting, as we employ the term, is voluntary and entire abstinence from all food except water. "Little driblet meals," says Dr. Chas. E. Page, "are not fasting. There should not be a mouthful or sip of anything but water, a few swallows of which would be taken from time to time, according to desire." We do not employ the word *fasting* to describe a diet of fruit juice, for example.

A writer speaks of fasting a child on fruits—but this means that the child was fed on fruits; that it was on a fruit diet. Fasting and feasting, no matter what one may feast upon, are not identical processes. We should be more careful of our use of terms.

Inanition is a technical term literally meaning emptiness, which is applied to all forms and stages of abstinence from food and to many forms of malnutrition due to various causes, even though the person is eating. If we keep the term *inanition* for all abstinence from food, the term *fasting* for that period of abstinence from the omission of the first meal to the recurrence of hunger, the term *starvation* for that period of abstinence from the return of hunger to death, we may avoid confusion. Prof. Morgulis classifies three types of inanition according to origin, as follows:

1. "Physiological inanition which is a normal, regular occurrence in nature. The inanition constitutes either a definite phase in the life cycle of the animal, it is a seasonal event, or it accompanies the periodic recurrence of sexual activity." The cases of the salmon and seal and of hibernating animals are examples of this. Voluntary fasting of normal subjects, either for exhibition purposes or for scientific study, Benedict calls "physiological fasting." Why this should be called "physiological fasting" and periods of enforced fasting, due to shipwreck, mine disasters, etc., should be called "starvation through accident," he does not explain, although the miners and shipwrecked sailors do not always starve. Often their periods of abstinence are relatively short and they live.

2. "Pathological inanition," which is in "various degrees of severity associated with different organic derangements"—obstruction of the alimentary canal (œsophageal stricture,) "inability to retain food (vomiting)." "excessive destruction of body tissues (infectious fevers)," and "refusal to take food either because of loss of appetite or mental disease." Benedict applies the phrase "pathological fasting" to disturbances of the digestive tract which preclude the taking of food.

3. "Accidental or Experimental Inanition." "In this category, of course, belong all individual experiences which have been the subject of carefully conducted scientific investigation."

To this should be added a fourth classification, a class with which Prof. Morgulis seems to be very largely unacquainted, which is largely or wholly voluntary but in which abstinence from food is not for mere experimental purposes, but for the promotion or restoration of health. I prefer to call this *hygienic fasting*. Others refer to it as *therapeutic fasting*. Fasting of this type is not wholly voluntary in acute "disease," except in the sense that all instinctive action is voluntary. It is the *hygienic fast* that we are chiefly concerned with in this volume, although we are going to make use of data gained from the other types of fasting that may be of service to us in better understanding and more intelligently conducting a fast.

Benedict mentions cases of fasting in hypnotic sleep, but provides no details. I have had no experience with such cases and have made no study of them. I should think that the phenomena in hypnotic sleep would follow the usual course. It may be possible that there would be more complete rest in hypnosis, although I am inclined to regard the state as one of tension. I certainly do not recommend hypnosis at any time for any purpose. I regard it as an unmixed evil.

In his *Inanition and Malnutrition*, Jackson says the term starvation "is more frequently used to indicate the extreme stages of inanition, leading to death." Unfortunately, this is too often not the case. Too often the term starvation is applied to the whole period of abstinence from food from the first day to the end in death.

Carrington says: "Many doctors speak of 'the fasting or starvation cure' — which simply shows that they don't know what they are talking about. Fasting is an absolutely different thing from starvation. One is beneficial; the other harmful. One is a valuable therapeutic measure; the other a death-dealing experiment." — *Physical Culture*, May, 1915.

A distinction must be made between fasting and starving, as will be seen as our study proceeds. Fasting is not starving. The difference between *fasting* and *starving* is immense and well demarcated. Dr. Hazzard expressed this fact in these words: "Starvation results from food denied, either by accident or design to a system clamoring for sustenance. Fasting consists in intentional abstinence from food by a system suffering from disease and non-desirous of sustenance until rested, cleansed, and ready for the labor of digestion."

Fasting is neither a "hunger cure" nor a "starvation cure," as it is sometimes called. Fasting is not starving. The fasting person is not hungry, and fasting is not a method of treating or *curing* "disease." Dr. Page says, "The term frequently applied—'starvation cure'—is both misleading and disheartening to the patient: the fact is he is both starved and poisoned by eating when the hope of digestion and assimilation is prohibited, as is, in great measure, the case in all acute attacks and more especially when there is nausea or lack of appetite."

Fasting is a rest—a physiological vacation. It is not an ordeal nor a penance. It is a house-cleaning measure which deserves to be better known and more widely used.

Fasting Among The Lower Animals

CHAPTER II

In the study of fasting it is necessary that we approach the subject from many angles. Perhaps no subject is less understood by the public and the "healing" professions than this oldest of means of caring for the sick body.

We are justified in studying every phenomenon which may throw light upon the subject and thus enable us to better apply the fast in our dealings with the sick. The fasting habits of man and animals are all legitimate objects of study. Not alone the fasting practices of sick animals, but fasting in healthy animals, whether voluntary or enforced, will aid us in more clearly understanding this subject. Particularly will such a study aid us in overcoming our cultivated fear of fasting. Hence the following studies.

The more one attempts to find out about the habits and modes of living of animals, the more one is impressed with the paucity of our dependable accumulated knowledge of the animal kingdom. Our biologists seem to be more intent upon classification than upon the important phases of life. If they study an animal, they prefer to kill it and dissect it, perhaps to mount it and place it in a case. They are more intent upon a study of death than of life. All unconsciously, perhaps, they have converted biology into necrology. I have, however, after much searching, succeeded in accumulating a considerable amount of material about the fasting habits of many animals. This I here propose to discuss under its various heads, as I have classified it.

FASTING WHEN NOT HUNGRY
Many animals normally go for long periods between feedings, not eating for the reason that they are not hungry. For example, there are many snakes that eat only at long intervals. Prolonged periods of abstinence from food and even water in some animals is compatible with both violent physical activity and unusual activity. In other animals it is compatible with reproductive processes, although physical activity is reduced to a minimum.

FOOD SCARCITY

I need devote but little space to the fact that animals fast for shorter or longer periods in times of food scarcity when floods, droughts, storms, etc., destroy their food supplies, or when snow has covered their food and rendered it temporarily inaccessible. It often happens in the lives of animals that they are forced to go for days at a time without food for the reason that they cannot find it. They sometimes, though relatively rarely, perhaps, go so long without food that they die of starvation. Luckily, they possess sufficient reserves to enable them to go without food for prolonged periods and survive. Animals that enter the winter season with considerable fat, commonly emerge from winter rather thin due to the fact that they are forced to subsist on greatly reduced food supplies and often have to go for days at a time without food. Even at the height of the food season insects may so completely destroy the food supply that many animals are forced to go for considerable periods without food.

FASTING IN ACCIDENTAL IMPRISONMENT

A number of accidental emergencies force both domestic and wild animals to fast at times. How frequently such accidents occur in nature we are not in a position to say, but they are probably more frequent than we may suppose.

In his *Curiosities of Instinct*, Karl Vogt tells of the case of a spaniel which visitors had accidentally locked up in the attic of an old castle-ruin. The dog had been able to secure a few drops of water by gnawing the edge of a cleft in a slate covered roof. A few heavy rain-showers had supplied him with water, but he had had no food of any kind—no grain, leather, rats or mice—during the whole summer and part of the autumn. A picnic on the castle mountain during the first week in October resulted in his rescue by a wandering party of sight-seers. The ribs of the little prisoner, who had been locked up since the middle of June, could be counted as easily as in a skeleton, but he was still able to drag himself across the floor and lick the hands of his deliverers.

The following account of "Bum" appeared in *Time* for April 27, 1931: "When Joseph Carroll, engineer of a Brooklyn laundry heard the Negro night watchman tell of a "ghost" he had heard one night last week, he walked into the engine room and straight to a boarded-up hole in the floor, relic of an unsuccessful well-digging. Stopping his ears, holding a knife in his teeth, he touched the knife to a pipe which went downward. Presently he could hear a distant moaning.

"He knew what was in the hole. Early in January he had found and adopted a mongrel puppy. But after a few days the puppy, which he called 'Bum,' disappeared. The same day, the hole over the excavation had been boarded up securely. The engine's noise must have drowned the dog's cries ever since.

'Hastily Engineer Carroll ripped up the board, descended, brought 'Bum', a skeletal dog, unable to stand alone, to the surface.

"No local veterinary would believe that a dog could have fasted for 14 weeks. Some thought 'Bum' must have lived by rat-catching; some cried: 'Impossible!' "

Local veterinarians were as ignorant of fasting as was a medical man who once roundly scored a woman who had undertaken to fast, under my direction, after he and several of his big priced colleagues (specialists and medical professors) had declared they did not know and could not find out what her trouble was and could do nothing for her. He declared that if she went six days without food her heart would collapse and she would die.

She had two fasts, one of twelve days, the other of thirteen, and recovered her health. The doctor came crawling back some three months later and apologized for his ungentlemanly and unprofessional conduct. "I have been reading up on these cases and I find that in Germany they are using fasting in them with excellent success," he said.

An Associated Press dispatch from Warsaw, Ind., dated Dec. 31, 1931, tells of a sow surviving four and a half months without food. Buried under an avalanche of straw on the Oscar Rebman farm, east of Warsaw, on July 15, while threshing was in progress, she remained buried until Dec. 30, when workmen who were pulling out straw heard a grunt and were surprised to see the sow walk out minus about half of her former weight. This was a period of 168 days without food and water.

A Reuters distpach from Durban, So. Africa, dated Nov. 3, 1955 tells of a cat that was found the day before by workers in an assembly plant, which had been accidentally sealed into a case of automobile parts, in Crowley, England, August 1. It had made the journey from England and had lived for three months without food. The news account said nothing of water, but, presumably the cat had also been all or most of this time without water. The cat died. It was stated that "a veterinarian treated the cat throughout the night, but it died of general exhaustion." It is possible that it died of the treatment. Few if any veterinarians would know how to properly care for an animal that had been so long without food. On the other hand, if the cat had been without water for three months, it is remarkable that it was still alive. It must have been almost completely dehydrated.

The "Great Blizzard of '49" was so terrible that many men, women and children and much livestock in the West froze to death. Many sheep froze around the haystacks. Unusually heavy snows fell and in some places remained for long periods. The snow was deep and animals were buried. Several reports of animals being buried deep in the snow for long periods were published. These are of special interest to us here, for the reason that these buried animals were deprived of food and of all possibility of obtaining food by the snow that covered them.

An Associated Press dispatch from Rapid City, S. D., tells of a pig found fifty-four days after the blizzard in that state. The dispatch says that before the blizzard of Jan. 2, 1949 struck, Jess Sparks, a farmer who lived northwest of Rapid City had twenty-one pigs. After the storm was over he could find but twenty of his pigs. He gave up, as lost, the missing pig. Forty-four days after the snow storm had buried the pig, Mr. Sparks heard a grunt. Digging through several feet of snow he soon released the pig, which walked out under its own power and, although very thin, did not resume eating at once.

A similar incident was reported by Jack Stotts of Cody, Wyo., who dug out a straw-stack that had been buried twenty feet deep for sixty-three days and found two Hereford heifers a little wobbly but otherwise in good condition. John Lemke, a farmer, in Dupress, S. D., dug out a sow that had been buried for three months. At the time of her burial she weighed three hundred pounds. She was skinny when rescued, but able to walk three quarters of a mile to a feed trough.

On the Wm. Brandt farm near Fort Morgan, Colo., a sheep was found alive on Feb. 12, 1949, after having been entombed in a snowdrift for forty days, having been hemmed against a board fence by the big blizzard that struck in early January. A companion sheep was dead. The two sheep had eaten away a small portion of a wooden fence. Other than this, they had no food while buried in the snow.

These are examples of burial of domestic animals. Wild animals must also frequently be buried by the snow and must remain for shorter or longer periods in their prisons. How many examples of burials similar to the foregoing burials of domestic animals that blizzard would have afforded, had they been recorded, we can only surmise. As the snow of the blizzard blanketed many thousands of square miles of territory, wild life could not have escaped it. Small animals especially were buried. They were forced to live without eating during their burial. The ability of an animal to fast for long periods under such conditions, means the difference between surviving and perishing.

Rabbits are well-known to be frequently buried in the snow. If we could know just how often such things occur in nature and how many hundreds of thousands of animals are thus forced to go without food for considerable periods each year, we would probably find that the ability to fast is a very important means of survival.

FASTING WHEN ANGRY OR EXCITED

An animal will refuse food when angry or excited. Indeed, an animal that is hungry and in the process of eating may be angered and will cease eating. Angry animals do not resume eating until their anger has subsided. Reports of dogs grieving over the absence or death of their owners, refusing food for long periods, are often carried by the press.

Of a similar character are those fasts undergone while standing guard. The polar bear, that is, the male, at least, will go without food for days, if his mate is wounded or killed. He stands guard over her and will attack with great ferocity any man or animal that comes near. Just how long he will stand guard over a dead female and go without food is unknown. But a few days of this hunger watch is all that have yet been verified.

FASTING IN CAPTIVITY

Some animals refuse to eat when held in captivity. They will starve to death rather than live as captives, thus making good Patrick Henry's ringing cry: "Give me liberty or give me death." One of these is the famous marine iguana, *Ambyrhymchus Cristatus*, a sea-shore lizard, of the Galapagos Islands, described as the "Vegetarian dragon" and "Fasting man." The iguana feeds on sea-weeds and can abstain from food for long periods—over a hundred days.

EXPERIMENTAL FASTS

Many thousands of animals of all kinds have been employed in experimental fasts. Insects, fishes, snakes, birds, rodents, rabbits, badgers, cows, horses, and many other types of animals have been used in fasts of varying lengths of time. In many of these fasts, the period of abstinence from food has been extended far beyond the normal limit of the fast into the period of starvation, some of them being ended before death occurred, others being carried on to death. While we are opposed to the suffering caused in animals by pushing the period of abstinence beyond the return of hunger, it has been done and the information thus obtained is available and we are at liberty to make use of it in our studies of the subject. Many of these experimental fasts will be referred to as we proceed in our study.

Writing of fasting experiments in animals, Benedict has the following to say about dogs and men: "The results obtained are of value to physiology in general, but of less value to human physiology. The metabolism of the dog is not that of man, for the nature of the food is such as to demand markedly different treatment in the alimentary tract. Both the stimuli to secretion and the composition of the digestive fluids are markedly different, and it seems probable that the deductions from the experiments with animals are of questionable value when applied to a man. This is perhaps even more noticeable in experimenting in pharmacology than in physiology, yet it is true that marked differences in physiological characteristics are observed between animals and men".

FASTING AFTER BIRTH

Fasts of longer or shorter duration are seen in many animals immediately after birth. For example, Fabre tells us that certain spiders eat no food for the first six months of their lives, but feast upon sunbeams. Chickens take neither food nor water for the first three days after they hatch from the egg. In most mammals there is no milk secreted for three or more days after their young are born. The fluid secreted during this period is devoid of food value.

PUPAL SLEEP

The *pupal* stage of insects which undergo metamorphosis, is that immediately following the larval stage. The term *chrysalis* has almost the same value as *pupa*. If the insect is not wholly quiescent during this *pupal* stage the word *nymph* is used. Since the larval stage of most insects differs so markedly from the adult stage, the pupal stage constitutes the intermediate stage in which the necessary bodily changes are effected. It is a period of internal transformation, during which most *pupa* are outwardly quiescent, they move very little, and do not eat at all. The marvelous structural and functional transformations take place during this period of abstinence from food, the *pupa* depending entirely upon its stored reserves for the accomplishment of its structural revolution. *Pupal* sleep may be artificially prolonged.

FASTING DURING THE MATING SEASON

That some animals fast during the mating season is well known, but our knowledge of the living habits of the animal kingdom is so meager that it is not known how many animals do so. So far as it is at present known, fasting during the breeding season is very rare among mammals and birds. Among mammals where there is keen competition between the males for possession of the females, feeding is curtailed, but this is hardly a fast.

Quite a number of fishes fast during the breeding season, the female of the *Cichlidae,* or mouth breeders, must fast at this time. *See History of Fishes,* by J. R. Norman. The best known example of fasting by fish during the mating season is that of the long fast of the male salmon. Prof. Morgulis describes in these words, the annual fast of the salmon: "At the time they commence to migrate from the sea towards the streams, their muscles are thoroughly encumbered with huge masses of fat. Fasting all their journey, which lasts many weeks and months, they are in a much emaciated condition when they get to the upper reaches of the rivers where the currents are rough and swift. Freed from the fat, however, their muscles are now agile and nimble, and it is at this time that the salmon displays the marvelous endurance and skill admired by all sportsmen, in progressing steadily against all odds of the tumultuous current, water-falls and obstructions."

Penguins and the male goose are the only birds I find mentioned as fasting during the mating season. The gander loses about one-fourth of his body-weight during this period. George G. Goodwin, Associate Curator, Department of Mammals, The American Museum of Natural History, New York, says: "It is questionable if any of the birds are capable of a prolonged fast—their rate of metabolism is too high. I have never heard that a gander fasted during the mating season and am inclined to question such a statement."

The basis of his questioning is not very solid; he has never heard of it. It may be assumed that if it were true he would have heard of it, but no man knows everything in biology and this is out of his special field. The other part of this objection, the high rate of metab-olism of birds, is no basis at all. It only reveals that he knows little of fasting. It is not likely that the rate of metabolism of the male salmon is low while he swims hundreds of miles up-stream. His *a priori* doubts must be considered, but they are not to be taken as final.

The Alaskan fur seal bull is the best known example of fasting by a mammal during the mating season. I have no information on the rate of metabolism in this mammal, but I think we are safe in assuming that, since he is a warm blooded animal and, at the same time, extremely active during the whole of the fasting period, his metabolic rate is high. During the entire three months breeding season of each year, the Alaskan fur seal bull does not eat nor drink (although within easy reach of abundant food) from May or the mid-dle of June to the end of July or early days of August. After fighting for his place on the shore and for his harem of from five to sixty fe-males, the male seal spends the summer fighting to keep his harem together and to keep his girls satisfied. Ray Chapman Andrews says, in his *End of the Earth*: "All through the summer he neither eats nor sleeps. It is just one long debauch of fighting and love-making and guarding his harem against unscrupulous invaders."

As a result of all this activity, Mr. Andrews says that "by Sep-tember he is a wreck of his former self. All his fat has disappeared, for that is what he has been living on by absorption all summer. His bones protrude, his side is torn and scarred, he is weary unto death. Blessed sleep is what he needs. Forsaking his harem, he waddles back into the long grass far away from the beach, there to stretch out in the warm sun. He will sleep for three weeks on end without waking, if undisturbed."

After long months of incessant physical and sexual activity, without food, the seal thinks first of rest and sleep. Food may be had after the long sleep. With man, also, despite popular prejudices to the contrary, there are times when rest is of more importance than food.

The sea lion also fasts during the mating season. Although less tempestuous, the domestic life of the sea lion is described as being very similar to that of the fur seals. Coming ashore sometime between the middle of May and early June, the summer is spent in fasting and sexual activities. By the end of summer, the master of the harem is exhausted and has lost much weight, but is still able to wearily slip down the sloping beach into the sea, where a few months of fat living restore his emaciated form. The exertions of these sea lions, both sexual and physical, as they fight much, is described as tremendous. I have no information as to whether they, like the fur-seal bull, go without water during this period.

What may be regarded as fasting during the mating season is the phenomenon seen among many insects which have but a short adult life. The caterpillar does little else than eat. In certain species, after it becomes a butterfly, it never eats at all. Fabre showed that some insects have no provision for hunger, the digestive organs being absent in the fullest developed insects. Perhaps such short-lived species as *ephemera* should not be considered in this connection. These insects come into the world in the evening, mate, the female lays her eggs and by morning both sexes are dead without ever having seen the sun. Destined for little else than reproduction, they have no mouth and do not eat, neither do they drink. But the peacock butterfly, which often travels for miles in search of a mate and lives for a few days, though it has the merest semblance of a digestive apparatus, does not eat. The insect world presents us with many examples of this kind.

Fasting during the mating season probably serves some very useful purpose. We know at least, that in the case of certain very low forms of life, it restores the male after several generations of parthenogenetic reproduction. For best results, animals that fast during the mating season seem to require a reduction of surfeit. They purchase rejuvenescence by curbing their anti-symbiotic propensities and abandoning conditions of surfeit. Instability resulting from surfeit and illegitimate food can be gotten rid of and stability regained only by a return to moderation and appropriate food. For immediate results abstinence from food is essential.

Reinheimer thinks that fasting has the effect of assisting towards a re-establishment of a tolerable degree of domestic symbiosis—both for ordinary physiological, as well as for genetic purposes—in those cases where domestic symbiosis is in danger of becoming perverted by the particular organism's transgressions against the laws of biological symbiosis.

HIBERNATION

All animals adapt themselves in some manner to the winter season. Winter is a difficult period for many plants and animals in northern countries. With its short days, low temperature, stormy weather, and scarcity of food both animals and plants are faced with the problem of keeping alive under very unfavorable circumstances. Both animals and plants have found many solutions to this problem, adapting themselves to winter in a wide variety of ways. Migration, as by birds, is but one of many solutions animals have found for this perplexing problem. Birds that migrate may lead a life as active in their southern homes as they do in their northern homes in the Spring and Summer. This is not so of animals that do not migrate.

Some animals store away supplies of food for this period. Bees store up honey, squirrels store away nuts, the mouse stores away food in various caches, the beaver stores twigs, gophers and chipmunks store up roots and nuts on which they feed when they awaken on an occasional warm day. On the colder days, these sleep and take no food. This is to say, many animals that store away food in various caches fast much during the winter months.

Other animals store their food supplies within themselves. These internal food supplies serve the animal as well as do the caches of food stored outside the body by other animals. We may say, then, that some animals store up their winter food supply within themselves. Hibernation by those animals that depend upon internal stores during the winter season is the solution for the exigencies of winter that has been adopted by more forms of life than any other solution. Bats, mice, hedgehogs, woodchucks, toads, newts, lizards, snakes, snails, flies, wasps, bees, and the great hosts of insects, bears, crocodiles, alligators, and many other animals do not migrate, but go into winter quarters. Animals that store up food outside themselves also carry internal supplies, for they, too, are often forced to go for extended periods without food. Squirrels, for example, frequently forget where they have buried their store of nuts.

Hibernation is a dormant state of existence, accompanied by greatly diminished respiration, circulation and metabolism, in which animals in the temperate regions spend the winter. During this period the animal functions are nearly suspended; the body heat is lowered to or nearly that of the air, the action of the heart is much reduced and the animal loses from thirty to forty percent of its weight. During hibernation the mammal may not feed, depending entirely on the stored food reserves within the body. The evidence at hand indicates that in such instances the body weight may drop as much as fifty per cent. Indeed, in bats, it drops more than this. In other animals food is stored within their winter nest and the hibernating animal awakens from time to time to consume its food.

Writing in *The National Geographic Magazine* (July 1946) under the title "Mystery Mammals of the Twilight," Donald R. Griffin says that hibernation of bats and other animals is still in many respects a "mystery to biologists." Mystery or not, it is a common fact of nature and represents one of the means adopted by animals to adapt them to the exigencies of winter.

Hibernation is most common in cold-blooded animals that are unable to leave regions of severe winters, but it is also practiced by numerous warm-blood animals. Some biologists say that the term hibernation should be restricted to a few mammals and prefer the phrase "lying low and saving nothing" for what they describe as the coma or lethargy of many of the lower animals, like some frogs and fishes, many snails and insects. Other biologists, although seeming to prefer to limit the term hibernation to the "winter sleep" of warm-blooded animals, also include under this term the "seasonal torpidity" of frogs, toads, reptiles, certain fishes, insects, the horseshoe crab and snails.

Among the many different forms of "lying low" seen in the winter life of animals are:

1. The relapsed life of some insect pupæ, where the body of the larva (*i.e.*, maggot) has become greatly simplified in structure; in fact almost embryonic again.

2. The arrested development of other insect larvæ, such as caterpillars and pupæ, where the metamorphosis into the winged form has ceased for the time being, like a stopped watch.

3. The suspended animation of small creatures, like bear animalcules (some of them quaintly like microscopic hippopotami) and wheel animalcules and small thread worms, in which we can detect no vitality for the time being.

4. The comatose state of snails and frogs, where we can see the heart beating, though the life of the body as a whole is at a very low ebb.

5. The state of true hibernation, restricted to a few mammals, such as hedgehog and dormouse, marmot and bat. This is a peculiar state very unlike normal sleep, with most of the vital functions, even excretion, in abeyance, with the heart beating very feebly and the breathing movements scarcely perceptible.

In all of these forms of "lying low" the animals hide away and cease their activities and approach a state of suspended animation during the winter months. Hibernation, so common among animals, appears, then, to be one aspect of the general tendency of animals to withdraw from an unfavorable environment. In hibernation the animal passes through the unfavorable period of low temperature and food scarcity in a dormant state. Thus hibernation, like migration, is one of the means of solving the food problem during the period of acute scarcity.

Mammals that hibernate are referred to by certain biologists as "imperfectly warm-blooded types," which are unable to produce enough animal heat to make good their losses in cold weather. It is doubtful if this is true of those species in which only the female hibernates. Food scarcity, rather than depressed temperature, seems to be the chief reason for hibernation. As æstivation is practically identical with hibernation, only taking place under certain opposite conditions (when it is hot rather than cold) but where, as in hibernation, there is food scarcity, those mammals that æstivate cannot be said to be "imperfectly warm-blooded types." The example of the tenree, that æstivates at the time for æstivation, even when far removed from its Madagascar home and placed where the temperature is warm and there is an abundance of food, would seem to indicate that there is more to this phenomenon than merely the external circumstances under which it occurs.

Hibernation resembles sleep and has been likened to a trance, but it is not sleep. The hibernating animal does sleep all or most of the time it hibernates, but hibernation is different from sleep. Sleep is not seasonal and is not occasioned by scarcity of food. Hibernation is prolonged and body temperature drops very low in this state whereas it tends to remain normal in sleep. Heart beat and respiration are very low in hibernation, they are reduced but slightly in sleep. Excretion is suspended in hibernation, it may be increased in sleep. There is great loss of weight during hibernation, in sleep there may be a gain of tissue. Hibernation is confined to the cold season, sleep takes place throughout the year, both at night and in the day time and lasts but a few minutes to a few hours at a time. Griffin says that the "torpor of hibernation is much more prolonged than ordinary sleep."

Is it correct to refer to hibernation as a comatose condition? Is the animal in a coma? Is the hibernation state one of torpor, lethargy, stupor? These terms are frequently used by biologists in describing the hibernation condition. Coma is defined as an "abnormal deep stupor occurring in illness or as a result of it," such as alcoholic coma, apoplectic coma, uremic coma, diabetic coma, coma vigil, etc. It would be interesting to know what a normal coma is. Stupor is defined as a "condition of unconsciousness, torpor, stupor. A state analogous to hypnotism, or the first stage of hypnotism." It is seen in African sleeping sickness, encyphalitis lethargica, hysteria and other pathological states. Torpor is "numbness, abnormal inactivity, dormancy, apathy." Torpid means "not acting vigorously, sluggish." Biologists use such terms as coma, comatose, lethargic, stupor, trance, etc., in describing hibernation as though there is something essentially pathological about it.

Dormant is perhaps the better word, as the root *dor* means sleep, although, as previously pointed out, hibernation is not synonymous with sleep. Dormant means "being in a state resembling sleep, inactive, unused." That hibernation does resemble sleep in many particulars is certain; that the hibernating animal is even more inactive than in sleep is equally true. Perhaps we can define hibernation as a dormant state of existence accompanied with greatly diminished respiration, circulation and metabolism in which many animals in the temperate regions pass the winter.

In hibernation the animal seeks out a secluded nook or burrow or a cave, where the temperature is higher than that outside and sinks into a strange reptile-like state. There it lies, or as in the case of the bat, hangs, in safety through the cold and storm. It eats nothing, it excretes nothing, the heart beats feebly, the breathing movements are scarcely perceptible—yet it survives. Indeed, it seems certain that it would not survive otherwise. Thus, hibernation viewed biologically, is seen to be an adaptation to the cold of winter by which the animal is enabled to survive.

Danger lies in sub-freezing weather for the hibernating mammal and many are frozen to death when their place of abode becomes too cold. Griffin says of the bat: "Another important requirement also usually satisfied by caves and burrows is that the temperature should not go below freezing. Apparently no mammal can survive freezing when it is hibernating and its body temperature is at the mercy of the surrounding air temperature." He tells of finding bats in caves, the openings of which are great enough to permit freezing, frozen up in huge ice stalactites. Most of the bats, he says, awaken and fly away to another and better sheltered cave, when the cave in which they are hibernating begins to get cold.

HIBERNATION IN PLANTS
Perhaps before we give further attention to hibernation among animals we may profitably take a hasty glance at the hibernating practice of plants. The "winter sleep" of trees, shrubs and many other plants is seen on every hand during winter. With the approach of Fall, these shed their leaves, their sap descends and they exist in a dormant state until the coming of Spring. In like manner bulbs, tubers, etc., undergo a prolonged "winter sleep." These plants fast through the whole of the winter months, taking no food during the

time. They take no carbon and nitrogen from the air and extract no minerals and nitrates from the soil. Metabolism is practically non-existent during this period. The cessation of the flow of sap in trees during the winter season is similar to the almost ceasing of circulation in hibernating animals. Plants like the daffodil, onion, beet, turnip, etc., store up large supplies of food in their roots—bulbs and tubers—during the Summer. Their tops die off in the late Fall or early Winter and they lie dormant during the long Winter, only to send up new stems and leaves when Spring arrives. This storing up of food in their roots is similar to the storing of fat by the bear.

HIBERNATION IN ANIMALS

Hibernation is common among insects and is seen in every group of vertebrates except birds, which substitute migration for hibernation. It is largely found in insect and vegetable eating species. Hibernation occurs regularly throughout the winter in such invertebrates as snails, crustaceans, myriapods, insects, arachnids, and the lower vertebrates, such as reptiles, amphibians and some fresh-water fishes. Many mammals inhabiting the colder regions, especially species living on the ground, or whose principle sources of food are unavailable in the winter, are known to hibernate. In such hibernating animals as the bat, ground-squirrel, marmot, hedgehog and dormouse, the temperature of the body drops from its typical warm condition to one or two degrees Centigrade above that of the surrounding air. In maximum dormancy the heart-rate is slowed considerably, sometimes to only one or two percent of the normal heart rate, the respiratory movements drop off to a similar extent and determination of oxygen consumption indicates a reduction to as low as three to five per cent of normal consumption.

During hibernation the animal may not feed, depending entirely upon the stored food reserves within his body. The evidence at hand indicates that in such cases the body weight may drop as much as fifty per cent. In other cases food is stored within the winter nest and the hibernating animal awakens from time to time to consume its food. In winter there are periods of fasting in those animals that hibernate only in a limited sense. Mice and squirrels, for example, that store food for the winter, often sleep for days at a time, without eating.

HIBERNATION BY BEARS

The bear is a typical hibernator, although not all bears hibernate. For example, the American grizzly bear does not. In the Himalayan or Asiatic black bear, hibernation is not complete as the bear comes out on warm winter days to feed. The brown bear, on the other hand, hibernates. In several species of bear only the female dens up in winter and appears to undergo a partial hibernation during which the young are born, the young cubs and the emaciated mother emerging in the Spring. The Polar bear is an example of this kind. The black bear, native to North America, gives birth to two or three cubs while hibernating. At birth these cubs are naked and and blind, and are but eight inches long. Hibernating bears are believed not to attain full dormancy.

The big black bear of northern Russia retires to a bed of leaves and moss about the end of November and "sleeps," if not disturbed, until about the middle of March; living during this time, upon the nutritive supplies stored in his own tissues. The fat, or well-fed bear will begin to fast some weeks before he retires to his den for his long winter's "sleep." Disturb him in the latter part of February and he will be instantly awake and alert, and will attack the intruder with a fury which has given rise to the expression, "as savage as a waked winter bear."

HIBERNATION IN RODENTS

Nearly all the burrowing rodents hibernate. Notable exceptions are gophers, chipmunks and squirrels which store up roots and nuts on which they feed when an occasional warm day induces them to arouse. On the colder days even these hibernate. The prairie dog and squirrel are said to be partial hibernators. In the northern part of his range the badger hibernates during the winter. He passes through a long winter without eating. After an absolute fast of ten weeks he will trot for miles in search of acorns or roots which he may then be forced to dig out of the half-frozen ground.

The dormouse (sleeping mouse) a term applied in the old world to a small squirrel-like rodent and in the U.S. to the common white-footed mouse is a long "sleeper' but seems not to "sleep" as deeply nor to be as far from consciousness as some other hibernating mammals. He makes himself very comfortable by weaving a thick network of dry grass into his winter bedclothes. This is so neatly and skillfully designed that it keeps in the heat and, yet permits a fair amount of air slowly to filter through. So carefully does he fill up the hole in his warm light wrapping, after he goes inside, there is no hint of a joint or a weak place. Here he spends a long winter of five months in deep "sleep" with no food and often loses more than forty per cent of his weight during this period.

The woodchuck is the most profound sleeper among the common mammals. Feeding on red clover, it goes to bed October 1, and does not come out until April 1. Its hibernation period is, therefore, six months. The bear does not sleep so profoundly and, if food is plentiful and the temperature mild, does not hibernate at all. The raccoon and gray squirrel sleep during the severest part of the winter; the skunk spends January and February in his hole; the chipmunk wakes up occasionally to eat; the red squirrel is abroad almost all winter. Many other mammals hibernate for a greater or lesser period of time.

HIBERNATION AMONG BATS

The hibernating habits of different species of bats differ so much that it is difficult to generalize. There is some evidence that some bats migrate upon the approach of winter, but most of them hibernate. Bats live on winged insects and must catch their prey in the air. Their feeding days are limited, except in the South, where insects fly about for a longer season. Indeed, their feeding days must be very short if frost comes early in Autumn. Their period of hibernation may be more than half a year. Their death-like inactivity is made necessary because of the need to make their meager supply of stored food hold out over such a long period of time. In the long winters of the north, hibernation often means going without food for five, six and seven months. If bats are to survive, it is essential that their food resources be made to hold out as long as possible.

Bats cluster in masses, usually in caves, old barns, and other places that offer protection from the inclemencies of winter. The hibernating bat appears in all respects dead. Its temperature sinks very low, its heart beats so feebly it is barely perceptible, and it takes long to awaken from its sleep. One naturalist describes the "winter sleep" of bats in the following words: "Most bats when fallen into their winter sleep look dead as nearly as may be. They grow cold, their heart beats feebly, and when they hang themselves head downward on some dusty beam or crouch in some smoldering wood, they might be taken for lumps of leather. Nothing about them suggests a living creature, and no one would imagine for a moment that they would presently be flying with a dash and a skill and a command of quick turns beyond the power of a bird."

Griffin says of the hibernating bat, "the heart rate slows to a point where it cannot be detected. Breathing almost ceases. The blood moves sluggishly. The body temperature falls almost to that of the surroundings.

"Bats hibernating in a cave where the air temperature is 33° F. may have a body temperature of 33.5° F. They feel cold to handle, and are stiff and unresponsive. It requires close observation to distinguish a hibernating bat from a dead one."

There is evidence that bats may awaken spontaneously during the winter and fly around in their cave, in rare instances flying considerable distances to other caves. Griffin says that "they are not continuously dormant throughout the whole winter. On successive visits to the same cave we usually found the bats in different parts of the passages, even when they were not disturbed on the previous visit. Probably they wake up from time to time and fly about a bit, perhaps occassionally wandering out of the cave to see whether spring has come yet, and then hang themselves up again for another long sleep." "Flying from cave to cave in winter seems to be a rare occurrence, but we obtained three returns of banded bats which had flown 55 to 125 miles from one cave to another during a single winter."

HIBERNATION IN COLD-BLOODED ANIMALS

While hibernating mammals seek caves, dens or hollow logs, usually making themselves dens of dry leaves or grass to sleep through the winter, the lower orders remain buried throughout the winter with the body temperature approximately that of the external environment, and with great decrease in metabolism. Reptiles hide away among stones or pits or caves, often coiling together, to form a huge, inert mass. Frogs, lizards, salamanders and certain fishes bury themselves in the earth below the reach of frost, the acquatic forms digging into the mud at the bottom of the stream. The few fishes which are known to lie dormant and take no food, sink into the mud of the streams or of the sea. Some fish, as the carp, lie quiet on mud bottoms. The horseshoe crab buries into the mud beyond the reach of oyster dredges in November, remaining in deep water until the middle of Spring. Because snakes hibernate so deeply below the ground that frost never reaches them, they live further north than any other reptile. Spiders and snails hibernate under stones, moss, etc., while slugs bury themselves in the mud and muscles and other mollusks living in the streams and lakes, descend into the mud.

As cold weather comes and winter approaches the purely acquatic species of frogs take to the water and burrow into the moist mud at the bottom of the ponds below the frost line. Here they hibernate throughout the winter, becoming cold and dormant, where the climate is severe, until revived in the Spring. Others bore into the soil, or beneath the fallen leaves, or into the rotting stumps, etc., and exist quietly and dormant until the coming of warm weather and food. During this period, most of the life activities of the frog cease. The heart beats very slowly and there is little evidence of life. The frog does not breathe through its lungs during this period but takes in oxygen through its skin. Toads also hibernate through the winter. Hibernating frogs and toads take no food, being dependent during this time on the food reserves stored in their bodies as fat and glycogen. All activities are suspended except those necessary to maintain life, such as the beating of the heart. Metabolism is much reduced, little oxygen is required, and respiration takes place entirely through the skin. Many other amphibians bury themselves in mud, this being particularly true of those that æstivate during the dry season.

Lizards residing in the temperate zones hibernate during the winter. Here in the Southwest, the great variety of lizards, some brilliantly colored, others dull and drab, like the noted horned toad, that one sees in the Summer months, is almost bewildering. Upon the approach of Winter they disappear. They may be found under boards, piles of straw, logs, etc., dormant and almost incapable of activity. If placed near a fire and made warm, they become as active as in the Summer months.

Newts are more difficult to find than lizards, but if one digs into the hole, often far down into the ground, where a newt is spending the winter, one may find a black shriveled object that is scarcely recognizable.

The snail prepares a really tough defense for itself. It seeks a hiding place, preferring a damp and rather warm atmosphere, and when ensconded in its new home, manufactures from its own juices a chalkly secretion covering the mouth of its shell. By puffing from its lungs it separates this covering from contact with itself. This defensive covering is porous to the air so that the sleeping snail can breathe. It then shrinks into the deep recesses of its shell instead of filling out the whole of it. Here it spends the winter in sleep; taking no food during the whole of this period.

HIBERNATION OF INSECTS

Most insects hibernate in the larval or pupal stage. The larvæ of many caterpillars hatch in Summer and sleep all Winter. A few insects, as certain moths, butterflies and beetles, hibernate in the adult stage. Caterpillars hide under moss, the bark of trees, etc., but they freeze solid and may be broken into pieces like an icicle; they gradually thaw out in the Spring, but when the changes are sudden, great numbers die. In Europe insects pass the winter, not as adults, but in the pupa stage, well wrapped up in a cocoon.

The queen bumble bee makes for herself a hole in the ground, the sides of which she polishes very thoroughly. She goes into this winter home in early October and does not come out for five months or more. She shifts her position and has moments of restlessness, but does not take food. She sleeps through all or most of her period of hibernation.

Queen wasps, though preferring a hole behind a piece of loose bark or in the wood of a decaying tree, employ a greater variety of hiding places than does the bumble bee, and retire in September. They are wide awake and active if the weather becomes warm.

INITIATION AND DURATION OF HIBERNATION

In general the time of the initiation of hibernation corresponds closely with the scarcity of food and lowering of temperature. The termination coincides with the return of favorable conditions. Some species, or some individuals, however, may commence the hibernating period while factors are still quite favorable, or may terminate the period at an unfavorable time. Modern theories of the mechanism stress the physiological sequence of events characteristic of the process. These events may apparently be set into activity under any one of several external conditions.

In temperate climates bears eat more, especially of flesh in the Fall, as they are laying up a store of food in preparation for their winter hibernation. They literally gorge themselves on foods which they convert into fat, but when they enter the dormancy period, stomach and intestines are empty.

Hibernating animals may be induced to awaken readily by "strong external conditions." Following awakening, there is gradual elevation of body temperature and a regaining of normal physiological activity and behavior. Lowering the temperature of the body to approximately 0° C. (32° F.) has been reported to awaken hibernating mammals, though some investigators report that animals may often be killed by freezing without awakening.

Just as there are some migratory birds that do not return home until May and leave again in August, so some hibernating animals do not come out of their dark quarters for as many as seven months. Their hibernating period is one of complete fasting. In general, the period of hibernation corresponds with the period of cold and food scarcity.

AESTIVATION

Aestivation is similar to hibernation, if, indeed, it is not identical with it. If hibernation is to be called "winter sleep," aestivation may be with equal propriety, called "summer sleep." In zoology, it is defined as a state of reduced metabolic activity in which certain animals become quiescent. It is a resting interval associated with warm, dry periods in areas that have alternating wet and dry seasons. Animals are induced to aestivate when drought and heat interfere with their activities. With their bent for pathological interpretations, biologists also define aestivation as "the state of torpidity induced in animals by excessive dry heat." Physiological and physical quiescence should not be mistaken for a state of torpor. The same objections to calling it sleep that we made in the case of hibernation are also valid with reference to aestivation.

Aestivation is seen chiefly in the tropics during the long, hot, dry season, when food is scarce and vegetation is taking a rest. A few animals in the temperate zones, especially in the desert regions, also aestivate. Alligators, snakes, certain mammals, as tauree, insects and land snails become dormant.

During the dry season in the tropics the pools and streams dry up. The crocodiles æstivate in Summer, "sleeping" through the dry season without feeding or emerging from the mud in which they have buried themselves. It is said that they are able to "sleep" in this almost "lifeless" state for a whole year. The alligators, the American division of the crocodile family, hibernate in this country very much like frogs, but in the tropics they æstivate. When water is no longer obtainable the South American alligator, and some other animals, bury themselves in the mud, reduce their physiological activities to a bare minimum, while the earth above them is baked into a hard crust. When the rains come again, they resume activity, and come forward renewed by their long fast and rest.

Certain fish are able, when the pools and streams dry up, to burrow deep down into the mud and lie there until the coming of the rainy season. The mud-fish of Australia is an example of these fish, but many examples exist in the dry countries where summer, rather than winter, is the "hard time." Indeed, if we are to judge by the fish that may be found in a dry pond after a heavy rain, we may have such fish in this country. The lungfishes, *Protoperis* of Africa and *Lipidosiren* of South America, live in mud cocoons during the dry season. When the rice fields which it inhabits dry up during the drought, the spearhead fish, *Opiocephidæ*, buries itself in the mud. Natives of Indo-Malaya "fish" for these animals with digging implements. The African lungfish digs into mud almost two feet, curls its tail around its body which becomes covered with mucus, and there exists, drawing air through a long tube and living on the breakdown of body fat and tail.

During droughts, planarians (*flatworms*) and leeches (*annelids*) bury themselves in mud. Small crustaceans, mollusks, etc., that are found in the pools and patches of water that frequently form in the desert, bury themselves deep in the clay or baked mud, when these pools dry up, and æstivate for long periods. Turtles aestivate in mud, while lizards and snakes retire to crevices. The Iberian water turtle hides under rocks.

Frogs burrow into mud and exist for months in its sunbaked hardness. During periods of æstivation frogs can survive the loss of half their body moisture. Certain Australian frogs become distended with water during the wet season and use this stored water during the æstivating period. This storing of water by these frogs is similar to the storage of fat by hibernating animals.

Birds are not known to æstivate, but a number of mammals, such as aardvark, *Orycteropus*, and some lemurs, *Chirogale millii* and *Microcebus*, undergo periods of quiescence.

Most prominent among æstivating animals of America are the land snails, although frogs, slugs, some fishes and other acquatic and semi-acquatic animals also æstivate. When the dry season comes, land snails secrete a membrane-like substance (epiphram), across the opening of their shells, leaving a small opening for the admission of air in breathing. Some snails secrete several epiphrams across the opening of their shells. There is an Australian snail that plugs the mouth of its shell with a morsel of clay before entering upon its period of æstivation. After a prolonged shower snails become active. Aestivating desert snails have been known to revive and crawl about after years in the dormant state. Records show that the African snail, *Helix desertorum*, may remain in æstivation as long as five years; the California desert snail, *Helix veatchii*, has become active after a six year æstivation period.

In the deserts of the world there are many plant-eating animals that lie dormant in times of drought, when vegetation is more scarce than during those periods when there is rainfall. There are many desert plants that also lie dormant during periods of drought. Both plants and animals fast during this period of dormancy.

In Australia the nymphs of a species of dragonflies æstivate in dry land. Slugs bury themselves in the ground and bivalve mollusks hide in the mud. Small crustaceans, mollusks, etc., that are found in the pools and patches of water that frequently form in the deserts, bury themselves deeply in the clay or baked mud, when these pools dry up and æstivate for long periods.

While it seems that heat, dryness, and lack of food are the factors that induce æstivation, as cold and famine seem to induce hibernation, there is reason to believe that there is more to the practice than the mere existence of certain external factors. For example, the persistence of the æstivating habit is illustrated by the *tenree*, which in temperate zoological gardens, where food and water are abundant, æstivates at the time of their scarcity in its native Madagascar. This would seem to indicate that something other than scarcity of food and high temperature is at work in æstivation, and, perhaps, also in hibernation.

A peculiar example of an animal that behaves opposite to æstivation is the Egyptian jerboa. It is said to be so closely adapted to dry conditions (of the desert) that rain or damp atmosphere induce it to pass into a dormant condition, in which state it does not eat.

Those animals that hibernate through the winter and æstivate through much of the summer, may and often do spend more of their life fasting than eating. The many examples of this kind that could be cited are enough to demonstrate conclusively that abstinence from food is not the natural calamity that we are taught to believe.

FASTING WHEN WOUNDED

Biologists, physiologists and research workers of all kinds are very fond of animal experimentation. But all of these workers are in the habit of ignoring important parts of the regular activities of animals. For example, they ignore, never mention, in fact, the numerous instances of dogs and other animals having fasted ten, twenty or more days when they have received internal injuries or a broken bone. That a sick animal refuses food is well known to all laymen, but physiologists and biologists seem to think that this fact is unworthy even of mentioning. Can we not learn from observing the normal and regular activities of animals living normal lives—must we assume that animals are capable of teaching us something only when under artificial conditions, and when subjected to processes that they never encounter in the normal course of their existence?

Dr. Oswald tells of a dog that had been put into the loft of a barn by the sergeant of a cavalry regiment. Losing its balance, while in the door of the loft and barking, it fell, turning a few somersaults as it came down, and landed on the hard pavement, "with a crack that seemed to have broken every bone in his body." He says "blood was trickling from his mouth and nose when we picked him up, and the troopers advised me to 'put him out of his misery,' but he was my little brother's pet, and, after some hesitation, I decided to take him home in a basket and give the problem of his care the benefit of a fractional chance. Investigation proved that he had broken two legs and three ribs, and judging by the way he raised his head and gasped for air, every now and then, it seemed probable that his lungs had been injured."

For twenty days and twenty nights the little terrier stuck to life in its cotton-lined basket without touching a crumb of solid food, but ever ready to take a few drops of water, in preference even to milk or soup. At the end of the third week it broke its fast with a saucerful of sweet milk, but only on the evening of the twenty-sixth day did it begin to betray any interest in a plateful of meat scraps.

Irwin Liek, noted German physician and surgeon, tells of instinctive fasting in three of his dogs. One of these had been run over by a truck which had broken several bones and injured it internally. The second had "devoured a considerable quantity of rat poison. It became very, very ill, suffered from diarrhea containing blood and pus" and "collapsed completely." The third lost an eye while "mixing it" with a cat. All three of these dogs fasted and recovered.

Physiologists have persistently ignored cases where dogs have voluntarily fasted for ten or twenty or more days when suffering from broken bones or internal injuries. Here is an action invariably pursued by nature which they persist in refusing to investigate.

It is said that the elephant, if wounded, and still able to travel, will go along with the rest of the herd and can be found supporting itself beside a tree while the remainder of the herd enjoys a hearty meal. The wounded elephant is totally oblivious of the excellent food all around him. He obeys an instinct as unerring as the one that brings the bee to his hive; an instinct which is common to the whole animal world, man included.

FASTING IN DISEASE

I need devote but little space to a discussion of what every one already knows; namely, that the sick animal refuses all food. The farmer knows that his "foundered" horse will not eat—is "off his feed," as he expresses it. The sick cat, dog, cow or other animal refuses food. Animals will abstain from food when sick for days and weeks, refusing all food that may be offered them until they are well.

Dr. Felix Oswald says: "Serious sickness prompts all animals to fast. Wounded deer will retire to some secluded den and starve for weeks together." Dr. Erwin Liek endorses fasting and observes that "small children and animals, guided by an infallible instinct, limit to the utmost their intake of food if they are sick or injured."

Arthur Brisbane disapproved of fasting and took Mr. Sinclair to task for advocating it. After a lengthy correspondence about the matter, Mr. Brisbane acknowledged that "even dogs fast when they are ill." Sinclair retorted, "I look forward to the time when human beings may be as wise as dogs."

A dog or cat, if sick or wounded, will crawl under the wood-shed or retire to some other secluded spot and rest and fast until well. Occasionally he will come out for water. These animals will, when wounded or sick, persistently refuse the most tempting food when offered to them. Physical and physiological rest and water are their remedies.

A sick cow or horse will also refuse food. The author has seen this in many hundreds of cases. In fact, all nature obeys this instinct. Thus does nature teach us that the way to feed in acute "disease" is not to do it.

Domestic cattle may often be found suffering from some chronic "disease." Such animals invariably consume less food than the normal animal. Every stock man knows that when a cow or horse or hog or sheep, etc., persistently refuses food, or day after day consumes much less than normally, there is something wrong with that animal.

NO FEAR OF FASTING

I have made no effort to exhaust the list of animals and plants that fast under conditions other than those of sickness or absence of food. The examples that have been given are sufficient to show that nature has no fear of prolonged abstinence from food and that abstinence is frequently made use of in nature, by animals in both the active and the dormant states, as a means of adapting the animal to various conditions of life, or as a means of internal alteration when this is needed. Under all conditions in which animals fast, the internal resources of the animal are drawn upon to nourish the vital tissues and carry on the indispensable functions of life.

In sickness, or when severely wounded, when no food can be digested, the organism also draws upon its internal store of supplies for these same purposes. Fever, pain, distress, inflammation suspend the secretion of the digestive juices, inhibit the muscular actions of the stomach and take away the desire for food. In such conditions there is but one source from which food can be drawn—the reserves.

In sickness, as in animals fasting through the mating period, there is much activity going on in the body. There is, therefore, much more rapid wasting of the body in these two conditions than is seen in hibernation and æstivation.

Viewing the wasted condition of animals at the end of their various fasting periods, it becomes very obvious that, while different species of animals vary in the amount of loss they can safely sustain, none of them are injured or endangered until after a large percentage of the normal weight of the body has been lost. There is, therefore, no danger in a fast of such lengths as are employed in sickness.

FASTING AS A MEANS OF SURVIVAL

After this survey of the many and varied conditions under which animals fast, and the different uses to which fasting is put, it becomes obvious that fasting is one of the most common phenomena in nature. It is second only to feeding and reproduction, with both of which phenomena it is allied, in importance and in breadth of application.

Fasting under so many different conditions is so common in nature and is employed as a means of meeting so many of the exigencies of life that I am forced to wonder why anyone is afraid to fast and why anyone should doubt its naturalness and helpfulness. It is one of nature's best established methods of dealing with certain physiological problems. The hibernating bear, the æstivating alligator, the sick elephant, the wounded dog—these all fast to meet the problems before them. Fasting in acute disease, when there is no digestive power, can be viewed only as a very useful means of adaptation.

As I have previously pointed out, biologically, hibernation is a means of adaptation to the conditions of winter which enables the animal to survive. The ability to go without food during this period is an important element in survival. Except for its ability to fast for extended periods, the hibernating animal would starve to death during the winter.

Our so-called scientists, sticklers as they are for classifications and minute differentiations, are still in the habit of referring to all abstinence from food as *starvation*. But they say of hibernation that it is a form of "starvation" that "spells survival instead of death." Strangely enough, these men refer to the abstinence of hibernation and that seen in the mating season in some animals as "physiological starvation." This is a misuse of terms. Starvation is at all times pathological or pathogenic.

The ability of an animal to fast, even for long periods, under many and varied conditions and circumstances of life, is a vitally important factor in survival. It is nature's best established method of dealing with certain physiological and biological problems. It may be properly regarded as a means of adjustment or adaptation—the hibernating bear, the æstivating alligator, the sick elephant all fasting to meet the problems before them.

If an animal can fast it is only because it can rely upon adequate internal resources and it can afford to fast precisely in so far and so long as it duly conserves these provisions. This is the reason hibernating and æstivating animals function on the lowest physiological level compatible with continued life. With no physical activity and only a bare minimum of physiological activity, their internal reserves are conserved and made to last for prolonged periods— months or a year.

Salmon and the fur-seal bull do not rest and they make no effort to conserve their resources. It would be interesting to know how long these animals could fast if they ceased their activity—physical and sexual.

HOW LONG CAN ANIMALS ABSTAIN FROM FOOD?
The most remarkable records of continued abstinence from food are to be found among the lower animals. Compared to some of these, man is a piker. It is often said that the marvels of long-continued abstinence from food reach their maximum in the "winter sleep" of several species of warm-blooded animals, but there are actually longer records than these present.

The recently produced *American People's Encyclopedia* tells us that the survival time in *acute starvation* (complete abstinence from all food save water) ranges from 21 to 117 days in dogs; rat 5 to 6 days; guinea pig 7 to 8 days; rabbit 15 days; cat 20 days; dog 38 days. There is some confusion about how long the dog may survive deprivation of food, although the matter of size may determine.

Reports of spiders undergoing incredibly long fasts, spinning webs daily, these made of substances within their bodies, until the weight of the webs so produced far outweigh the weights of the spiders at the beginning of the fast, cause me to suspect that the spiders had sources of food supply of which the observers were unaware. I find it difficult to believe that spiders have mastered the art of making something out of nothing.

Even one-celled organisms (amœba, paramecia, etc.) can exist without food for from four to twenty-one days. Like muscle cells in a fasting man, fasting one-celled organisms only undergo a diminution in the size of the cell. These die only after the cellular reserve is exhausted. These little beings possess a food reserve which they can live on in emergencies. In the same way, each cell in the bodies of the higher animals possesses its own private food reserve.

Among vertebrates the time they can subsist without food ranges from a few days in small birds and mammals to possibly years in some reptiles. The time they can go without food depends on the amount of reserve possessed and the rate at which it is consumed. In cold-blooded animals, the reserves are usually plentiful and the demand made upon them is small, so that they may fast for long intervals, without being forced to renew their stores. In warm-blooded animals, whose reserves are frequently lower and whose great activities make a greater demand upon these, the reserves are more rapidly depleted.

Among cold-blooded animals the survival time without food is usually much greater than among warm-blooded animals, since the former do not have to "burn fuel" in order to maintain a high body temperature. Snakes and other reptiles easily go for long periods without food. Snakes have been kept alive without food for almost two years. A python in captivity has been observed to go without food for a period of thirteen months. Frogs have survived sixteen months and fishes twenty months without food. Invertebrates can stand even longer periods of deprivation; the larva of the beetle

Trogderma tarsale living for five years, during which time they lost 99.8 percent of their body substance. Spiders have been observed to exist without food for seventeen months and more. Fabre tells us of certain spiders that they eat no food of any kind for the first six months of their lives but feast upon sunbeams. Goldfishes have been known to go for long periods without food, while *proteus angeainus,* an amphibian, has been known to live for years without food. In his *Researches sur L'Inanition,* Chossat tells us that the land tortoise of southern France, can "starve" for a year without betraying a reduction of vital energy, and that *Proteus anguinus,* the serpent salamander, even for a year and a half, providing the temperature of its cage is kept above the freezing point. Rhine salmon have been known to go without food for eight to fifteen months.

Oswald says: "Reptiles, with their small expenditure of vital energy, can easily survive dietetic deprivations; but bears and badgers, with an organization essentially analogous to that of the human species, and with a circulation of blood active enough to maintain the temperature of their bodies more than a hundred degrees above that of the winter storms, dispense with food for periods varying from three to five months, and at the termination of their ordeal emerge from their dens in the full possession of their physical and mental energies."—*Fasting Hydropathy and Exercise,* pp. 60-61. The condor, like all other vultures, is able to fast for days. It usually gorges itself, however, when it does get food.

Edwin E. Slossom, M.S., Ph. D., Director of Science Service, Washington, says in his *Keeping Up With Science* (Page 261): "Among the lower animals existence under inanition may extend over incredibly protracted periods. Scorpions are known to have starved for 368 days, and spiders have survived starvation for seventeen months. The larvæ of small beetles have been known to live through more than five years without food, their body mass being reduced in this time to only one-sixth-hundred of what it was at the start. There is a unique record of a fresh water fish, *Amia Calva,* which fasted twenty months and even then had not apparently reached the end of the rope but was killed. Frogs survive starvation for sixteen months, and snakes remain alive even after two years of fasting. The longest recorded fast endured by a dog was 117 days, or nearly four months." A. S. Pearse, Professor of Zoology at Duke University, tells us that "certain ticks can exist in an active state for as long as four years without eating anything."

Perhaps the longest periods of abstinence are seen in æstivating animals of the deserts. It should not be overlooked, also, that snails and other animals of northern deserts, that æstivate in the dry season and hibernate through the winter, spend most of their lives fasting.

Fasting in Man

CHAPTER III

Man is an animal and, as such, is subject to the same laws of existence and the same conditions of living, as are other animals. As a part of the great organic world, he is not a being that is set apart from the ordinary and regular conditions of life, governed by different laws and requirements of existence. It is not surprising, therefore, that we find man not only able to fast for prolonged periods and able to do so with benefit, but also find him fasting under a wide variety of circumstances and for a wide variety of purposes. In the following pages, we shall briefly review the most important of the conditions under which man fasts and the purposes for which he fasts.

RELIGIOUS FASTING

Fasting as a religious observance, has long been practiced for the accomplishment of certain goods. Religious fasting is of early origin, antedating recorded history. Partial or entire abstinence from food, or from certain kinds of foods, at stated seasons, prevailed in Assyria, Persia, Babylon, Scythia, Greece, Rome, India, Ninevah, Palestine, China, in northern Europe among the Druids, and in America among the Indians. It was a widely diffused practice, often indulged as a means of penitence, in mourning and as a preparation for participation in religious rites, such as baptism and communion.

At the very dawn of civilization the Ancient Mysteries, a secret worship or wisdom religion that flourished for thousands of years in Egypt, India, Greece, Persia, Thrace, Scandinavia and the Gothic and Celtic nations, prescribed and practiced fasting. The Druidical religion among the Celtic peoples required a long probationary period of fasting and prayer before the candidate could advance. A fast of fifty days was required in the Mithriac religion in Persia. Indeed, fasting was common to all the mysteries, which were all quite similar to the Egyptian mysteries and were probably derived from these. Moses, who was learned in "all the wisdom of Egypt," is said to have fasted for more than 120 days on Mount Sinai.

The mysteries of Tyre, which were represented in Judea in the days of Jesus, in a secret society known as the Essenes, also prescribed fasting. In the first century A.D., there existed in Alexandria, Egypt, an ascetic sect of Jews, called Therapeutæ, who resembled the Essenes and who borrowed much from the Kabala and from the Pythagorian and Orphic systems. These Therapeutæ gave great attention to the sick and held fasting in high esteem as a *curative* measure.

Fasting is mentioned quite frequently in the *Bible* while several fasts of considerable duration are recorded therein, as, Moses forty days (Ex. 24:18; Exodus 34:28); Elijah forty days (1st Kings, 19:8); David seven days (2 Sam. 12:20); Jesus forty days (Matthew 4:2); Luke, "I fast twice in the week" (Luke 18:12); "This kind cometh not out save by prayer and fasting" (Matt. 17.21); a fast throughout all Judea (2 Chronicles 20:8). The *Bible* cautions against fasting for mere notoriety (Matt. 6:17, 18). It also advises fasters not to wear a sad countenance (Matt. 6:16); but to find pleasure in fasting and to perform one's work (Isa. 58:3), and that certain fasts shall be fasts of gladness (Zech. 8.19).

We may very properly assume that some great good was the object of the many fasts mentioned in the *Bible* even though we may be sure that they were not always intended for the *"cure"* of *"dis-ease."* We may also be sure that the ancients had no fear of starving to death by missing a few meals.

For two thousand years the Christian religion has recommended "prayer and fasting" and the story of the forty day's fast in the wilderness has been told from thousands of pulpits. Religious fasts were frequently practised in the early days of Christianity and during the Middle Ages. Thomas Campanella tells us that frail nuns often sought relief from periods of hysteria by fasting "seven times seventy hours," or twenty and one half days. John Calvin and John Wesley both strongly urged fasting as a beneficial measure for both ministers and people.

Among the early Christians, fasting was among the rites of purification. Fasting is yet a regular practice among the nations of the Far East, especially among the East Indians. The many fasts of Gandhi are generally known.

Penance-worn members of the early church frequently retired to the desert for a month or two to fight down temptations. They would drink water from some dilapidated old cistern during the period, but to eat so much as a millet-seed was considered a breach of their vows and destroyed the merits of their penance. At the end of the second month the "gaunt world-renouncers" generally had sufficient strength to return home unassisted.

The writer of *Peregrinato Silviæ*, in describing how Lent was observed in Jerusalem, when she was there about 386 A.D., says: "They abstained entirely from all food during Lent, except on Saturdays and Sundays. They took a meal about midday on Sunday, and after that they took nothing until Saturday morning. This was their rule through Lent."

Although the Catholic Church has no law requiring fasting, as we use the term, it was voluntarily practiced by many individuals in the past. Fasting, whether total abstinence from food or abstinence from proscribed foods, is regarded by this Church as a penance. The Catholic Church also teaches that Jesus fasted in order to instruct and encourage belief in the practice of penance.

The Roman Church has both "fast-days" and "abstinence-days," though they are not necessarily the same. The "law of abstinence" is on a different basis and "is regulated, not by the quantity, but by the quality of food" permitted. "The law of abstinence forbids the use of meat or meat broth, but not eggs, 'lacticinia' (milk) or condiments of any kind even from 'the fat of animals'." The rule of the church in fasting is: "What constitutes fasting is the taking of only one full meal in a day." "In earlier times a strict fast was kept until sunset. Now this full meal may be taken any time after mid-day, or, as the church's approved authors hold, shortly before. Some even hold that the full meal may be taken at any time during the 24 hours." But this "one full meal in twenty-four hours" does not prohibit the taking of some food in the morning and evening. Indeed, "local custom," which is often a somewhat undefined phrase, as determined by the local bishop, determines what extra food may be taken daily. In America the rule is that the morning meal should not exceed two ounces of bread; in Westminster (England) the limit is three ounces. Obviously a "fast" of this nature is not what we mean by fasting, for a man may eat enough in this manner to grow fat. Nor can *Hygienists* accept the so-called moral principle of the Roman Church—"parvum pro nihilo reputatur" and "ne potus noceat"—"a little is reckoned as nothing," "lest drink unaccompanied by anything solid should be harmful." We hold, as Page expressed it, that little driblet meals are not fasting.

The Lenten fast of Catholics is also merely a period of abstinence from certain proscribed foods, although there are Catholics who take advantage of the period for a real fast. The early practice of fasting until sundown, then feasting, is similar to the practice of Moham-medans in their so-called fast of Ramadan. During this season the people do not eat and cannot drink wine nor smoke cigarettes from sunrise to sunset, but they have their cigarettes handy, ready to begin smoking as soon as the sun goes down and they enjoy a night of feasting. A grand carouse at night makes up for their abstinence during the day. Their cities hold nightly carnivals, the restaurants are lighted and the streets are filled with revelers, the bazaars are well illuminated and the peddlers of lemonade and sweetmeats are in their glory. The wealthy sit up all night receiving and returning calls and giving dinner parties. After days of this feasting and revelling, the people celebrate the end of their month of "fasting" with the feasting of *Bairam*.

When we are informed that the Archangel Michael appeared to a certain priest of Sipponte, after the latter had spent a year in fasting, we are not to think of the priest as having abstained from all food, but from certain foods during this period. This is a religious use of the term fasting that clouds many of the stories we receive of religious fasts. We are not always certain that the individual abstained from food. He may have merely abstained from certain proscribed foods.

When people are commanded by religion to abstain from flesh on certain days of the week, as a means of subduing their "animal appetites," but are permitted to drink wine, eat liberally of fish (which is also flesh), to which are added *rich* and *stimulating* sauces, such as they add to eggs, lobsters, and various shell-fish, we have an obvious abandonment of what may have been, originally, a sound view of dietetics and the observance of a mere superstitious rite. When the Mohammedans are forbidden to drink wine, but are permitted to intoxicate themselves by unrestrained use of coffee, tobacco and opium, there is an obvious departure from a former rule against inebriation of all kinds. When, during Ramadan, the Mohammedan is commanded to touch neither solid nor liquid food from sunrise to sunset, but is permitted to revel in gluttony, inebriety and debauchery from sunset to sunrise, where is the gain? We have but a symbolic abstinence, a mere rite or ceremonial that feebly imitates what may have been, originally, a wholesome practice.

The fact is, and this should be obvious to the least intelligent, that there is nothing in natural law that sanctions any interruptions of or departures from sobriety, abstinence, moderation and right conduct. Natural laws indicate no specific days and no special number of days for special fasts or for special periods of abstinence from any food or indulgence. A fast is to be taken under natural law when there is a need for it and it is to be abstained from when there is no need for it. Hunger and thirst are to be satisfied on all days and at all times of the year and should at all times be satisfied with wholesome food and pure water. The man who refuses to satisfy the normal needs of the body, as indicated by thirst and hunger, is as guilty of a breach of natural law as is the man who abuses his body by overindulgence.

At the present time Christians of all sects and denominations rarely undergo a real fast. Most fasts of Roman, Eastern Orthodox and Protestant communicants are merely periods of abstinence from flesh foods. Abstinence from flesh foods other than fish on "fast" days appears to have been enjoined merely to aid the fishing and shipbuilding industries. Among the Jews fasting always means entire abstinence from food, and at least one of their fast days carries with it abstinence from water, also. Their periods of fasting are commonly only short ones.

While the Hindu Nationalists' leader, Gandhi, fully understood the hygienic value of the fast, and often fasted for hygienic purposes, most of his fasts were "purification" or penance fasts and political weapons by which he compelled England to accede to his demands. He even fasted for the purification of India, and not merely for his own cleansing. "Self-purification fasts" of several days are of frequent occurrence in India. A few years ago Jayaprakash Narayan, leader of the Indian Socialist party, underwent a fast of twenty-one days to enable him to fulfill better his public tasks in the future. He underwent this purification fast in a nature cure clinic under the supervision of the man who had supervised several of Gandhi's fasts.

Fasting formed part of the religious observances of the Aztecs and Toltecs of Mexico, the Incas of Peru and of other American tribes. Fasting was also practiced by the Pacific Islanders; while there are traces of fasting in China and Japan, even before their contact with Buddhism. In Eastern Asia and wherever Brahmanism and Buddhism have spread, fasting has been kept alive.

Benedict says that the many recorded instances of prolonged and more or less complete religious fasts are "so clouded by superstition and show such a lack of accurate observation that they are without value to science." While I agree that their value to science is limited, I do not agree that they are devoid of all value. They are certainly of value in confirming the possibility of abstaining from food for long periods of time under varying circumstances of life.

The fact is that scientists have made so few observations of fasters that they are still as clouded in their views of the process as are the accounts of religious fasters.

FASTING AS MAGIC

With fasting as magic we have nothing to do, except to study the phenomenon. Tribal fasts, as seen among the American Indians, to avert some threatened calamity, or fasting, as by Gandhi, to purify India, is the use of fasting as magic. Fasting was widely observed, both in private and in public ceremonials by the American Indians. Fathers of newborn children are required to fast among the Melanesians. Fasting was often part of the rite of initiation into manhood and womanhood or for sacred and ritual acts among many tribes of people. David's seven days' fast, as recorded in the *Bible*, while his son was ill, was a magic fast. Ceremonial fasting carried out in several religions may properly be classed as magic fasting. If we carefully distinguished between magic fasting and protest fasting, as in hunger strikes, we may say that magic fasting is fasting undergone to achieve some desired end outside the person of the faster. We are interested in such fasts, simply as another part of the evidence that man, like the lower animals, may fast for extended periods and may do so, not only without harm, but with positive benefit.

DISCIPLINARY FASTS

Major W. C. Gotschall, M.S., says: "There is nothing new about fasting. Among the ancients it was recognized as a sovereign method of attaining and maintaining marked mental and physical efficiency. Socrates and Plato, two of the greatest of the Greek philosophers and teachers, fasted regularly for a period of ten days at a time. Pythagoras, another of the Greek philosophers, was also a regular faster, and before he took an examination at the University of Alexandria, fasted for forty days. He required his pupils to fast for forty days before they could enter his class." H. B. Cushman tells us in his *History of the Choctaw, Chickasaw and Natchez Indians*, that the Choctaw warrior and hunter "often indulged in protracted fasts" to train him to "endure hunger."

PERIODIC AND YEARLY FASTS

Luke mentions in his *Gospel* the practice of fasting one day out of each week, which seems to have been very general in his day. Periodic fasting has been practiced by many different peoples and by many different individuals. It is asserted that the ancient Egyptians were accustomed to fasting for a brief period, about two weeks each summer. Many people of today do this same thing. They have a fast or two fasts each year. Others follow the custom referred to by Luke and fast one day out of each week. Others fast three to five days out of each month. The practice of periodic fasting takes many forms with many different individuals. These fasts are usually of but short duration, but they are always of distinct benefit.

HUNGER STRIKES

Hunger strikes have become very frequent during the past forty years. Perhaps the most famous of these have been the protest fasts of Gandhi and the hunger strike of McSwiney and his co-political prisoners in Cork, Ireland, in 1920. Joseph Murphy, who went on the hunger strike with McSwiney, died on the 68th day of his fast; McSwiney on the 74th day.

Older readers will recall that some years ago when the sufragettes of England would go on hunger strikes, they would be forcibly fed by a painful process, while, at the same time, there was much talk of letting them "starve" in prison.

The number of men and women who have fasted in India, largely in protest against some grievance, since Gandhi popularized the practice, runs into many thousands. Mass fasting has been practiced on a large scale in several instances. Most of these fasts have been for but a few days, but in some instances they were announced to be "unto death" unless their aim was achieved. So far, each case of fasting has been broken short of death, usually upon importunings of family, friends or physician. One of the "unto death" fasts, which did not go so far, was that of Shibban Lal Saksena, leader of the Peasants, Workers and Peoples Party. A fast of forty days was undergone by Ramchandra Sharma while a fast of thirty-six days was undergone by Swami Sitaram, all three of these fasts being of a political nature—hunger strikes.

Political fasting is not without its humorous side. The news of October 2, 1961 carried the story of the breaking of a 46-day fast undertaken by Master Tara Singh, Sikh leader, to dramatize his demand for a separate Sikh state in the Punjab. On the same day 76-year-old Hogiraj Suryadey, ascetic and religious leader, started his fast in protest against the Sikh's having their own state. The fasts neutralized each other, although it would seem that by maintaining the status quo, Suryadey won the contest. It must be conceded, however, I think, that a fight of this nature is less taxing on the resources of the people and results in less bloodshed than does an old-fashioned shooting revolution.

Gandhi's frequent fasts were usually protests against some British policy, although sometimes he fasted to purify India because of some wrongs she had committed. He was, however, fully acquainted with the *Hygienic* value of the fast and was fully conversant with the literature on the subject. His longest fast seems to have been about twenty-one days. Many men and women in all parts of the world have staged hunger-strikes of longer or shorter duration.

EXHIBITION OR STUNT FASTS
There have been a number of fasters who were more or less professional fasters, fasting largely for show and making money out of the process. These have fasted publicly and have charged admission to the public to get in to see them. Of such were Succi and Merlatti, two Italian exhibition fasters, and Jacques. Jacques fasted 42 days in London in 1890 and 50 days in the same city in 1891. He fasted

30 days in Edinburgh, in 1889. Merlatti fasted 50 days in Paris in 1885. Succi took several long fasts ranging from 21 to 46 days. One of his fasts was carefully studied by Prof. Luciani, famous Italian authority on nutrition.

EXPERIMENTAL FASTS

Experimental fasts in which men and women have taken part are, perhaps, more numerous than we think. Profs. Carlson and Kunde, of the University of Chicago, made a few experiments of this nature a few years ago. Their fasts were of relatively short duration. Before his death Dr. Carlson conducted several experiments with the fast and he took short fasts himself. But few experimental fasts of considerable duration have been made in man. Dr. Luigi Luciani, professor of Physiology in the University of Rome, studied a thirty days fast undergone by Succi in 1889.

Victor Pashutin, director of the Imperial Military Medical Academy, Petrograd, Russia, performed a number of experiments upon animals, and investigated cases of death from starvation in man and published the results of his researches in his *Pathological Physiology of Inanition.*

Dr. Francis Gano Benedict, of the Carnegie Institute at Roxbury, Mass., published a book some years ago, entitled the *Metabolism of Inanition.* In spite of the care observed in the conduct of his fasting experiments and the skill with which the various tests and measurements were carried out, very few decisive results came from these experiments, for they were based on short fasts, the longest one of seven days having been that of a hypochondriac, who, according to Tucsek, being abnormal, could not produce normal physiological results. It is also true that the first few days of the fast witness the worst troubles, so that the results of these short fasts were very misleading or, as Prof. Levanzin says, "that great book on which the Carnegie Institute squandered six thousand dollars is not worth the paper on which it was printed." Benedict's discussion of past experiments with the fast is devoted to fasts in healthy subjects and this can throw but little light on the importance of the fast in disease.

In 1912 Professor Agostino Levanzin, of Malta, came to America to be studied by Prof. Benedict, while he underwent a fast of thirty-one day's duration. His fast was commenced on April 13, 1912 at a weight of "less than two pounds over 132 pounds, normal weight, according to the Yale University measurements, my height being five feet, six and one-half inches." Levanzin thinks that this is an important point in every fast. He points out that professional fasters, like hibernating animals, generally overeat before they start fasting and accumulate a good store of fat and other reserves. He thinks that, due to this fact, the long fasts previously studied were of the destruction of adipose tissue and not of the whole body. He attempted to avoid this "mistake" by starting his fast at "normal" body weight. It was his opinion that the length of the fast is of no importance if it is not started from normal body weight. He was of the opinion that man can lose sixty percent of his normal body-weight without any risk of death or damage to his health. He says that the greatest part of the normal body weight is also a storage of food.

"At the outset of my fast my exact weight was a shade over 133½ pounds (60.6 kilograms). At the conclusion of the thirty-one days of my fast, I weighed barely 104½ pounds (47.4 kilograms), a total loss of twenty-one pounds during the fast. Throughout the fast tests were taken of my pulse rate, blood pressure, respiration rate, respiration volume, blood examination, anthropometrical measurements, urine analysis, and growth of hair, not to mention innumerable other observations of my mental and physical condition from day to day."

FASTING WHEN EATING IS IMPOSSIBLE
There are pathological conditions under which eating is impossible. Such conditions as cancer of the stomach, destruction of the stomach by acids, and by other causes, renders it no longer possible to take food. Persons in this condition often go for extended periods without food, before they finally die. A few such cases will be mentioned in the text as we proceed with our studies. In certain conditions of gastric neurosis food is vomited about as fast as it is swallowed, or it is passed into the small intestine with almost equal rapidity and hurried to the exit and expelled without being digested. Such an individual, though eating, is to all practical purposes, going without food. Such a state of affairs may last for an extended period.

SHIPWRECKED SAILORS AND PASSENGERS
Shipwrecked sailors and aviators forced down at sea have, in many instances, been forced to exist for long periods without food,

and often without water. Many have survived long periods without food under the many severe conditions that the sea offers. During the recent war many instances of this nature received much publicity.

In *My Debut As A Literary Person*, Mark Twain, seriously in this instance, records some of his experiences with and observations of fasting: He says: "A little starvation can really do more for the average sick man than can the best of medicines and the best of doctors. I do not mean a restricted diet, I mean total abstinence from food for one or two days. I speak from experience; starvation has been my cold and fever doctor for fifteen years, and has accomplished a cure in all instances. The third mate told me in Honolulu that the 'portyghee' had lain in his hammock for months, raising his family of abscesses and feeding like a cannibal. We have seen that in spite of dreadful weather, deprivation of sleep, scorching, drenching, and all manner of miseries, thirteen days of starvation 'wonderfully recovered' him. There were four sailors down sick when the ship was burned. Twenty-five days of pitiless starvation have followed, and now we have this curious record: 'all men are hearty and strong, even the ones that were down sick are well, except poor Peter.' When I wrote an article some months ago urging temporary abstinence from food, as a remedy for an inactive appetite and for disease, I was accused of jesting, but I was in earnest. 'We are all wonderfully well and strong, comparatively speaking.' On this day the starvation regimen drew its belt a couple of buckle-holes tighter; the bread ration was reduced from the usual piece of cracker the size of a silver dollar to the half of that, and one meal was abolished from the daily three. This will weaken the men physically, but if there are any diseases of the ordinary sort left in them they will disappear."

ENTOMBED MINERS

Frequently, when there are mine cave-ins, one or more miners are entombed for shorter or longer periods, during which time they are without food and often without water. Their survival until they can be rescued depends not upon food, but upon air. If the oxygen supply is exhausted before rescuers reach them they perish, otherwise, they survive days without food. The entombed miner is like the animal buried for days and weeks under a snow-drift. He is able to go for prolonged periods without food and survive, just as are these animals.

FASTING IN ILLNESS

It is estimated that fasting for the alleviation of human suffering has been practiced uninterruptedly for 10,000 years. No doubt it has been employed from the time man first began to get sick. Fasting was part of the methods of healing practiced in the Ancient Aesculapian Temples of Toscurd Guido, 1300 years before the time of Jesus. Hippocrates, the mythical Greek "Father of Physic," seems to have prescribed total abstinence from food while a "disease" was on the increase, and especially at the critical period, and a spare diet on other occasions. Tertullian has left us a treatise on fasting written about 200 A.D. Plutarch said: "Instead of using medicine rather fast a day." Avicenna, the great Arab physician, often prescribed fasting for three weeks or more.

I think that there is no room to doubt that man, like the lower animals, has always fasted when acutely ill. In more modern times the medical profession has taught the sick that they must eat to keep up their strength and that if they do not eat their resistance will be lowered and they will lose strength. The thought behind all of this is that unless the sick eat they are likely to die. The reverse of this is the truth—the more they eat, the more likely are they to die. In his *Eating for Strength*, M. L. Holbrook, an outstanding *Hygienist* of the last century, says: "Fasting is no cunning trick of priestcraft, but the most powerful and safest of all medicines."

When animals are sick they refuse food. Only when they are well, and not before, will they resume eating. It is as natural or normal for man to refuse food when sick as for animals to do so. His natural repulsion to food is a safe guide to not eating. The aversions and dislikes of the sick, especially to food, noise, motion, light, close air, etc., are not to be lightly dismissed. They express protective measures of the sick body.

FAMINE AND WAR

War and famine, whether the famine has been produced by drought, insect pests, floods, tornadoes, earthquakes, freezes, snows, etc., have frequently deprived whole populations of food for extended periods, so that they have been forced to fast. In many of these instances they have had limited food supplies, but in others no food has been available for long periods. The ability of man to fast, even for long periods, proves to be, as with the lower animals, an important means of survival under such circumstances. Such prolonged periods of deprivation were much more frequent in past ages than today, when rapid transportation and modern means of communication make it possible to get food to people in famine districts in a very short time.

FASTING UNDER EMOTIONAL STRESS

Grief, worry, anger, shock and other emotional irritations are almost as potent in suspending the desire for food and in rendering digestion practically impossible as are pain, fever and severe inflammation. An excellent example of this is that of the young lady, in New York, who a few years ago attempted to drown herself and who explained, when rescued by two sailors, that when her sweetheart who had been in port two days had not called to see her nor communicated with her, she thought she had been jilted. Her sailor friend, kept on duty and not having opportunity to communicate with her, was permitted to see her. He asked when she had eaten and she replied: "Not since yesterday, Bill, I couldn't." Her grief or sense of loss had resulted in a suspension of digestive secretions and a loss of desire for food.

FASTING BY THE INSANE

The insane commonly manifest a strong aversion to food and, unless forcibly fed, will often go for extended periods without eating. It is customary in institutions devoted to the care of the mentally ill, to force-feed such patients, often by very cruel means. This aversion to food by the insane is undoubtedly an instinctive move in the right direction. In his *Natural Cure*, pp. 140-143, Dr. Page presents a very interesting account of a patient that recovered normal mental health by fasting forty-one days, after other treatment had miserably failed. One case of insanity in a young man who came under my care refused food for thirty-nine days, resuming eating on the morning of the fortieth day of fasting, greatly improved in mental condition. I have used fasting in other cases of mental disease and have no doubt that fasting is distinctly beneficial and, I am convinced that when the insane patient refuses food, this is an instinctive measure designed to assist the body in its reconstructive work.

HIBERNATION IN MAN

Of possible human hibernation, it has been said that it is "a condition utterly inexplicable on any principle taught in the schools." Nonetheless, there are a number of peoples who practice a near approach to hibernation during the winter season. This is true of the Eskimos of northern Canada, as well as of certain tribes of northern Russia. By putting on fat and wintering very much as does the bear, only much less completely, the Eskimo reveals that man has some hibernating power. By keeping warm, usually by huddling together in the home, and moving very little, he goes through the long winter on half the usual food. At the onset of winter, the Eskimo will sew himself up in his fur-lined parka, leaving accessible openings for certain physiological necessities, and will stay in his hut for the duration of the winter, existing on dried salmon, hard-tack, ground corn cakes and water. The fact that he undertakes very little physical activity reduces the amount of energy spent, thus aiding him in sustaining the food reserves accumulated in his body at a level at which there is no danger of systemic detriment.

Certain Russian peasants of the Pskoy region have been known to sleep around a fire during most of the winter, awakening once daily to eat. There is no evidence that this is anything other than a quasi-hibernation, as they employ fire to keep themselves warm, awaken daily to eat and, it should not be forgotten, it is easily possible to take all the food required by an even active life in one daily meal. Reports that certain Indian fakirs have been able to assume a dormant state and survive burial for a year or more must be treated with skepticism.

INSTINCTIVE FASTING

Fasting above all other measures can lay claim to being a strictly natural method. There can be no doubt that it is the oldest of all measures of meeting those crises in the organism called "disease." It is much older than the human race itself, since it is resorted to instinctively by sick and wounded animals.

"The fasting-cure instinct," says Oswald, "is not limited to our dumb fellow-creatures. It is common experience that pain, fevers, gastric congestions, and even mental afflictions 'take away the appetite,' and only unwise nurses will try to thwart the purpose of nature in this respect."

The doctrine of total depravity taught men to distrust the promptings of their natural instincts, and while the doctrine is slowly fading from religion, it is as strong as ever in medicine. The promptings of instinct are ignored and the sick are stuffed with "good nourishing food" to "keep up their strength."

"There is a very general concurrence of opinion," says Jennings, "that the aversion to food that characterizes all cases of acute disease, which is fully in proportion to the severity of the symptoms, is one of Nature's blunders that require the intervention of art and hence enforced feeding regardless of aversion." Dr. Shew declared: "Abstinence is by far too much feared in the treatment of disease generally. We have good reason for believing that many a life has been destroyed by the indiscriminate feeding which is so often practiced among the sick."

In the human realm, instinct prevails only to the extent that we permit. Although one of the first things Nature does to the person with acute "disease" is to stop all desire for food, the well-meaning friends of the sick man encourage him to eat. These may bring in tasty and tempting dishes designed to please his taste and excite an appetite but the most they ever succeed in doing is to get the patient to nibble a few bites. The ignorant physician may insist that he must "eat to keep up strength," but Mother Nature, who is wiser than any physician who ever lived, continues to say, "do not eat."

The man who is sick, but who is able to be about his work, complains of having lost his appetite. He no longer enjoys his food. This is because his organic instincts know that to eat in the usual way is to increase the "disease." The man thinks the loss of appetite is a great calamity and seeks a way to restore it. In this he is encouraged by physician and friends, who, alike, erroneously think that the sick man must eat to keep up his strength. The physician prescribes a tonic and stuffing and, of course, the patient is made worse.

LONG FASTS IN MAN

In the preceding chapter it was shown that animals may go without food for prolonged periods without damage to their bodies or to individual organs. The objection is often raised that, while some animals may do this, man cannot. For, there are still those who would place man outside of the uniformities of Nature and make him an exception. Nevertheless, the facts prove that man may go for long periods without food, not alone without injury to himself, but with positive benefit.

Old mistakes are repeated year after year in reference works, so that the public is at all times misinformed. The *New Standard Encyclopedia* (1931) says: "Generally death occurs after eight days of deprivation of food." This encyclopedia mentions the fifteen men survivors of the frigate Medusa (1876), who were thirteen days on an open raft without food, and also a case instanced by Bernard which was "sustained on water alone for 63 days." Succi's forty days fast is also mentioned. No mention is made of fasting as a *Hygienic* or remedial measure, and not a single scientific and up-to-date book on fasting is included in the bibliography.

Until the 1921 revisions of that work were made, the *Encyclopedia Britanica* and similar works, carried articles on inanition and fasting, stating, over the signatures of eminent medical authorities, that from ten to fourteen days marked the extreme limit which the human body could endure without food.

Thousands of fasts of much longer duration, even up to 70 and 90 days, had been recorded; but the medical profession and scientists gave no attention to them. The "authorities" gave up their false notions only after the McSwiney hunger strike forced them to do so.

That "common sense" may still be arrayed against the demonstrated facts of experiment and experience, and that men who pose as scientists, may deny what may be known about the body because it does not seem to them to harmonize with what they think they now know about the body is amazing proof that there have been ignorant bigots and that they are not all dead.

Sinclair says he talked with a well-known and successful physician, "who refused point-blank to believe that a human being could live for more than five days without any sort of nutriment. There was no use talking to him about it—it was a physiological impossibility." He refused to investigate the evidence offered that it could be done. Bigotry we have with us always. Men who form their opinions in advance of investigation and, then refuse to investigate, lest they have their opinions swept away, are all too common.

The *American People's Encyclopedia* says that the survival time of acute "starvation" (complete abstinence from all food save water) is forty days in man. It says that in individual men the survival time (as determined in laboratory "starvation" experiments) ranges from 17 to 76 days. It is not likely that any such laboratory experiments have ever been made. One thing we may be certain of; namely, the survival times given are not accurate. A baby may survive more than seventeen days of fasting. Numerous fasters have not only survived but benefitted by fasts lasting longer than 76 days.

While man is, apparently, not capable of fasting for such long periods as are many of the lower animals, many long fasts have been recorded in man. "Modern science" is said to be very skeptical of these reported long fasts; but "modern science," despite its proud boasting of its experimental methods and its readiness to investigate, is not willing to investigate fasting. If any of the nit-wits who are called scientists really desire to observe and study long fasts at first-hand, it may be easily arranged. There is no excuse for either doubt or incredulity when knowledge may be had.

In this connection, it should be noted that the so-called author-ities look well upon the reported fast of 65 days underwent by Marion Crabtree, of Savanna, Ill., in 1911 at the age of 101, because, they say, old people need much less energy than younger ones; according-ly, they say, old people would be the best of all people to take long fasts.

Many reports are on record of people fasting for many years. These fasts never took place and may all be set down as frauds. Although most of these "fasts" have been in women, there is one instance of a man who is reported to have lived for an incredibly long time without food. This man, Hermolus, is reported to have lived for forty years on the odors of flowers and the assistance of the saints and without taking a morsel of food. Then there is the famous case of Mary J. Fancher, of Brooklyn, N. Y., who was reported to have fasted for thirteen years, beginning in 1866. Clergy-men, physicians and many famous figures visited her, in 1866 a New York magistrate reported that this fast had not affected her health at all.

Among the reported long fasts that never took place was that of Ann Moore, the "Staffordshire Wonder," who was reported to have gone without food for more than two years. Skeptical physicians proposed a test to which she readily consented. The test lasted thirteen days and was successful. Still skeptical, the physicians proposed a more stringent test to which she assented. After nine days of actually fasting, she gave up and confessed that in her previous fasts, food had been smuggled in to her.

Miss Maria de Conceicas, a young girl of about seventeen years of age, of Mendes, Brazil, fasted some years ago for the "cure" of epilepsy. At the time her fast was reported in the *New York Journal*, she was said to have fasted for six months, greatly puzzling her physicians. Her fast continued for some time thereafter. After six months without food a medical examination, showed: "Pulse, temperature and respiration normal, complete vacuity of the bowels; all organs perfect; repugnance to all kinds of food." At one time previous to this she is reported to have fasted for two months. A two month's fast is entirely possible, but I have doubts about her fast of more than six months, despite the medical report.

In the mid-nineteenth century Louise Latean claimed that she had neither eaten, drunk, nor slept for four years. Her story was attested to by five physicians. Religious folks thought she was a miracle. Other physicians were skeptical and pointed out that she was subject to paroxysms and other nervous symptoms. Finally, a physician sent by the Belgian Royal Academy of Medicine searched her room and disclosed a store of food in a cupboard. Louise then confessed that she had nocturnal periods of forgetfulness. Another case of this kind was the "fast" of Sarah Jacob, a Welsh girl, who was reported to have lived for two years, two months and a week without food. Under test conditions she died in eight days. Her speedy death (of starvation, it is said) would seem to indicate that she had actually been fasting previous to the test, but not for more than two years.

There is the now famous case of the Bavarian girl, Therese Newman, who maintains that for several years she has eaten nothing but a tiny portion of the Sacred Host taken each morning. The Sacred Host is the wafer eaten by Catholics in "holy communion." A tiny portion would be but a fragment of this. In 1927 a German physician and a team of nurses studied her for two weeks maintaining strict watch to guarantee that she had no food. Her weight dropped in this time from 121 to 112 pounds. She is reported to have lost almost nine pounds on Friday, an incredible loss in one day. She rapidly regained her weight after the watch was discontinued. Physicians who have studied this case, fearing to tell the truth, merely say that they are unable to explain it. They merely point out that she has a history of nervous hysteria.

Anyone who has had extensive experience with fasting knows that fasters invariably lose weight and that a time is reached, after variable periods of abstinence, when to go longer without food is to result in death. Four months may be somewhere about the extreme limit that a human being can go without food and still live, and this is possible only in a relatively few individuals. To fast for such an extended period, one must begin the fast with an abundant reserve of food stores and one must conserve this reserve to make it hold out as long as possible. Certainly nervous individuals (epileptics, hysterics, etc.) would use up their meager reserves in far less time than this. Most, if not all of these reported long fasts, have been in cases of hysteria and investigations of them have revealed that they were getting food on the sly. The fasts have been fakes and under test conditions have proved to be so.

The fact that fakers have pretended to fast for such incredibly long times, and have been revealed as frauds, however, is not evidence that real fasting for prolonged periods has not been done. A brief mention of a few fasts in men and women will help to dispel the lingering doubts about the ability of man to go without food for long periods of time. Muni Shri Misrilji, a member of the Jan religious sect, underwent a fast which lasted 132 days, to impress upon his co-religionists the need for unity. Although this fast was not carefully watched, there seems to be no doubt that the man actually fasted this long. In 1828 the Parisian medical journals reported the case of a young girl who had typhoid fever and who took no food for 110 days.

Robert de Malone, founder of the Cistercian brotherhood, being overcome with grief upon hearing of the death of a female friend, decided to follow her into the henceforth. His religion forbade direct suicide, so he retired to a mountain-lodge of a relative, and abstained from food, hoping that one of his frequent fainting fits would result in death. After seventy days without food, he began to suspect the miraculous interposition of Providence, reconsidered his resolution and resumed eating. He began taking his food in half ounce installments and soon recovered from his great emaciation.

He led an active life for the next fourteen years, supervising an ever-increasing number of scattered monasteries.

Augusta Kerner, of Ingolstadt, a trance faster, survived in a semi-conscious condition nearly a quarter of a year without food.

Dr. Dewey tells of two children, of about four years, one of them his patient, whose stomachs were destroyed by drinking a solution of caustic potash. The patient of Dr. Dewey was "a delicate boy of spare-make." It required seventy-five days for the body to exhaust its reserves, and "there seemed to be only a skin and a skeleton when the last breath was drawn." Dr. Dewey tells us that "not one light drink of water was retained during life and yet the mind was clear up to even the last half hour." "The other child (with a larger supply of reserves) lived three months."

Dr. Hazzard tells us of an emaciated patient who had been bed-ridden for years, because of chronic functional "disease," the muscles being greatly wasted from lack of use, who fasted a total of 118 days out of a period of 140 days with practically complete recovery of health as a result.

Mr. Macfadden had one man to fast for ninety days in his institution. While the McSwiney hunger strike was in progress, I heard Dr. Lindlahr tell of one man who fasted seventy days in his institution. The longest fast I have ever personally conducted up to the present writing was one of ninety days. Long fasts in men and women have been numerous. Literally, thousands of them have gone beyond forty days, some of them going beyond a hundred days. The hunger strike of McSwiney, Lord Mayor of Cork, and his companions attracted a goodly amount of attention in 1920. Nine of these strikers kept up their fast for ninety-four days, and then returned to eating, and to health and strength. Although these men fasted longer than did McSwiney, they all recuperated rapidly, after their return to normal feeding, and are reported to have acquired a condition of body superior to that existing before the fast.

On the 47th day of his fast, McSwiney's sister addressed a letter to Cardinal Bourne in which she said: "Those of us who have been watching him through all these weary days have come to the inevitable conclusion that he has been supernaturally sustained in his struggles." Archbishop Mannix of Australia said of him: "I find him to be a veritable miracle."

No assumption of divine intervention in such cases is needed to explain them. God does not intervene in the cases of fasting worms, hibernating bears, and sexually active seals or salmon. Man is sustained while fasting as these animals are sustained. No miraculous element enters into a long fast. The whole thing may be explained by ordinary natural causes.

Strychnine was injected into the veins of McSwiney after food and alcohol were forced upon him. Undoubtedly he would have lived longer except for this and the nervous tension under which he was kept throughout his "strike." One of his colleagues died after 68 days of fasting.

Pashutin records the case of a youth, age eighteen, who took a spoonful of sulphuric acid after which he was unable to take any food at all for the first week, took only a little liquid food for the next four weeks and the last ten weeks no food but water. He reports that there was no albumen or sugar in the urine and that the man vomited after every attempt to eat. He died at the end of three months and twenty days.

He records the case of a man, age forty-two, who died in four months and twelve days after drinking some sulphuric acid. Pashutin says of this case "starvation appears complete," but informs us that two days before death the blood contained 4,849,000 red and 7,852 white cells per cu. mm.

A third case recorded by Pashutin is that of a young girl, age nineteen, who drank sulphuric acid. He says: "Some liquid food was given for four months but not believed absorbed as it was eliminated too rapidly and no chlorides in urine at all." Her "dead body was like a skeleton, but mammary glands remained unaffected." Her body temperature began to decrease only during the last eight days of her life. The girl complained only of thirst, not of hunger.

Dr. Hazzard describes a sixty day's fast by a woman, age 38, who suffered with obesity and Bright's "disease". The woman recovered health, and though she had been married twenty years, had her first baby one year after the fast. She records the case of another woman, age 41, with heart trouble, who fasted sixty-three days and attended her home duties and visited Dr. Hazzard's office daily.

In January, 1931, the press carried the following account of a woman in Africa, who fasted 101 days to reduce her weight:

"Cape Town, South Africa, Jan. 31—Authentic reports from Salisbury, South Rhodesia, state that Mrs. A. G. Walker, a noted Rhodesian singer, has been fasting 101 days, during which time she has consumed only two or three pints of cold and hot water daily.

"Last October Mrs. Walker weighed 232 pounds, so she desided to fast. She has lost sixty-three pounds. She says that she is in perfect health, goes out to parties and carries on with her public singing."

At noon, Oct. 31, 1932, an English businessman (age 53 years) of Leeds, London, who refuses to permit his name to be published, but who freely discussed his fast with reporters, began a fast under the direction of Mr. John W. Armstrong, who, though not a doctor of any school, has conducted hundreds of fasts and has been very successful in his work.

This man received nothing but water until 6:30 P.M., Feb. 8, 1933, when he was given the juice of one orange. Thereafter he received nothing but water until noon of Feb. 9. He weighed 191 lbs. (13 st. 9 lb.) at the beginning of the fast; 132 lbs. (9 st. 6 lb.) at the end of fifty days of fasting and 102 lbs. (7 st. 4 lb.) at the close of the 101 days without food—a loss of 89 lbs.

Before going on the fast the patient was blind (cataract in both eyes), had no sense of smell, had hardening of the arteries and heart trouble. He had previously been treated with iodine, aspirin, atropin and other drugs. In August before commencing the fast he was unable to tell night from day.

Mr. Armstrong reports that by the fifty-sixth day of the fast the cataracts had ceased to exist and the patient was able to see a little. Thereafter, sight improved gradually until vision again became normal. His sense of smell returned, heart improved and arteries became better.

To newspaper reporters, who interviewed the patient on the last day of the fast, the patient stated, "I was on my last legs. Nothing did me any good and I tried fasting as a last resort." "I would have tried anything in the hope of getting better again. I started the fast as an experiment for 10 days, then, as I seemed a little better, I went on from day to day.

"I stopped at 101 days. But I could have gone on for another 10 days or so easily if I had wished."

He said, "It *is* easy to fast after the first fortnight," but during the first fortnight he was forced to use great will power to resist food.

In a letter to me dated April 12, 1933, Armstrong informs me that his patient was able to walk about daily during the whole of the fast and talked rapidly to reporters for two hours on the 101st day. The patient was in first class condition at the time of writing the aforementioned letter. He also reports that up to the fiftieth day of the fast there were "no visible favourable results except that his skin was more natural in appearance and his arteries were softer."

These cases should convince any fair-minded and intelligent person that there is no immediate danger of starvation when a patient is placed upon a fast. If the pathological condition is remediable, the body will remedy it before any danger of starvation threatens.

A J. Carlson, Prof. of Physiology, University of Chicago, holds that a healthy, well-nourished man can live from fifty to seventy-five days without food, provided he is not exposed to severe cold, avoids physical work and maintains emotional calm. His maximum period of seventy-five days has been surpassed several times.

Luciani found that Succi lost 19 per cent in weight during his thirty days' fast and was otherwise in good health. With the gradually lowering rate of daily loss of weight as the fast progresses, it would probably have required another fifty days for Succi to have lost the forty per cent of his weight that some physiologists now consider the limit of safety.

Terence McSwiney died after seventy-eight days of fasting. On Sept. 14, 1929, Jatindranath Das, arrested along with fifteen others in the Lahore Conspiracy, died after sixty-one days without food— a hunger strike. Assuming that the conditions surrounding the two prisoners were similar, and that the emotional struggle in each of these men was not greatly different, the difference in time required for these two men to reach the end was due to the differences in the amounts of stored food reserves each carried.

Pashutin records the case of a criminal who died on the sixty-fourth day of a hunger strike and says of the case: "It indicates that in a man there are no less reserves than in animals." The amount of reserves carried by man varies in individual cases and this is the biggest determining factor in deciding how long one may safely go without food.

In over forty-four years of conducting fasts, I have conducted nearly thirty-five thousand fasts, ranging in duration from three days to three months. I have conducted about six fasts that have gone sixty or more days, one of sixty-eight days and one of ninety days. I have had literally hundreds of fasts that have lasted from forty to fifty and more days, and one of seventy-two days.

The statement has been made by certain religious authorities, in discussions of religious fasts, that the ancients could withstand fasting better than man of today. Such statements have been based on ignorance. There is no reason why the American of today cannot fast as long and with as much benefit as could the ancient Roman, Greek or Hebrew. There is no physiological, biological or other evidence that nature favored those ancient peoples more than she has us. They were not better constructed than are we.

A few years ago a mountainer preacher, Jackson Whitlow, of Stooping Oak, Tenn. went upon a fast, which he said had been ordered by Jehovah, who told him to eat nothing until further orders. He went for fifty-one days without food and then, having received instructions from on high to terminate the fast, broke it. Shortly before this time a report came from India of a fast, also undertaken from religious motives of 132 days, which, so the news accounts said, was apparently honestly undergone. A Russian medical volunteer is reported to have fasted sixty days to provide the profession with useful biological information.

Although there is little skepticism of the reality of that 132 days fast undergone by Muni Shri Misrilalji, a member of the Jain religious sect, there is no undeniable proof that he actually fasted this long. Numerous fasts of variable durations are on record in which the fasters died, most of them in medical hands. None of them have been fasts of exceptional length and it is probable that if they had been correctly handled, few if any of these fasters would have died.

It is generally assumed by popular or newspaper writers on fasting that, if a fast has not been observed by a medical man, its duration is not "scientifically" established. I have, for example, conducted fasts for over forty years and I have had most of my fasting patients under my direct supervision in institutional care. When I state that a certain man fasted for forty or fifty days, I know that he received no food during this period. But my fasts, not being supervised by a medical man, are not "scientifically" established. Actually, this is of no consequence. A fast of forty days is a fast of forty days whether the so-called "scientific" world accepts it or not. "Science" is pedantic, arrogant, esoteric and often insane.

I have had many people tell me that the forty day's fast of Jesus was a miracle. It has also been asserted that the long fasts of Moses and Elijah were miracles. Tanner's two fasts, one of forty days and the other of forty-two days, are frequently referred to as "unusual." Such fasts, of which there have been many, are often set down as historical oddities or eccentricities. They are thought of as isolated and extra-ordinary facts that have occurred from time to time, but as being without the limits of possibility for the average man or woman. Jesus or Tanner may have fasted for forty days and lived, and Tanner may have secured distinct benefits from his fast, but I could not go without food for even a day, is the statement of many when the fast is under discussion. As Dr. Page puts it in *The Natural Cure*, "It is commonly supposed that these are uncommon men; they are uncommon only in possessing a knowledge as to the power of the living organism to withstand abstinence from food, and in having the courage of their opinions."

The facts presented in this chapter prove conclusively that nature has no fear of a fast, even a long fast, and that the danger of starvation is very remote. We may enter upon a prolonged fast, in most instances, with perfect confidence that we are not going to perish of starvation in a few days, or even in a few weeks. This, of course, is not sufficient reason for us to fast. If fasting is not productive of positive benefit, the mere fact that it is not essentially dangerous is not enough to cause us to abstain from food. It shall be the purpose of the succeeding pages of this book, not alone to point out the many and varied benefits that may be derived from judicious fasting, but how to fast to secure maximum benefits.

FASTING ABILITY AND SURVIVAL

From the foregoing parts of this chapter it will be seen that fasting in man is practiced under about as wide a variety of circumstances as among the lower orders of life and for about as many purposes of adjustment and survival. Fasting is a vitally important part of man's life and, until modern times, when we have made a fetish of eating and have developed a ridiculous fear of going without food, even for a day, has played a major role in many of his activities.

It is very obvious that the ability to go for prolonged periods without food is as important a means of survival under many conditions in the life of man as it is in the lower animals. It is quite probable that primitive man was forced even more often than modern man to rely upon this ability in order to survive periods of food scarcity. In acute disease, in particular, the ability to go for prolonged periods without eating is very important in man, for the reason that he seems to suffer far more with disease than do the lower animals. In this condition, in which, as will be shown later, there is no power to digest and assimilate food, he is forced to rely upon his internal stores.

If man can fast, this is because he, like the lower forms of life, carries within himself a store of reserve food that may be utilized in cases of emergency or when raw materials are not available.

A Bill-of-Fare For The Sick

CHAPTER IV

Organisms capitalize the results of the joint work of their several organs and physiological systems in the form of capacities and valuable stored substances. They may learn to use this stored capital, this biological raw material which they have woven into their fabric and built into their flesh and blood, in the interest of the whole organism or in doing useful work; or they may consume it in wasteful expenditures of one kind or another, or they may use it under circumstances, such as "disease" or famine, when food cannot be digested or is not to be had.

When we go without food, no matter what the reason, nor how long the period of abstinence, the functioning tissues must live upon something. Berg says that when the food supply is completely cut off, the functions of circulation, respiration, etc., can still be carried out, "so that in the organs of most vital necessity the processes of assimilation continue even though the organism as a whole is foredoomed to death from a lack of the intake of energy." Surpluses of stored materials (stored for just such emergencies) are called upon to supply nutriment for these functioning, therefore hungry tissues. Some of these are oxidized to provide heat. This not only provides nutriment for functioning tissue, but it results in a removal of surpluses that may be cluttering up the avenues of life.

It is highly important that the body shall have some reserve supplies at all times to be drawn upon in case of need, for the ability to go for prolonged periods without eating is an important factor in survival and is made use of under a wide variety of circumstances and conditions in wild nature. Hence it is that we find that the body's economical tendency causes it to accumulate reserve stores, so that under stress and strain and in periods of scarcity, it will be able to go for more or less extended periods of time without the ordinary and regular food supplies. We note that the female cat, nursing several kittens, although eating regularly, loses much weight during her period of nursing. Her reserve stores are drawn upon almost as much as if she were fasting. These are replenished after the nursing period is over. There are many other circumstances in life in which these reserves are requisitioned for supplies.

Nutrition does not cease during a fast, for "nutrition is life." The purpose of the fast is not to suspend metabolism, but to free it. Working tissues must eat and as, when no food is eaten, the only sources of nutriment for these tissues is the internal stores of the organism, these are necessarily drawn upon for supplies. Jennings correctly explained the support of the vital tissues during the fast at a time when but little or no scientific investigations of the matter had been made. Well or sick, the functioning tissues of the animal that is not eating, draws upon its reserves.

While all animals lay up reserves of food for emergencies and these are commonly more or less generally stored in the organism, there are some animals that possess specialized stores in addition to the general stores. These specialized reserves have been appropriately called "built-in pantries." An excellent example of such "built-in pantries" is the big tail of the Gila Monster, a lizard of our southwestern desert and of Mexico. This poisonous reptile is able to live for several months without any food except what it draws from its heavy tail.

The well-fed Gila Monster possesses a thick, heavy tail. In barren years the Monster may be found with its tail thinned down almost to the spine, it having drawn upon this store of nutritive material for sustenance. It stores up food in the tail when food is plentiful and subsists on the tail when food is scarce. The Monster is capable of going for long periods without food, specimens having been kept in cages without food for upwards of six weeks.

An unusual type of "built-in pantry" is seen in the young of the Amazonian tree frog or, rather, its tadpoles. They possess an extra heavy tail and, instead of feeding upon algae (vegetables) as do other tadpoles, they gradually absorb the tail and utilize this as food as they undergo the changes and developments that constitute metamorphosis. No other food is required for their growing and developing bodies until they are sufficiently matured to hop about and search for food. The ordinary tadpole also absorbs its tail during the period when its legs are developing, at which time it also abstains from eating.

The hump or humps on the back of camels constitute stored food made up of fat. The size, plumpness and erectness of the hump are indications of the camel's ability to go without food. When his food supply runs low, as he trudges through the desert, he draws upon his hump or humps for food. (A similar hump of fat that represents stored food is seen in the Brahma cattle, of which we have a large supply here in the southwest). If the camel is forced to draw heavily upon his hump, it becomes empty and falls over on the side of his spinal column and hangs like an empty bag until replenished.

The penguin, which has a long winter fast, stores up food for lean times. To sustain him during his seasonal fast, the emperor penguin stores up twelve or more pounds of fat, chiefly about the stomach region. The huge buttocks of Hottentot women have been listed as "built-in pantries," but to class steatopagy as a "portable pantry" is, perhaps, to wrongly designate this deformity, although certainly the fat may be drawn upon in case of need. There seems to me, however, to be no more reason to think of the huge buttocks of the Hottentot as a specialized reserve than there is to think of the equally huge abdomens of many European and American men and women as such.

The fact is that all fat represents stored food supplies, but, except in cases of really healthy animals that have been feeding on adequate food supplies, there is little reason to think that it is adequate to meet all of the nutritive needs of the fasting animal for more than a brief period. It is more than likely that in all of these animals, there are stores of sugar, minerals, vitamins, etc., in the liver, and other glands and in the muscles. There are, of course, the usual reserves in the blood, bones, bone marrow and in other tissues. Fat, alone is not adequate food for a fasting animal.

In Persia, there exists a variety of sheep called fat-tailed sheep, that has an enormous tail made up of fat and other stored food elements. During seasons of plenty the sheep stores up large quantities of food in its tail—prize specimens often developing such heavy tails that their owners provide them with small carts which are placed under the tails and fastened to prevent the tails from dragging the ground. When pasturage becomes scarce the sheep draw upon the food reserves stored in their tails for nutriment. This is a literal example of "cutting off the tail of a hungry dog and feeding it to him."

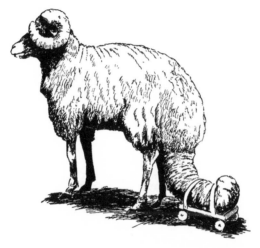

These specialized provisions for storing food reserves are analogous to the provision possessed by the camel for storing water. There are other animals which have other specialized storages for food reserves upon which they may draw in times of food scarcity. Although such specialized structures are not universal in the animal kingdom, nature provides in all animals for the storing of food reserves, even though there is no specialized structure provided for this purpose; for food is as likely to be scarce for one animal as for another. All hibernating animals are equipped with specialized apparatus for storing up food reserves. It has been urged against fasting by man that he is not a hibernating animal. It is quite true that man possesses no specialized food reserves, as does the Russian bear, for example; but he does possess generalized food reserves, like all animals. The dog, cat, cow, horse, elephant, etc., are not hibernating animals, yet all of these instinctively refuse food when ill or wounded. Hibernating animals are inactive and have stored food reserves which have been put away for just this period; but there are other animals which go for long periods of time without food and which are vigorously active at the same time. The Alaskan fur-seal bull and the salmon are remarkable examples of this. The fact is that, all animals, man included, are provided with food reserves which are held in store against a period of forced or necessary abstinence from food.

As in all animals that periodically fast, fat is stored in large quantities during the periods between fasts and is used during the fast with which to supply the nutritive needs of the working tissues, both the fear of acidosis from the rapid breaking down of fat, and the supposed demand for larger quantities of protein seem to me to be greatly exaggerated. It is, of course, true, that all of these animals possess sugar, mineral, protein and vitamin stores, but fat seems to be the preferred storage material. In the fat are also minerals and vitamins.

Those marine monsters to which the name whale has been given are veritable gluttons. We are told that in the South Atlantic the humpbacks, blue whales and the fin whale live almost exclusively upon the plankton shrimp which they eat in "astronomical quantities." These whales fatten on the enormous sholes of shrimp that exist near the surface during the summer. In winter these whales eat little so that their blubber is greatly reduced in quantity. I have never seen it stated that whales ever fast for extended periods; only that they eat little. During these periods of restricted eating, their store of fat serves them as food with which to supply their functioning tissues.

There is something wrong with the reasoning of a man who urges the eating of liver, heart, spleen, intestines, and other internal organs, the taking of cod-liver oil, etc., as sources of vitamins, and then declares in the next breath that the body does not store up vitamins. He may declare that fasting should not be undergone because there is not sufficient vitamins in the body to sustain the nutritional processes through a fast of more than a few days and he will assert the truth of this proposition in the face of the examples of thousands of men and women who have undergone long fasts with great benefit.

Bees not only store up honey for winter use, but they also carry food reserves stored within themselves. The same thing may be said for squirrels which store nuts for winter use. These and many other animals have two sources of supply in case of need. Of a slightly different character is the way in which fasting female birds and fish will absorb the eggs stored in their bodies and utilize these as food. Morgulis, experimenting with the newt, *Duemyctium*, found that the "ripe" female withstands abstinence best, because she actually absorbs and utilizes the large reserve of stored food in the mature eggs and thereby saves her other organs and tissues from wasting. Heidkamp found, in experiments with *Tritoncristattus*, a fresh water salmon, that when the female is denied food, the fully developed eggs in her body are the first to be absorbed.

Prof. Morgulis further says: "Active growth and regeneration are not incompatible with inanition, and the wear and tear, at least in some organs, is so completely repaired as to evade for a long time the effect of a nutritional stringency. Inanition does not preclude the ability for extreme and sustained exertion."

Under ordinary circumstances, the generalized food reserves of man and animal are capable of sustaining functional and structural integrity for a considerable time without more food being consumed. Under the most favorable circumstances of quiet, rest and mental poise, these reserves are capable of holding out much longer. There is a sense in which the utilization of these reserves is analogous to cutting off the tail of a hungry dog and feeding it to him, but the analogy will not go on all fours. These reserves are stored up for just such uses and there are times and conditions when they must be used. Indeed there are conditions of "disease" in which it is impossible to make use of food from any other source—conditions in which the body is unable to take the raw materials and make use of them.

Not only are these food reserves capable of nourishing the vital tissues of the body for long periods, but the body does not permit any of its vital tissues to be damaged or consumed so long as these stores hold out. It is only after these reserves have been exhausted that nature will permit any of the vital or functioning tissues of the body to be damaged. There is no danger of damage to the vital organs from a prolonged fast. Fear of fasting is unfounded and based on ignorance or misinformation.

Abstaining from all food except water until these food reserves are consumed, is *fasting*. Abstaining from food after these food reserves have been consumed, is *starving*.

Discussing the death of president Garfield, who lived eighty days after he was shot, and who wasted until "all that seemed to be left of the great president when he drew his last breath on the night of the 80th day at Elberson was a thin skin covering a skeleton," Dr. Dewey asks: "What became of the tissues in this case? Did they evaporate?"

When food is withdrawn from man or animal, the demand for substance with which to maintain the structures and functions of the vital tissues is thrown upon the reserves of the fasting organism. The fasting organism makes the most of the material at hand—it spins out the inevitable loss as far as possible, indeed, those substances which are absolutely essential for the preservation of the vital spark or for the continuance of the motion of such necessary organs as the heart and central nervous system, are only used up when the supply from other organs has almost entirely failed. Fats and any store of glycogen are first used up, along with part of the proteins, until, when from a quarter to a half of the total body weight has been lost, the machine stops for want of motive power.

If the fasting continues, readjustments are made to secure minimum demands upon the nutritive stores; as the fast progresses, the body tends to conserve its supplies by lessening activity both physical and physiological, so that the rate of loss gradually diminishes.

In cold-blooded animals, in which fasting is a regular physiological occurrence in the life-cycle, the reserves are usually plentiful and the demand made upon them is small, so that they may fast for long intervals without being forced to renew their stores. In warm-blooded animals, whose reserves are frequently lower and whose greater activities make greater demands upon these, the reserves are more rapidly depleted. However, it is only after all these reserves are exhausted that the organized tissues are requisitioned as nutritive substances.

The reserves last much longer if the faster rests, than if he is active during the fast. Better results are achieved in the fast if rest is observed. Work, long walks, strenuous exercise, etc., waste the body's reserves without producing any compensating benefits.

Physical effort, external cold, worry and strong emotions increase the rate with which the body's reserves are utilized. Fever, perhaps does the same, at least in most if not all acute diseases.

Nelson's Encyclopedia says: "The observations made during the fast of Succi and others show that the body wastes less rapidly when the patient is kept warm and at rest. The fatty tissues are the first to be used up, and later the proteids of the skeletal and intestinal muscles. The heart muscle does not diminish appreciably and probably it derives its substance from the less essential muscles. In long continued fasts the tissues waste more rapidly during the first few days. Later the body uses its reserves of nourishment more economically."

Previous fasting seems to train the body to a more economical use of its reserves. The enormous economy of an educated disposal of the body's forces is thus seen. A second or third fast is also almost always more comfortable than the first fast, although in many first fasts there is no discomfort at all.

"Human flesh," says Dr. Page (*The Natural Cure*, page 73), "by absorption, constitutes a most appropriate diet in certain conditions of disease. The absorption and excretion of diseased tissue is, under some circumstances, the only work that nature can with safety undertake, and in these cases, no building up can be accomplished until a solid foundation is reached and the debris removed; and not then, unless while this good work is going on, the nutritive organs are given an opportunity to virtually renew themselves."

Human flesh, by absorption, becomes the bill-of-fare of the sick and in all serious acute illness the only possible bill-of-fare. Dr. Dewey was Acting Assistant Surgeon, U.S.A., in charge of a ward in the Chattanooga Field Hospital in 1864, where, he says, "postmortems were the rule" and that they were numerous. In discussing these post-mortems he says, "there was one fact revealed in every post-mortem of tremendous significance, that failed to make any impression on my mind other than to remember it. The fact that no matter how emaciated the body, even if the skeleton condition had been reached, the brain, the heart, the lungs, except themselves diseased, never received any loss."

These soldiers according to the theories of the time were fed "plenty of good nourishing food," to "keep up their strength." They "wasted" as do all such patients, because the vital tissues of their bodies were feeding off the less vital or non-vital tissues. The vital tissues so fed themselves because there was no other possible way for them to feed.

These studies reveal to us that there are alimentary reserve stores in the body gathered to guard against times of need. These nutritive reserves are ready for use at short notice and with little energy expenditure by the body. They are capable of supplying all essential needs for the time being, and can be replenished at leisure, after the work of reconstruction has been completed.

If the adipose tissue and other reserves are abundantly present, one may fast thirty to ninety or more days without consuming one cell of the essential tissues of the body.

"With no digestive drudgery on hand," says Oswald, "Nature employs the long-desired leisure for general house-cleaning purposes. The accumulations of superfluous tissues are overhauled and analyzed; the available component parts are turned over to the department of nutrition, the refuse to be thoroughly and permanently removed."

Organisms capitalize the results of the joint work of their several organs both in the form of increased capacities and valuable stored substances and are able to use their stored capital as though to some extent independent of immediate external supply. This stored capital, or biological raw material, is woven into the inner fabric of organisms by the reciprocal labors of their various parts and is ready for instant utilization when need arises.

The aggregate tissues of the organism may be regarded as a reservoir of nutriment capable of being called in any direction or to any point, as needed. The ability of the body to nourish its vital tissues off its food reserves and its less vital tissues, is of extreme importance to the sick man who is unable to digest and absorb food. Except for this ability, the acutely ill would perish of starvation.

Pashutin records the case of a girl 19 years old who starved to death after ruining her digestive tract by drinking some sulphuric acid. He says "her dead body was like a skeleton, but mammary glands remained unaffected." He also records that in cases of hibernating animals, the growth of granulation tissue in wounds continues during the deepest slumber, even when every other function seems almost to have ceased. The heart may beat as slow as one beat in five to eight minutes, and the blood circulation be so slow that cuts made in the flesh bleed very slightly, yet the cuts heal.

Contrary to popular (and even professional) opinion, the vital tissues of the fasting organism do not begin to break down from starvation immediately upon the withdrawal of food. Ths fasting body does lose weight, but "live weight" losses are not reliable indications of tissue changes within the organism. The largest draft upon the body stores during a fast is made upon the fat and in both man and animals the rapid loss of weight during the first one to four days of a fast, particularly noticeable in the fat person, is due to the tendency of fat to fall off rapidly.

Thus, it is seen that the vital tissues are nourished first off the food reserves and when these are exhausted, off the less vital tissues. No damage will or can occur in any of the vital tissues of the body so long as its reserves are adequate to meet the nutritive needs of these tissues. This varies from a few days in very emaciated people to a few months in very fat individuals. There need be no fear of fasting, even the most prolonged fasting, under experienced and intelligent guidance. The human body may have stored within it such enormous resources of energy that it will be able to fast many days.

Because they are ignorant of the reserves of the animal body, which are available for sustenance, when, for any reason it is denied food, physicians, nurses, patients, their relatives and friends, are afraid of fasting and insist that the sick must eat to "keep up their strength." Never was there a greater fallacy entertained.

One important feature about fasting has been entirely overlooked by all the so-called scientific investigators of fasting. I refer to the manner in which it causes the breaking down, absorption and elimination or use of abnormal growths, effusions, exudates, deposits, etc. The scientists have conducted all their experiments on healthy animals or healthy men and are, for this reason, in no position to know its effects in the sick body.

They learned that useless fat and the less essential tissues are consumed first, and the most essential tissues of the body are hardly touched, even where death from starvation results. But never having watched the process they cannot know anything of the rapidity with which dropsical fluid, for example, is absorbed from the cavities or tissues and utilized as food. They cannot know how tumor-like growths are often rapidly absorbed and how, even large tumors are reduced in size. Resolution in pneumonia is hastened, the process taking place so rapidly, often that it would be difficult to believe unless one should see it. "Diseased" tissues are broken down, exudates, effusions and deposits are absorbed and either used or eliminated.

The body utilizes everything it can dispense with during a fast in order to preserve the integrity of the essential tissues. The useless and least essential things are sacrificed first.

The fat man, fasting, is eating all through his fast; he is eating a lot of surplus tissue that he has been carrying around as dead weight. But we do not have to be fat to be able to fast. Even the underweight person carries a store of food reserve. I have often been amazed at the ability of skinny patients to fast and to maintain their strength while doing so. I have seen them go without food for as much as twenty-two days when I had judged by their appearance that three to four days would be their safe limit. We go without food, and while we do this, we eat what surplus tissue (fat, etc.) that we have. After our reserves are exhausted or nearly so, we must resume eating, else we begin to break down and consume our essential tissues and this means that we begin to die. We should never be reduced to the necessity of "eating" ourselves—our reserves should constitute our bill-of-fare while we abstain from food.

There is an economical tendency of the organism to accumulate reserve stores in the body so that under stress or strain or deprivation and want, it shall be able to go on for sometime without the ordinary supplies of food. Man or animal in case of famine, shipwreck, or under other circumstances in which food cannot be secured, would perish forthwith, except for these generalized food reserves stored in the body.

We saw in a previous chapter that each cell and each organ has its own private food reserve. In addition to this there is a considerable quantity of glycogen stored in the liver, much surplus protein and other food substances carried in the blood and lymph, several pounds of fat in the body (even thin people have considerable fat) and much food reserve in the marrow of the bones. In the glands there is stored a considerable supply of vitamins. It is possible that the body can retain and re-use its vitamins as it can its iron and certain other minerals. Collectively, the above stores constitute a reserve food store that is capable of sustaining the vital organs and their functions through an emergency of considerable length. The ensemble of the body's food reserves is well balanced with respect to the various nutritive elements, salts, vitamins, etc. They are capable of meeting the nutritive needs of the vital tissues for long periods.

There is still another source of foods, which, in some animals may amount to several days' supply. In ruminants the food residues (undigested food) in the intestinal tract are usually very large (so large, indeed, that the variability in "fill" contained in the digestive canal disguises the true body weight and has been a constant cause of uncertainty in determining changes in the body tissues, and amounting often in the case of the steer to one-fifth of the entire body weight) and serve as a source of food for a considerable period after food has been withdrawn, so that the immediate demands upon the body's actual reserves are not great.

The alimentary reserves of omnivorous animals, although usually plentiful, are quickly exhausted when food is denied. In dogs and man the alvine canal is almost immediately exhausted of its food supply, so that the true fasting period is more quickly reached. The whole expense of fasting is thrown upon the food reserves in their bodies almost from the outset.

Hibernation differs from ordinary fasting in that the hibernating animal possesses special stores for the period, and in that the metabolic rate is decreased much more in hibernation, thus lessening the need for food.

The fasting organism subsists on materials previously stored in its tissues. It would be erroneous to suppose that during a fast, under whatever condition, the processes of nutrition are suspended. Only those concerned with the digestion and absorption of raw materials are interrupted.

The fasting organism is nourished as truly off its accumulated reserves as if it daily consumed an abundance from the fat of the land. Prof. Morgulis says, indeed, that "inanition must be regarded as a special—perhaps, the simplest—form of nutrition." He adds that materials for growth and repair of tissue, energy for maintenance and energy for work, are supplied "under the conditions of inanition" from the "rich deposit of nutritive substances" which "every organism contains in its tissues" and "which constitute the common foods when they serve to nourish another organism."

Autolysis

CHAPTER V

In order that we may comprehend much that takes place within the fasting organism, it is necessary that we have an understanding of the process of *autolysis*, which, although very common in nature, has been all but overlooked by physiologists generally. We have previously mentioned the fact that the vital or functioning tissues of the fasting organism are nourished off the food reserves stored in the body. These reserves are stored as rather complex substances, such as sugar (glycogen), fat, protein, etc., and are no more fitted for entrance into the bloodstream and use by the cells than are the fats, proteins and carbohydrates of another animal or another food. Before they can be taken up by the circulation and assimilated by the cells, they must first be digested.

Let us begin with a familiar example of the digestion and absorption of a part of a living organism by the organism itself. In the process of becoming a frog the tadpole grows four legs. After these are fully formed, it no longer has use for the tail that served so well in the tadpole stage, so it proceeds to get rid of it, not by shedding it as is popularly supposed, but by absorbing it. The tail is made up of muscle, fat, nerves, skin, etc. To absorb these structures, they are digested in the same way that fat and muscle are digested in the digestive tract. By the action of the appropriate enzymes the proteins and fats are broken down into their constituent amino and fatty acids. Only thus are they fit to re-enter the circulation. Only as fatty acids and amino acids can they be re-used with which to nourish other structures of the body of the frog.

During the period when the tail of the ex-tadpole is being absorbed, the young frog does not eat. Indeed, it ceases to eat when the forelegs come into view. Fasting may be essential to the absorption of the tail, at least it hastens the process, for it compels the utilization of the tail as food with which to nourish the vital tissues of the fasting frog.

We may liken this process to that of the eating of its skin by the toad. Toads molt several times yearly. They swallow their molted skin after they emerge from it. To make use of the molted skin, the toad must first digest it. Its proteins and fats must be reduced to simple acceptable compounds, such as amino acids and fatty acids. This is done in this instance in the stomach and intestine of the toad. But in the case of the fasting frog digesting its tail, the work is done within the tail itself.

The thymus gland, which controls the growth of the young, is absorbed after its work is completed. Noting the manner in which the body rids itself of non-functioning or no-longer-needed structures, as in the case of this gland, it would be extraordinary were it to really turn out that there are structures in the body that are truly functionless and have been so for ages. At this point, however, our interest in this gland and its absorption is for a different lesson. It is referred to here to point out that it is broken down and absorbed by the process of autolysis. There can be no doubt that the materials of which it is composed are re-used by the organism.

The word autolysis (a-tol-i-sis) is derived from the Greek and means, literally, self-loosing. It is used in physiology to designate the process of digestion or disintegration of tissue by ferments (enzymes) generated in the cells themselves. It is a process of self-digestion — intra-cellular digestion.

A number of autolytic (a-to-lit-ik) enzymes are known and are included under the general terms, *oxidases* and *peroxidases*. Physiologists know that proteolytic (protein digesting) enzymes are formed within many, if not in all living tissues. Apparently every tissue turns out its own enzyme, which, probably, under all ordinary circumstances of life, is employed in the regular processes of metabolism. Under other conditions the enzymes may be employed to digest the substances of the cells themselves. In their *Textbook of Physiology* (1946 edition) Zoethout and Tuttle mention that under certain experimental conditions the unrestrained activities of the enzymes normally present in the liver (proteases, lipases, carbohydrases) digest the proteins, carbohydrates, and fats of the liver. In normal life this digestion of the liver does not occur. These various intra-cellular enzymes play a conspicuous part in the metabolism of food substances; that is, in the normal or regular function of nutrition or metabolism.

A few familiar examples of autolysis will prepare the reader to understand its use in "disease." The phenomena of fasting supply many examples of the control the body exercises over its autolytic processes. For example, tissues are lost in the inverse order of their usefulness — fat and morbid growths first, and then the other tissues. These tissues (fatty tissue, bone marrow, etc.) and food substances (glycogen) are not fit to enter the blood stream before they are acted upon by enzymes. Indeed, human fat, or human muscle, is no more fitted to enter the circulation without first being digested, than is fat or muscle from the cow or sheep. Glycogen (animal starch), stored in the liver, must be converted into a simple sugar before it can be released into the blood stream. This conversion is accomplished by enzymic action.

The manner in which an abscess "points" on the surface of the body and drains its septic contents on the outside is well known to every one of my readers. What is not generally known, is that this "pointing" on the surface is possible only because the flesh between the abscess and the surface is digested by enzymes; that is, it is autolyzed and removed.

The absorption of the bone-ring support established about the ends of a fracture is made possible by the autolytic disintegration of the bone-ring. The re-arrangement of materials in pieces of planaria and the dissolution of the pharynx in the piece containing this, to form a new one to fit the new size, as described elsewhere, is made possible by autolysis.

Sylvester Graham had some conception of the process of autolysis and of its use in disease. He thought that it is a general law of organic life that, when, by any means or from any cause, the catabolic processes exceed those of anabolism, the body always lays hold of and removes those substances which are of least use to the organism. For this reason, he said, all the morbid accumulations, such as wens (cysts), tumors, abscesses, etc., are rapidly diminished and often wholly removed under severe and protracted abstinence and fasting.

The view of many physiologists of Graham's era was that the lymphatics throughout the body, like the lacteals in the intestines, possess, to a high degree, the power to take up from the tissues, food substances, which they convert into a chyle-like substance, but of a more refined and sublimated quality, and that this pre-digested material is returned to the general circulation to be used in all parts of the body as nutriment. Although Graham thought that the "assimilating power" of the lymphatics (or, as they often called them, the *absorbents*) was real, he was of the opinion that the physiologists had magnified it. Nonetheless, he said that "when supplies of food in the alimentary canal are exceedingly small or entirely cut off for a considerable time, the lymphatics unquestionably become much more active than usual, and prey upon the adipose and other substances of the body, forming a lymph which has many of the characteristics of chyle and blood, and which may, to some extent, in such an emergency, serve the purpose of nutrition." He said that this does not occur in the ordinary and undisturbed operations of the organism when the digestive tract supplies adequate food materials. He, along with many other physiologists of the period, thought of lymph, under these circumstances, as being "mainly if not entirely an excrementitious substance."

He did not think that there are any facts to justify the assumption that the fat thus converted into lymph is used as nutriment during a fast. He regarded fat as being more or less in the nature of uneliminated surpluses (largely of an undesirable character) that the body was forced to store because it was unable to excrete. For this reason, it is unfit for food. His view was that in a perfectly healthy state of the body, a perfect equilibrium between the processes of assimilation and disassimilation is maintained so that no fat accumulates.

AUTOLYSIS IN PLANTS

The plant kingdom teems with examples of autolysis, but a few familiar examples will suffice for our present purpose. All bulbs, of which the onion will serve as an example, maintain within themselves a new plant surrounded by sufficient food to tide it over during a period of rest, during which period it does not take up food from the soil and air. Indeed, it may be taken out of the ground and stored for long periods. The onion may begin to grow in the bin or bag in which it is stored. It sends up stems and soon almost the whole of the bulb of the onion is transformed into green blades. The bulb gradually becomes soft, and finally, there is left a mere shell, as the growing plant digests and utilizes the substance of the onion. Beets, turnips and many other tubers will grow in the same manner. By autolytic digestion of the substances in the tuber, material is provided for growth and even while out of the ground, these plants will put forth stems and leaves and grow.

Who has not seen the housewife put a sweet potato in a jar of water and hang it up and watch it grow. It sends out stems which grow to great lengths and puts out many green leaves. Such a potato plant will continue to grow so long as there remains any of the food that was stored as sweet potato. The so-called Irish potato will also put forth stems and leaves and these will grow, drawing upon the substances stored in the potato as their sole source of food. If there is light, the leaves and stems of the potato will be green; if they are kept in the dark, the stems and leaves will be white. If there is a crack several feet away through which a little light enters, these stems will grow in the direction of the source of light and will grow several feet long, if the light is that far away. By *autolysis* the stored food substances in the tubers are broken up and made usable by the young plant.

The early growth of all plants from seed involves digestion of food stored in the seed. Seed, like the eggs of animals, are chiefly storehouses of food. The actual living part of the seed is almost microscopic in size.

A rose cutting or a fig cutting placed in the soil and watered, will put forth roots and leaves and grow. Both the leaves and the roots are grown from materials within the cutting. Cut a begonia leaf into small pieces and properly tend these and each piece will grow into a new begonia plant. The substances of the fragment of the leaf are used out of which to build a new plant. These are instances of the autolysis, redistribution and reorganization of materials contained within the part.

AUTOLYSIS IN ANIMALS

At the very commencement of life *autolysis* is an essential process. The embryonic development of animals in eggs involves digestion of the food stored in the eggs. Eggs, however large or small, contain a living germ that is microscopic in size which is the only living part of the egg. The remainder of the egg consists of stored food material out of which the evolving animal constructs its organs and parts. This food substance is no more suited to the use of the evolving embryo than it is suited to the use of the adult animal. Before it can be used in making tissue, it must be digested. This digestion is achieved by enzymes produced by the embryo.

The fasting salamander, the tail of which has been cut off, grows a new tail. It draws upon its general food stores for materials out of which to construct the new tail. These materials must first be broken down (digested) by the process of autolysis and then transferred to the growing tail. Here we watch a process that is somewhat the reverse of that seen in the frog that is absorbing its tail. Here materials are taken from the body and used in producing a tail; there materials are taken from the tail and used with which to nourish the body.

The enormous growth of the gonads of fasting salmon is accomplished by transferring materials from the body of the salmon to the testicles. Autolysis is necessarily the first step in this transfer of materials. The body is not only able to build tissue, it can also destroy tissue. It can not only digest and utilize the tissues of other organisms, it can digest and use its own tissue.

AUTOLYSIS DURING PUPAL SLEEP

The period of *pupal sleep* in the life of insects is a period of great and complex organizational changes, resulting in a new and radically different insect. The larvæ of insects devote their whole attention to growing and moulting. They eat enormous quantities of food and grow large and fat. The silk worm, for example, during its thirty-day period of growth, increases its weight fifteen thousand times. At the end of its larval stage the silkworm spins for itself a cocoon by which it protects itself in the pupa stage. There emerges from the cocoon, not a worm but a silkfly. The caterpillar of the butterfly changes to a chrysalis. The outer covering of the chrysalis is a hardened shell, usually brown in color. There emerges from this, not a worm, but a butterfly. Whereas, the worm-like larva enters the cocoon or chrysalis, it emerges an adult butterfly or moth, totally changed, both in internal and external structures, with different functions to perform and a different life to lead.

It is during the stage of pupal sleep that the entire organism of the insect undergoes a complete and radical metamorphosis, there is a tearing down of old structures, a re-shuffling of materials, the creation and re-aggregation of parts, so that what emerges from the pupa, when the transformation is complete, is an organism so unlike either the pupa or the larva that it may easily be mistaken for a totally new and distinct species.

It is interesting to note that during the pupal stage of insect life no food is taken. During this period of outward quiescence, all of the material stored up by the gluttonous larva is used out of which to construct a totally new and different organism. By autolysis old structures are torn down, stored materials are digested and prepared for new use, the materials are shifted from one part of the organism to another. All of this marvelous process of metamorphosis takes place while the animal is fasting. Here is a striking example of the constructive work that the organism may carry on while abstaining from food. But it should be understood that materials could not be shifted from one part of the body to another and no-longer-needed structures could not be torn down and the materials of which they are composed could not be used out of which to construct new structures, except that they are first digested. *Autolysis* is as essential at this stage of the insect's life as the ability to construct new parts.

Metamorphosis in insects supplies us with one of the most remarkable examples of both autolysis and the distribution and reorganization of materials that go on in living organisms as regular parts of the process of living. The maggot of the common housefly dissolves into a creamy liquid seemingly as structureless as the yolk of an egg. The original organs are destroyed and new ones are fashioned. No new materials, except, perhaps, air and moisture, are employed in this creation of the new form. During fifteen days of fasting, the pupa of the honey bee metamorphoses into a full grown bee, the changes undergone amounting to a transformation of one form of life into another form, with different organs, different functions and a radically different way of life.

The overfed caterpillar wraps itself in a hermetically sealed cocoon and goes to sleep and, during its sleep, it transforms itself into a gorgeous butterfly with bright wings that flash in the sun. As it undergoes metamorphosis, its muscles and its organs undergo dissolution into a substance that resembles a sort of pus. All of its internal structures are torn down by autolytic processes and are distributed to different parts to be completely reorganized. The metamorphosis of chrysalis into butterfly is as though some fairy with a magic wand stood by and directed operations. Here we observe no mere chemical process; here is organization and prevision; here is controlled tearing down and rebuilding; here is no mere turning out of compounds, but the construction of complex organs that are to function in the future.

The cocoon takes no food during this period of metamorphosis; the whole reorganization process is done while fasting and the materials that are stored in the body of the caterpillar, while it is eating its way through the world, are used for the transformation of the "worm" into a butterfly. As remarkable as is the process of metamorphosis itself, is the fact that practically no material is left over. The material in one caterpillar is just sufficient to make one butterfly.

DISTRIBUTION OF MATERIALS

The severely wounded animal refuses to eat, yet its wound heals. Great quantities of blood are sent to the site of the wound. This represents a great quantity of food taken to the part. The blood is the distributing agent in all higher forms of life. The fasting animal draws upon its reserves of food materials out of which to repair its torn, cut or broken tissues. These are first autolyzed and then carried to the part of the body where they are needed. The body can not only distribute its nutritive supplies; it can also re-distribute them. It possesses the ability to shift its chemicals and fasting supplies many examples of this. Autolysis makes re-distribution possible.

The ability to re-distribute substances and supplies is common to all forms of life. This ability is an ever-present protection against injury, except under the most prolonged deprivation. The digestion and re-organization of parts seen in worms and other animals, when deprived of food, the digestion and re-distribution of reserves, surpluses and non-vital tissues, as seen in all animals, when forced to go without food, constitute, for the writer, some of the most marvelous phenomena in the whole realm of biology.

AUTOLYSIS IS CONTROLLED

Autolysis is a rigidly controlled process; it is no blind, undirected bull-in-a-china-shop affair. Not only throughout the fasting period, but also throughout the starvation process, as well, the body exercises control over autolysis. The most rigid economy is exercised throughout both periods in the digestion and utilization, not only of the vital and most vital tissues, but of the dispensable and expendable tissues. In a later chapter we shall study the control of the autolytic process during fasting. Here I wish to call attention to the fact that in starvation there is no indiscriminate wasting of the body, but rather the same safeguarding of the more vital tissues and a slow sacrifice of the less vital tissues that is seen in the fasting period.

When the frog fasts during the time it is consuming its tail, only the tail disappears. Never does one of the legs of the frog undergo autolytic disintegration. No needed structure is digested and absorbed. If planaria or flat worms, are cut in small pieces and placed where they can absorb nourishment, each piece will grow into a small worm. If they cannot get nourishment, they cannot grow. Each piece, therefore, completely re-arranges its materials and becomes a perfect, but very minute worm. The piece that contains the pharynx, finding this too large for its diminished size, will dissolve it and make a new one that fits its new size. We have here a process similar to the metamorphosis of insects that goes on in the pupal stage. Here is manifest the ability to tear down a part and shift its constituent materials. The same thing is seen in the softening and absorption of the bone-ring support around a point of fracture. Only part of the bone-ring is digested, the remainder is retained to reinforce the weakened structure.

Zoethout and Tuttle point out that autolysis is a controlled process and mention the following examples of carefully controlled autolysis that normally occur at certain periods of life: "atrophy of the mammary glands at the close of lactation, of the uterus after parturition, the general atrophy of old age, and the resolution (dissolution) of the exudate formed in the lungs during pneumonia." The atrophy of the thymus gland at puberty should also be included in this list.

These authors offer other examples of controlled autolysis, saying: "During starvation some organs (heart and brain) are absolutely necessary and their activity cannot be dispensed with; hence they must be supplied with proteins. These proteins are obtained from the skeletal muscles, which must be looked upon not only as organs of contraction but also as storehouses for proteins. The proteins of the muscles and other organs are digested by the intracellular proteases (enzymes) into soluble proteins, amino acids, which are then carried by the blood stream to the vital organs. Another striking illustration of the transfer of protein from one organ to another is seen in the tremendous development, in the spawning and fasting salmon, of the ovaries at the expense of the muscles, which lose as much as 30 per cent of their weight."

Neither the ovaries, nor the heart, nor the brain can live, grow and function on a diet of amino acids. They need minerals, carbohydrates, fats and vitamins. Fasting salmon lose more than weight of muscle; they also lose fat and glycogen. There is great accumulation of phosphorus in the gonads of fasting salmon.

It is interesting to note that this control of autolysis extends also to pathological tissues, such as tumors, deposits, effusions, etc., and is not confined to the normal tissues of the body. Examples of this will be given later.

The fact that autolysis is a rigidly controlled and not a haphazard process, is our guarantee that the vital tissues of the body will not be sacrificed during even prolonged abstinence from food. It guarantees us that only the non-vital tissues will be digested and their constituents carried throughout the body to nourish the vital tissues.

Three important facts stand out clearly in what has gone before:

1. By reason of its possession of intracellular enzymes the body is capable of digesting its own proteins, fats and carbohydrates.

2. It is fully capable of controlling the self-digesting process and rigidly limits it to the non-essential and less essential tissues. Even in starvation, when vital tissues are destroyed, there is rigid control of the process and the tissues continue to be drawn upon according to their relative importance.

3. The body is capable of utilizing the end-products of autolytic disintegration of its own tissues to nourish its most vital and most essential parts.

THE AUTOLYTIC DISINTEGRATION OF TUMORS

Trall asserted that all abnormal growths possess a lower grade of vitality than normal growths, hence are easier to destroy. I think it may be equally true that they do not command the support of the organism as do normal growths, as they are deficient in nerve and blood supply. This lack of support makes them the ready victims of the autolytic processes of the body. It is generally held by men with wide experience with the fast that abnormal tissues are broken down and eliminated more rapidly than normal tissue during periods of abstinence. Physiologists have studied the process of autolysis, although they have suggested no practical use that may be made of it save that of employing it to reduce weight. It now remains for physiologists to learn that by means of rigidly controlled autolysis, the body is able to digest tumors and utilize the proteins and other food elements contained in them to nourish its vital tissues. Why have they not investigated this vitally important subject? The facts have been before the world for more than a hundred years.

Over a hundred and thirty years ago Sylvester Graham wrote: "It is a general law of the vital economy, that when, by any means, the general function of decomposition exceeds that of composition or nutrition, the decomposing absorbents always first lay hold of and remove those substances which are of least use to the economy; and hence, all morbid accumulations such as wens, tumors, abscesses, etc., are rapidly diminished and often wholy removed under severe and protracted abstinence or fasting."—*Science of Life*, pp. 194-195.

The process of autolysis may be put to great practical use and may be made to serve in getting rid of tumors and other growths. To fully understand this, it is necessary for the reader to know that tumors are made up of flesh and blood and bone. There are many names for the different kinds of tumors, but the names all indicate the kind of tissue of which the tumor is composed. For example, an *osteoma* is made up of bone tissue; a *myoma* is composed of muscular tissue; a *neuroma* is constituted of nerve tissue; a *lipoma* consists of fatty tissue; a *fibroma* is composed of fibrous tissues; an *epithelioma* is composed of epithelial tissue, etc. Growths of this nature are known, technically, as *neoplasms* (new growth) to distinguish them from mere swellings or enlargements. A large lump in the breast may be nothing more than an enlarged lymphatic gland or an enlarged mammary gland. Such an enlarged gland may be very painful, but it is no *neoplasm*.

Tumors being composed of tissues, the same kind of tissues as the other structures of the body, are susceptible of autolytic distintegration, the same as normal tissue, and do, as a matter of experience, undergo dissolution and absorption under a variety of circumstances, but especially during a fast. The reader who can understand how fasting reduces the amount of fat in the body and how it reduces the size of the mucles, can also understand how it will reduce the size of a tumor, or cause it to disappear altogether. He needs, then, only to realize that the process of disintegrating (autolyzing) the tumor takes place much more rapidly than it does in the normal tissues.

In his *Notes On Tumors*, a work for students of pathology, Francis Carter Wood says: "In a very small proportion of human malignant tumors spontaneous disappearance for longer or shorter periods has been noted. The greater number of such disappearances has followed incomplete surgical removal of the tumor; they have occurred next in order of frequency during some acute febrile process, and less frequently in connection with some profound alteration of the metabolic processes of the organism, such as extreme cachexia, artificial menopause, or the puerperium."

No more profound change in metabolism is possible than that produced by fasting and the change is of a character best suited to bring about the autolysis of a tumor, malignant or otherwise.

The conditions Wood mentions as causing spontaneous disappearance of tumors are, for the most part, "accidents" and are not within the range of voluntary control. Fasting, on the other hand, may be instituted and carried out under control and at any time desired. It is the rule that operations are followed by increased growth in the tumor. Spontaneous disappearance following incomplete removal is rare. The same may be said for extreme cachexia and artificial menopause. In fevers we have rapid antolysis in many tissues of the body and much reparative work going on, but we cannot develop a fever at will. Pregnancy and childbirth occasion many profound changes in the body, but they are certainly not to be recommended to sick women as *cures* for their tumors. Even if this were desirable, it would be a hit-or-miss process. The effects of fasting are certain. There is nothing hit-or-miss about the process. It works always in the same general direction.

Fever is a remedial process and does help to remove the cause of the tumor. None of Wood's other causes of spontaneous disappearance assist in removing the cause of tumors. Fasting does assist greatly in the removal of such cause.

During a fast the accumulations of superfluous tissues are overhauled and analyzed; the available component parts are turned over to the department of nutrition to be utilized in nourishing the essential tissues; the refuse is thoroughly and permanently removed.

Due to a variety of circumstances, some known, others unknown, the rate of absorption of tumors in fasting individuals varies. The general condition of the patient, the amount of surplus contained in his body, the kind of tumor, the hardness or softness of the tumor, the location of the tumor and the age of the patient are all known to influence the rate of tumor absorption. Let me cite two extreme cases to show the wide range of variation in this respect.

A woman, under forty, had a uterine fibroid about the size of an average grapefruit. It was completely absorbed in twenty-eight days of total abstinence from all food but water. This was an unusually rapid rate of absorption. Another case is that of a similar tumor in a woman of about the same age. In this case the growth was about the size of a goose egg. One fast of twenty-one days reduced the tumor to the size of an English walnut. The fast was broken due to the return of hunger. Another fast a few weeks subsequent, of seventeen days, was required to complete the absorption of the tumor. This was an unusually slow rate of tumor-absorption.

Tumor-like lumps in female breasts ranging from the size of a pea to that of a goose egg will disappear in from three days to as many weeks. Here is a remarkable case of this kind that will prove both interesting and instructive to the reader. A young lady, age 21, had a large, hard lump—a little smaller than a billiard ball—in her right breast. For four months it had caused her considerable pain. Finally she consulted a physician who diagnosed the condition, cancer, and urged immediate removal. She went to another, and another and still another physician, and each made the same diagnosis and each urged immediate removal. Instead of resorting to surgery the young lady resorted to fasting and in exactly three days without food, the "cancer" and all its attendant pain were gone. There had been no recurrence after thirteen years and I think that we are justified in considering the condition remedied.

Hundreds of such occurrences under fasting have convinced me that many "tumors" and "cancers" are removed by surgeons that are not tumors or cancers. They cause me to be very skeptical of the statistics issued to show that early operation prevents or *cures* cancer.

Let me cite a comparatively recent instance from my own practice. A manufacturer brought his wife to me from Los Angeles. A growth in one of her breasts had caused her to consult two or three physicians in that city. Each of them had insisted upon the immediate removal of her breast. I placed her upon a fast which was continued for thirty days. At the end of the fast, the tumor, which was about the size of an English walnut at its beginning, had been reduced to the size of a pea. In less than a month on a vegetable and fruit diet this small remainder disappeared.

Subsequently the woman gave birth to five children at about two year intervals. She nursed each of the first three children for two years and the last two for eighteen months each and during each of these nursing periods the formerly tumorous breast functioned well. The health and vigor of the children presented unequivocal evidence of the quality of the mother's milk. Was this not better than removal of the breast? Was this an exceptional case? By no means. I see them regularly. Such cases are seen daily in institutions in various parts of the world where fasting is employed.

The removal of tumors by autolysis has several advantages over their surgical removal. Surgery is always dangerous; autolysis is a physiological process and carries no danger. Surgery always lowers vitality and thus adds to the metabolic perversion that is back of the tumor. Fasting, by which autolysis of tumors is accelerated, normalizes nutrition and permits the elimination of accumulated toxins, thus helping to remove the cause of the tumor. After surgical removal tumors tend to recur. After their autolytic removal, there is little tendency to recurrence. Tumors often recur in malignant form after their operative removal. The tendency to malignancy is removed by fasting.

John W. Armstrong (England) says: "I have seen lumps in female breasts treated to fast, some of them after diagnosis by 'experts,' the bulk after self-diagnosis and to disappear, on water only, in from four to twenty days."

Bernarr Macfadden says: "My experience of fasting has shown me beyond all possible doubt that a foreign growth of any kind can be absorbed into the circulation by simply compelling the body to use every unnecessary element contained within it for food. When a foreign growth has become hardened, sometimes one long fast will not accomplish the result, but where they are soft, the fast will usually cause them to be absorbed."

A small tumorous growth which had existed for more than twenty years was absorbed during Mr. Pearson's longest fast and did not return thereafter. Dr. Hazzard records the recovery, during a fifty-five day's fast, of a case diagnosed by physicians as cancer of the stomach. Tilden, Weger, Rabagliati and many others record many such cases.

I have seen repeated instances of the absorption of tumors in my own patients. I had one complete recovery in the case of a uterine "cancer" during a thirty day's fast. I have seen numerous small tumors completely absorbed and large ones greatly reduced in size.

In Europe and America, literally thousands of tumors have been autolyzed during the past fifty years, and the effectiveness of the method is beyond doubt. I can give no definite information about bone tumors and nerve tumors; but, since these are subject to the same laws of nutrition as all other tumors, I am disposed to think that they may be autolyzed as effectively as other tumors.

In my own experience I have seen numerous fibroid tumors of the uterus and breast, lipomas in various parts of the body, a few epitheliomas, a whole group of myomas and a number of tumors that were apparently early cancer autolyzed and absorbed while the patient fasted. I have seen many warts disappear during fasting and I have seen many warts on which the fasting process seemed to have no effect. I have never seen a mole affected by the fasting process. I have seen a number of cysts completely destroyed by fasting and others that were merely reduced in size. It will be recalled that Graham mentions having seen cysts (wens) absorbed during fasting.

LIMITATIONS

It is certain that the autolyzing process has its limitations, for example, a tumor that has been permitted to grow to such enormous size that several long fasts during the course of two years or more, with a rigid feeding schedule between fasts, would be required to break it down and absorb it, if, indeed, it could be done. There was a school in Chicago some years ago that taught that "the normal tissue may be consumed before the morbid tissues are used up," in fasting. While this school did not confine this statement to tumors, there are a few conditions in which this can be a fact, and in large tumors it may be so. Aside from large tumors, it is hardly probable that this is so in any recoverable cases. Only in rare instances, where the amount of morbid tissue is very great, and these are probably all irremediable, can this occur.

In general, good tissue is not used up as fast as bad and the tumor will "starve" before the body. Except where it is very large, we may be sure that in all cases, hunger will return before any damage is done to the vital tissues. In more than one case of cancer, where opiates had been used to relieve pain, I have seen three or four days' fasting bring relief.

One other limitation must be noted; namely, tumors that are so situated that they dam-up the lymph stream will continue to grow (feeding upon the excess of lymph behind them) despite fasting. In cases where complete absorption is not obtained, the tumor is sufficiently reduced in size not to constitute a menace. Thereafter proper living will prevent added growth. Indeed, we have seen a number of cases where a further decrease in size followed right living subsequent to fasting.

OBJECTION

Dr. James C. Thomson, a prominent Natural Therapist, of Edinburgh, Scotland, has offered an objection to the use of the fast to cause the autolytic disintegration of tumors. He says that "if the autolysis is being carried forward in a satisfactory manner, *i.e.*, with vigor and completeness, then during the fasting period *the patient will be living on bad meat,* that is, on his own long-established tumor which is made up of unwholesome materials, otherwise they would not have been built into a tumor. Accordingly the better the work that is being done during a fast the more certain it is that during that phase the person will be irritable, restless and at times depressed."

While I doubt that the flesh that makes up most human tumors is as bad as much of the flesh foods that are regularly taken by flesh-eaters, there is a small modicum of truth in what Dr. Thomson says. It should be pointed out, however, that most tumors are small and that days and weeks are often involved in their absorption, so that the amount of material they supply for any single day is very small. A few grams a day would be all that they would yield. The bad portions of this would be excreted. The food upon which the vital tissues are nourished during this period is derived from the stored food reserves and not from the tissues of the tumor—the amount the tumor supplying being so small as to be negligible.

I doubt that the irritableness, restlessness and depression that only occasionally accompany the process of autolytic disintegration of a tumor, are due to the exceedingly small amount of unsuitable food material derived from the tumor. These states are most likely to be due to the toxins the autolytic process releases from the tumorous and other tissues, for, not only is the tumor unsuitable for food, but much of the other tissues of the body have been requisition-ed as storage places for unexcreted waste and drugs. One of the most important processes that the body carries out during a fast is that of clearing out all this general unsuitability. The tumorous tissue is not the only tissue that is autolyzed and disposed of. If the process results in some discomfort, even actual pain, it is certainly worth going through for the benefits that accrue.

Fasting is Not Starving

CHAPTER VI

The word *starvation* is derived from the Old English *steorfan*, meaning to die. Today it is used almost wholly to designate death from lack of food. When we mention fasting to the average person and even the average physician, he immediately pictures to himself, the dire consequences that he thinks must inevitably result from going for even a few days without food. To him to fast is to *starve*—that is, die. Physiologists, physicians, biologists and other professionals, who should know better and who should be more precise in their use of terms, are also guilty of confusing the terms *fasting* and *starvation*. Members of the "learned professions" habitually employ the two terms synonymously, thus helping to perpetuate the delusion. This is not only true, but I have found, in discussing the matter with physiologists and others, that they are short-sightedly incapable of making a distinction between the two processes.

The fear of fasting is kept alive by the press, which, ever so often carries the story of somebody dying while fasting, and invariably death is attributed to starvation. These deaths are presented as "horrible examples" of the "evils of fasting." How rare are these deaths! But it would be enlightening if we could have all the details of each of these deaths. No doubt, we would find that most of them are not due to abstinence from food at all. Most of these deaths have been due to irreparable damage to some vital organ (organic disease), an occasional one may have been due to pushing the period of abstinence beyond the fasting period, a few have been due to injudicious breaking of the fast, some of them have been due to drugs. But every day people die from unnecessary and "unsuccessful" operations and the press keeps quiet. Every day people die from drugging and the editors and newsmen ignore such deaths. Fasting is their target.

The uninformed physician imagines that the blood and the vital or functioning tissues of the body begin to break down the moment food is withdrawn; that organic destruction sets in immediately and that every day the fast is prolonged means a greater destruction of the vital tissues. That this idea is false will become apparent presently.

In previous chapters it was shown that the body, at all times, has stored within itself reserves of food sufficient to last for considerable time in the event of scarcity of food or of sickness, when food cannot be digested. We saw how the body feeds upon this food reserve and how the vital tissues of the body feed upon the least essential, so that even if actual starvation occurs, there is almost no damage to the vital organs.

So long as the body's food reserves last, the individual abstaining from food is fasting. When this reserve has been consumed to the point where it is no longer able to sustain the functions of life, further abstinence becomes dangerous, starvation begins. It is only after this point is reached that any real damage is sustained by the vital organs and their functions. As a general rule, under proper conditions of environment, one may fast for weeks, and even months, before the starvation point is reached. "It is perfectly true," says Sinclair, "that men have died of starvation in three or four days; but the starvation existed in their minds—it was fright that killed them."

Laboratory workers describe destructive changes in the pancreas, supra-renal glands and other organs and glands of the body, as a result of starvation. But these changes occur after the period of fasting proper has been passed. The vital cells of the organs and glands—those doing the actual physical and chemical work of these organs—do not begin to break down until actual starvation begins.

Morgulis says: "Apart from the purely pathological phenomena occurring in the terminal stages (the starvation period) of fasting, it should be mentioned that the histological peculiarities appearing in the very beginning of inanition are associated with changes in the colloidal condition of the protoplasm and are not at all degenerative in kind. The progressive atrophic changes coincident with inanition are simply due to the gradual withdrawal of metaplasmic inclusions which represent the nutritive reserves of the cells. The atrophic diminution of both cells and nuclei does not, therefore, present a pathological phenomenon either. Moreover, the morphological processes in inanition are not invariably destructive, cell proliferation going on even when the organism has been deprived of nourishment for a long time."

This means that, except during the actual starvation period, the wasting of parts during a fast is the result of the using up of those portions of the protoplasm of the cells containing the products of their secretions and not of an actual destruction of the cell proper. The metaplasm is slowly used as the fast progresses, so that the size of the cells and, consequently, of the organ is gradually reduced, but there is no actual deterioration in structure of the cells, tissues and organs.

Dr. Morgulis makes the cautious, perhaps over-cautious, estimate that a fast which involves a body loss of ten to fifteen per cent is harmless and usually beneficial; and that the danger point in fasting begins when from twenty-five to thirty per cent has been lost. He has had animals recover normal health after a weight loss of sixty per cent. We have seen the same thing in more than one man and woman.

A number of people have died of serious organic "disease" while fasting, and autopsies have been performed in many of these. In every case there was still considerable subcutaneous fat, whereas, this is always entirely absent where death has been caused by starvation. Except in a case or two where the heart had never sufficiently developed or where there was previous heart "disease," the heart was found to be normal in all cases; while in actual starvation, the heart is always contracted or markedly atrophied. The pancreas is little, if at all affected, in death during the fast, whereas in death from starvation, this gland is almost entirely absent. In these cases the blood was normal in amount with no anemia present; while in starvation, the relative blood volume is reduced and there is usually marked anemia.

In starvation the tongue remains coated, the breath offensive, the pulse and temperature sub-normal and hunger may disappear for days at a time.

Death may result at any time, feeding or fasting, due to the failure of some particular vital organ, which is so far destroyed that a fatal ending cannot be prevented by any means, but death from abstinence from food cannot occur until all possible nutritive material has been exhausted. "True starvation begins," says Sinclair, "only when the body has been reduced to the skeleton and the viscera."

Fortunately we are not left unprotected and unwarned in this matter. Before the danger point is reached an imperious demand for food will be made. We say, then, that so long as hunger is lacking, the patient is fasting; but after hunger returns, if he continues to abstain from food, he is starving. Besides the return of hunger, there are other indications that the body is ready to take food, as stated elsewhere.

Carrington has well summed up the matter in these words: "Fasting is a scientific method of ridding the system of diseased tissue, and morbid matter, and is invariably accompanied by beneficial results. Starving is the deprivation of the tissues from nutriment which they require, and is invariably accompanied by disastrous consequences. The whole secret is this: fasting commences with the omission of the first meal and ends with the return of natural hunger, while starvation only begins with the return of natural hunger and terminates in death. Where the one ends the other begins. Whereas the latter process wastes the healthy tissues, emaciates the body, and depletes the vitality; the former process merely expels corrupt matter and useless fatty tissue, thereby elevating the energy, and eventually restoring the organism that just balance we term health."

Prof. Morgulis divides what he calls starvation, or *inanition*, into four periods—"each period comprising approximately one-fourth of the total loss in weight sustained at the time of death."

The first of these periods of "every complete inanition," (by "complete inanition" is meant abstinence from all food until death occurs) is a "transition from the condition of adequate feeding to the basal metabolism of fasting"—"the organism is readjusting itself from the prefasting metabolic level to the level of the true physiological minimum characteristic for the particular individual."

The division between the next two periods is not well marked or defined. They constitute one period divided into "early and late phases" and "are not very distinct but merge gradually one into the other." During these "two periods," physiological activities are at a minimum peculiar to this individual. The length of these two periods will be determined by the size of the animal or man or the surplus food reserves on hand.

The final or fourth stage of inanition "is characterized by the predominance of pathological phenomena caused by the prolonged stringency of nourishment and exhaustion of the tissues." This is the true starvation period and sets in when the body's nutritive stores are practically exhausted.

—118—

Prof. Morgulis refers to the whole period, from the omission of the first meal until death finally ends the scene, as starvation and as fasting. He uses the two words synonymously and does not distinguish between fasting and starvation as we do. It will be noted that all pathological phenomena, of which we are so frequently warned, belong to the fourth stage of inanition; or, to the period of starvation proper, as distinct from fasting, as we employ these terms.

Morgulis points out that "the morphological changes observable in advanced starvation are practically identical with those generally found in every pathological condition and present nothing peculiar" and suggests that perhaps all "pathological changes of tissues are primarily inanition effects."

Further applying his division of "starvation" into four periods, Prof. Morgulis says: "All scientifically studied fasts of men have been of relatively short duration. In the longest fast of this kind lasting 40 days Succi lost only 25 per cent of his original weight. Judging by the loss of weight, therefore, the experiments on inanition with human subjects have not extended far beyond what may be regarded as the second stage of inanition and, regardless of the length of time of the abstinence, had no deleterious effect whatever upon the subjects because the fasts were invariably discontinued long before the exhaustion stage had been reached."

Taking up the study of Levanzin's fast of 31 days, undergone at Carnegie Institute, Morgulis says that this fast extended over the first two inanition periods. The first of these periods, lasting fifteen days saw a loss of ten per cent of Levanzin's weight and represents "the transition from the metabolism of the well nourished condition to that of the fasting condition."

By the end of his 31 days' fast, Levanzin lost about 20 per cent of his weight. "Assuming the maximum loss he could possibly have survived 40 per cent," says Morgulis, "it is clear that the fast could have extended another month before a fatal termination. In other words, the fast was broken at a relatively early stage." If we take into consideration the fact that the second 20 per cent of Levanzin's weight would not have been lost nearly so rapidly as the first 20 per cent, it is very certain that he could have fasted much more than another month before a fatal termination.

The rule that man or animal can sustain a loss of 40 per cent of his or its body weight before death results must not be taken too seriously in practice. Obviously an emaciated man or woman weighing only 90 or 100 pounds cannot afford to lose 40 per cent of his or her weight. On the other hand a man who ought to weigh about 150 pounds, but who actually weighs 350 pounds, can afford to lose much over 50 per cent of his weight. Exhibition fasters have survived a reduction of body weight of thirty per cent without anything like a total collapse of vital vigor.

Within recent years physiologists have tried to determine how long man can live without food by figuring on a basis of the period of time required for animals, particularly mammals, to starve to death. Their experiments indicate that the period in which death from starvation ensues is proportionate to the cube root of the body weight.

A mouse weighing 18.0 grams dies after five or six days without food. The corresponding "starvation period" in man would be 15.6 times as long or 96.5 to 109 days. A dog weighing twenty kilograms dies in sixty days; the corresponding period for man is eighty-nine days. A cat weighing twenty-one kilograms can live eighteen days without food; the corresponding period for man would be fifty-five days. A rabbit weighing 24.22 kilograms dies after twenty-six days; the corresponding period in man would be seventy-nine days.

From these figures, A. Putter, M.D., a German physician, who has made a study of fasting, concludes that there is nothing in comparative physiology to show that man cannot live from ninety to a hundred days without food, if he were kept under proper conditions of warmth, rest, fresh air, water and emotional poise.

Sylvester Graham denied that the fat man lives longer in prolonged abstinence from food than does a thin one. He says, "If the fat be designed for the nourishment of the body during protracted fasts, etc., then if a very fat man, in the enjoyment of what is ordinarily considered good health, and a lean man in good health, be shut up together, and condemned to die of starvation, the fat man ought to diminish in weight much more slowly, and to live considerably longer than the lean man; but directly the contrary to this is true. The lean man will lose in weight much more slowly, and live several days longer than the fat man, in spite of all the nourishment which the latter may derive from his adipose deposits"—*Science of Human Life*, pp. 193-194.

Trall took a similar view, as does Carrington, who says of Graham's statement: "I may say that this has been my own experience, precisely." The explanation offered is that, while the fat person has a large store of fat on his frame, he is deficient in other food requisites. Fatty tissue, these man think, is invariably diseased and deficient tissue. Trall said, "Feed a dog on butter, starch, or sugar alone, and you will save in him the consumption of fat, but the dog will die of starvation. He will be plump, round, *embonpoint,* and yet die of inanition"—*Alcoholic Controversy*, pp. 148-149. This seems to be what they thought will take place in the fasting fat man.

This is an *a priori* conclusion, since the experiment has never been made, and it is not borne out by animal experimentation. There is, as I have emphasized elsewhere, a vast difference between a fast and a very deficient diet, such as the diets described by Trall. The ultimate results of the two types of nutrition are very different. Nevertheless, there may be cases of fat individuals who would actually starve to death before a thinner person does so, for the reason that the nutritive reserves in the fat person may be so unbalanced that he cannot go long without food. I have, myself, cared for fat men and women who did not fast well and who did not hold up under fasting as well as do many who are actually skinny. But I have never been sure that in these patients, the trouble was not largely if not wholly mental. In view of the fat person's love of food and his worrying and fretting when deprived of it, he may actually kill himself while the thin man is still philosophizing about life and death.

If there can be such a thing as unbalanced reserves, and I presume that such may exist, there is as much reason why the thin man, eating the same type of diet as that eaten by the fat man, may have an unbalanced reserve as there is that the fat man may have this. The greatest losses in the fast, however, are in those very nutritive factors that are most abundant in the diet of most people, while the body clings to the factors that are commonly lacking. The tendency is for nutritive balance to be restored. The fact that the fat man who does not fast well, loses all of the difficulties that appear to have come from fasting, as soon as he gets his first half-a-glass of fruit juice, indicates that his troubles are mental.

Graham's statement that the fat man will lose weight much faster than the thin one is literally true, but what he overlooked is that this rapid loss of weight is not continued. Indeed, we often see fat women who undertake a fast to reduce, lose twenty to twenty-five pounds the first two weeks, but six pounds the third week and two pounds the fourth week. The rapid rate of loss does not continue. It should be observed at this point, also, that some thin people lose rapidly the first few days of their fast.

A fast of a hundred days or more can be survived even under the most favorable conditions, only by the individual who possesses sufficient food reserves to sustain his vital organs and vital functions for this period of time. The smaller the amount of food stores one has in reserve, all things else being equal, the earlier is the starvation period reached.

What Morgulis classes as the first three stages of starvation, we class as the period of fasting; while his fourth period of starvation is classed by us as the starvation period. Fasting begins with the omission of the first meal and ends with the return of natural hunger. Starvation begins with the return of hunger and terminates in death. Fasting is distinctly beneficial; starvation is distinctly harmful. It is precisely because the average medical man does not distinguish between these two major phases of abstinence from food, and because he imagines that the pathology developed during the starvation period belongs, also, to the fasting period, that he offers his false objections to fasting.

It was conclusively demonstrated in the laboratory, by Lasarev, that the changes in the various organs of the body are definitely related to particular stages of fasting and starvation. Vital organs do not begin to break down as soon as the first meal is omitted. Fasting belongs to that period during which there are ample food reserves to maintain vital integrity. The fasting period is, therefore, determined by the amount of reserves the body has on hand. Starvation sets in after the reserve stores have been sufficiently exhausted that they are no longer adequate to maintain functional and structural integrity.

Thousands of fasts, ranging from a few days to three months in duration, in men, old and young and both sexes, in all conditions of life, have demonstrated not only that man can go for long periods without food and not be harmed thereby, but also, that he will receive great benefit from a rationally conducted fast. To *starve* is to die; to *fast* is to live.

There is no sense in the panicky fear of missing a few meals that is so prevalent in both lay and professional circles today. The fear of starvation expressed on every hand is a foolish fear. "I am not going to starve," says a long-suffering invalid upon being advised to fast. "I am not going to starve to death," says Mr. Average Man, when advised to fast. They warn others, who are fasting, that they will starve to death. Physicians conjure into being (in their imaginations) the dire consequences of going without food for a few days or a few weeks. They refer to men who employ fasting as "starve-to-death doctors." Although we oppose letting people "starve to death," we take no decided stand against them stuffing themselves to death: instead, we rather encourage it.

Several years ago a number of English soldiers died at Aldershot after eight hours of maneuvers in an English summer, and after being deprived of food for eight hours, and it was actually asserted that they died of starvation. A British physician, A. Rabagliati, M.A., M.D., F.R.C.S., asserted that "they did not and could not have died of starvation," and contrasted these soldiers with patients of his who had fasted and whose fasts "have lasted not for hours or days, but for weeks; after which, in numerous cases patients have recovered from severe and long-continued illnesses." It is more than likely that these soldiers were killed by the fatigue and heat because they had previously been heavy eaters and heavy drinkers, hence, were without stamina and resistance.

My opinion, based on more than forty years of experience in conducting many thousands of fasts, in all ages and conditions, many of them very long fasts, is that fasting is never the cause of death. In evaluating this opinion the reader is asked to keep in mind the definition of fasting given in a preceding chapter and the distinction there made between *fasting* and *starving*. He should also bear in mind that death may occur during a fast from causes other than lack of food, as it may occur when the patient is being fed regularly.

A man may fast in the last stages of cancer and die of cancer without reference to the fast. He will also die, and in most instances just as quickly or more so, if eating. To say that the feeding cancer patient dies of cancer and the fasting cancer patient dies of starvation is to stretch popular prejudice to the breaking point.

The frequency with which "sudden death" from heart disease follows an unusually heavy meal in men and women who have been eating regularly and have not fasted a single day, should be sufficient to cause the thinking man or woman to pause before attributing death of the fasting heart patient to the fast. I do not recall ever seeing a heart patient die while fasting, although I have seen a number of them die while eating. I have seen them undergo long fasts to recovery and I have seen others die shortly after breaking a short fast. The fact is common knowledge that the man with a serious heart disease is likely to die apparently suddenly, even though he is eating regularly; such a man may also die while fasting. It would be inaccurate to say that the man who died while fasting was killed by fasting while the man who dies while eating, dies of heart disease.

I was called to see one case in which the man, in the last stages of pulmonary tuberculosis, had undertaken a fast on his own responsibility. I gave it as my opinion that he had already carried the abstinence too far. I doubted that he could make a come-back. He died two days later. Did he die of tuberculosis or of starvation? I think that he died of both. His statement to me was that he had suffered so much and so long that he had undertaken the fast with the determination to either get well or to die in the process and that it was a matter of indifference to him whether he lived or died.

I am convinced, from a few experiences I have had, that fasting hastens the fatal termination in cancer of the liver and cancer of the pancreas. Certainly there are conditions in which fasting or extended fasting are inadvisable. The fast should not be misused, but the results of its misuse should not be used to condemn the whole process.

In 1906 C. P. Newcom, a youthful octogenarian vegetarian of England, who dedicated the last years of his life to the search for a *cure* for cancer and who claimed to have succeeded in *curing* one case of cancer by fasting, stated that *starvation* is the correct word when applied to cancer: "The patient *fasted*, but the cancer *perished* for want of nutriment."

The opinion has been expressed that "natural death" should be assisted by total abstinence from solid food, for it is a cruel practice to stuff the dying. The stuffing program increases and produces agonies, hastens death and "makes immediate burial a necessity." It is true that the dying patient who is not fed is more comfortable and is more likely to have a clear head up to the end.   It is not likely that, in fatal cases, abstinence will end life sooner.   Indeed, with few exceptions, it would be more likely to prolong life.

Chemical And Organic Changes During Fasting

CHAPTER VII

Abstinence from food may mean missing one meal or it may mean going without food until death results from starvation. Missing one meal produces no organic or chemical changes in the body; in starvation, many changes occur. It is necessary to know that different changes occur at different stages of the period of abstinence and that the changes at different stages are of different, even opposite character. For example, in women and female animals, atrophy of the mammary glands is seen in starvation, but in fasting, there is only a loss of fat. In the early stages of abstinence in young guinea pigs, the pancreas, like the other internal organs, is in general more resistant to loss of weight. Pancreatic losses in the early stages of abstinence are relatively slight, while in advanced stages, that is, in starvation, pancreatic loss (atrophy) is extreme, being, as a rule, relatively greater than that of the entire body. Many examples of similar differences will be given throughout the pages of this book.

There is naturally and necessarily a loss of weight when man or animal ceases to eat and if food is abstained from long enough, death results from too great loss. In discussing the differences between *fasting* and *starving* we made use of Morgulis' four stages of the inanition period—from the omission of the first meal until its ending in death. In general, in both birds and mammals, the loss of weight is greatest during the first fourth of the inanition period, least in the second and third, and intermediate in the fourth, although this final acceleration of loss is variable or even absent.

In all animals, from worms to man, the various organs and tissues of the body differ very greatly in their rates of loss while *fasting* and *starving*. In general, it may be said that most of the soft tissues of the body lose weight during a fast, but they lose at varying rates. Instead of a uniform wasting of the body's resources, biologically important organs are sustained at the expense of less important ones.

Structural changes during fasting are largely those that result from loss of weight. At death from starvation the amount of weight lost may be fifty to sixty per cent. No such losses are registered in a fast. Succi lost 25 per cent of his weight in forty days of fasting. As before pointed out, individual organs or tissues, show a very unequal emaciation, some living at the expense of others. It will be interesting to note some of the losses and changes which occur during the fast. In death by starvation the following losses have been observed by different investigators:—

	Yeo's Physiology	Chossat	Voit	Gross
Fat	97	93	97	97
Muscles	30	43	31	30.5
Blood	17	75	27	27
Liver	56	52	54	53.7
Spleen	63	70	67	66.7
Pancreas	--	64	17	17
Skin	--	--	21	--
Intestines	--	--	18	18
Kidneys	--	--	26	25.9
Lungs	--	--	18	17.7
Testes	--	--	40	40
Heart	--	--	3	2.6
Brain and Spinal Cord	00	2	3	3.2
Nerves	00	2	--	--
Bones	--	--	14	13.9

* Nerve centers.

Chossat's table was made from animal experimentation, and agrees very well with the observations of others, except in the loss of blood. Others have given this as less than twenty per cent. The *International Encyclopedia*, under "fasting," gives a table showing the losses sustained by an animal while fasting for thirteen days. This table gives the loss of blood for this times as 17% and the loss to the brain and nerves as none.

As not all of these losses were recorded on the same types of animals, some using cats, others using other animals, the variations in the figures may be the results of different rates of losses in different species and not the results of inaccuracies in measuring the losses. Had the testes of the salmon been observed, a great gain rather than a loss would have been observed. There are doubtless other animals in which the testicles gain while fasting, although, as we have defined fasting, most of these losses took place after the end of the fast and in the starvation period. It will be noted that Chossat's table gives a very high loss of blood, a figure that no other investigator agrees with. Best and Taylor, in their Physiology text say that the central nervous system loses, in "prolonged starvation," five per cent, as estimated from "normal standards," and that, contrary to general belief, the loss to the heart is but little less than that sustained by the skeletal muscles. They neither define "prolonged starvation," nor "normal standards," nor do they tell how they arrived at their figures. These physiologists point out that the different tissues are lost in fasting at different rates and that, despite great losses of weight, considerable activity may still be engaged in. For example, "a dog has been starved for 117 days. By the end of this time it had lost 63 per cent of its weight, but was fairly active." This is a greater loss of weight than is commonly considered safe, yet we often see men and women who are eating regularly and who are so thin that they are under half what should be their normal weight by any reasonable standard.

It will be observed that during the fast the tissues do not all waste at an equal rate; those that are not essential are utilized most rapidly, those least essential less rapidly and those most essential not at all at first and only slowly at the last. Nature always favors the most vital organs. The fat disappears first, and then the other tissues in the inverse order of their usefulness. The essential tissues obtain their nourishment from the less essential, by enzymic action, a process which we studied under *autolysis*.

From these tables it will be seen that the brain and nervous system continue intact (retain their structural and functional integrity) until the last and retain the inherent power to maintain their nutrition unimpaired, although every other tissue has wasted beyond repair; and that the blood, even in the most extreme cases, does not show extraordinary depletion. Such physiological facts would seem to argue that nerve and blood supply throughout the body are virtually normal during a fast; and that the human body is, in reality, a veritable organization of assimilable food elements dominated by a self-maintaining intelligence which is capable of preserving relative structural integrity and physiologic functional balance even when all food is withheld for considerable intervals.

Only in a very special sense does the body "start eating itself" when one begins to fast. It never consumes its tissues indiscriminately, but, true to its rule of always favoring its most vital organs, it uses up the least useful tissues first. Selective action is exercised from the beginning and the most rigid economy is exercised in appropriating its food reserves in sustaining the heart, lungs, brain, nerves and other vital organs. Even the respiratory muscles are more carefully guarded than the other muscles of the skeleton.

The accompanying two diagrams, Nos. 1 and 2, are after Voit. Diagram 1 shows the percentage of the total loss of the body borne by each organ in death by starvation, while diagram 2 shows the percentage of loss in each organ under the same circumstances. These tables also include the proportion which the loss in each bears to the weight of a similar animal killed in good condition. The careful student will bear in mind that most of the actual tissue losses shown by these tables occurred in the fourth of the inanition periods—the period of starvation proper—and do not occur during the fasting period.

While table 1 shows that the musculature of the body supplies the greatest loss of weight, the actual loss to the muscles only reaches 21 per cent of the total muscular substance (chiefly the superficial muscles), while, though the actual proportion of weight lost is less, 97 per cent of the fat present is used up. The other organs which lose much of their weight are the spleen with 67 per cent; the liver with 54 per cent, and the testes with 40 per cent. The central nervous tissue and the heart supply only 0.1 per cent of the total loss, and 3 per cent of their actual substance. A closer and more detailed view of the losses of the more important organs and tissues will help us to better understand the subjects we are here dealing with.

BLOOD CHANGES

The blood diminishes in volume in proportion to the decrease in the size of the body so that the relative blood-volume remains practically unchanged during a fast. The quality of the blood is not impaired; indeed, an actual rejuvenation of the blood may occur.

Dr. Rabagliati pointed out that the first effect of the fast is to increase the number of red blood corpuscles, but if persisted in suffi-

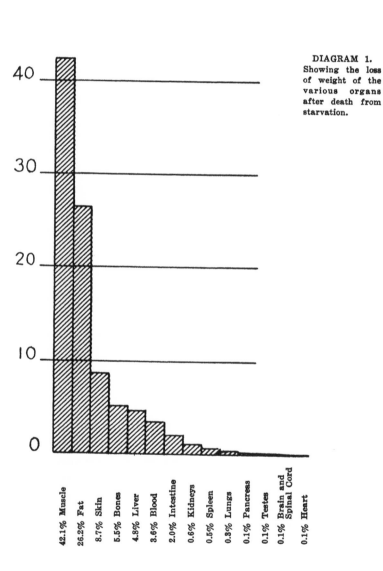

1. Percentage of Total Loss Borne by Each Organ.

DIAGRAM 1.
Showing the loss
of weight of the
various organs
after death from
starvation.

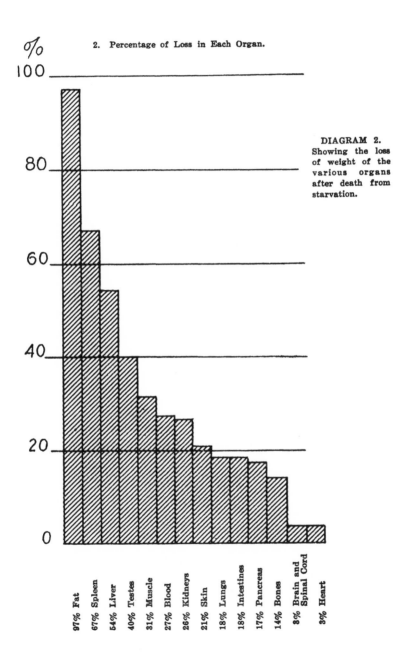

2. Percentage of Loss in Each Organ.

%
100

80

60

40

20

0

DIAGRAM 2.
Showing the loss
of weight of the
various organs
after death from
starvation.

97% Fat
67% Spleen
54% Liver
40% Testes
31% Muscle
27% Blood
26% Kidneys
21% Skin
18% Lungs
18% Intestines
17% Pancreas
14% Bones
8% Brain and Spinal Cord
3% Heart

ciently long decreases them. The increase of erethrocytes, during the early part of the fast, he regarded as due to improved nutrition resulting from a cessation of overeating. This increase in red blood cells has been repeatedly noted in anemia. The decrease is seen only after the starvation period is reached.

Prof. Benedict says: "Senator and Mueller in reporting the results of their examinations of the blood of Celti and Briethaupt, noted an increase in the red blood corpuscles with both subjects. In later examination of Succi's blood, by Tauszk, the conclusions reached were (1) that after a short period of diminution in the number of red blood corpuscles there is a slight increase; (2) that the number of white blood corpuscles decreases as the fast progresses; (3) the number of mononuclear corpuscles decreases; (4) the number of eosinophiles and polynuclear cells increases; and finally (5) that the alkalinescence of the blood diminishes."

Later experiments agree almost entirely with these results. The *Carnegie Institute Bulletin, 203,* pages 156-157 says: "The results of the above studies (of fasting) are conspicuous rather from the absence than the presence of striking alterations in the blood picture," and adds: "The final conclusions as to the effects of uncomplicated starvation on the blood to be drawn from the results óf examination of Levanzin, are: "In an otherwise normal individual, whose mental and physical activities are restricted, the blood as a whole is able to withstand the effects of complete abstinence from food for a period of at least 31 days (the length of Levanzin's fast), without displaying any essentially pathological change." Structural and morphological changes do not occur in normal blood cells during a fast.

Pashutin records the case of a man who died after four months and twelve days (132 days) without food and says that two days before death the blood contained 4,849,400 red and 7,852 white corpuscles in one cu. mm. Prof. Stengel says: "The blood in starvation preserves its corpuscular richness surprisingly, even after prolonged abstinence."

Fasting for only one week will increase the number of red cells in an anemic person. Medical and laboratory experimenters have conducted all their experiments on healthy men and animals, hence they have not been permitted to observe the regenerating effects of fasting upon the blood. Their statement that "human blood is relatively resistant during fasting" is true, but it does not tell the whole truth. Their statement that "there is a tendency to increase in the red cell count" is also true, but even this does not tell the whole truth.

Jackson says: "During human inanition, the erythrocyte (red cell) count is often within normal limits, but sometimes increased (especially in total inanition and earlier stages), or decreased (especially in chronic and late stages). In animals, the red cell count appears more frequently increased in the earlier stages of total inanition, often decreasing later. In hibernation, the erythrocyte count is variable."—*Inanition and Malnutrition*—p. 239.

Normal blood contains from 4,500,000 to 5,000,000 and as high as 6,000,000 in healthy young men, red cells per cu. mm. and 3,000 to 10,500, with a probable average of 5,000 to 7,000 white cells per cu. mm. Dr. Eales' blood was examined June 20, 1907, the first day of his fast, by Dr. P. G. Hurford, House Physician to Washington University Hospital, St. Louis. It showed the following:

Leucocytes 5,300 per cubic millimeter.

Erethrocytes 4,900,000 per cubic millimeter.

Hemoglobin 90%.

A blood test was again made on July 3, the 14th day of his fast, by Dr. S. B. Strong, House Physician, Cook County Hospital, which showed:

Leucocytes 7,000 per cu. mm.

Erethrocytes 5,528,000 per cu. mm.

Hemoglobin 90%.

It will be noted that the blood has materially improved on the fast.

A third examination of Dr. Eale's blood made by Dr. R. A. Jettis, of Centralia, Ill., on August 2, showed:

Leucocytes 7,328 per cu. mm.

Erethrocytes 5,870,000 per cu. mm.

Hemoglobin 90%.

A further improvement in the condition of his blood is here seen.

Laboratory investigators have reported an increase in the red cells of healthy fasters with a decrease in white cells. In anemia, fasting often results in an increase in the number of red blood corpuscles to more than twice their former number, with a concomitant decrease in the number of white blood cells. In a talk in Chicago a few years ago, Dr. Tilden said: "Cases of pernicious anemia taken off their food will double their blood count in one week." Dr. Weger reports a case of anemia in which a 12 days' fast resulted in an increase of the number of red cells from 1,500,000, to 3,000,000; hemoglobin increased fifty percent, and white cells were reduced from 37,000 to 14,000.

Wm. H. Hay, M.D., in his *Health Via Diet*, tells of caring for 101 cases of progressive pernicious anemia, during twenty-one years by fasting, correct diet and colonic irrigation. Of these 101 cases he says that 8 failed of initial recovery. Part of the recoveries were made permanent by right living. Some of those who relapsed resorted once more to the fast and again recovered.

The first 13 cases of progressive pernicious anemia which Dr. Hay placed upon a fast recovered in from two weeks to longer. The fourteenth case, being in a dying condition when she arrived, did not recover. Dr. Hay says: "The blood during a fast undergoes no visible changes as to cell count unless markedly abnormal when the fast is begun in which case there is a return to normal." * * * "For most of two weeks (in progressive pernicious anemia) the red erethrocyte, count continues to fall before there is a regeneration in the blood-making organs; then gradually the microscopic picture begins to show round erethrocytes with regular edges, no crenations or irregularities, and soon there is noticeable increase in number of these with gradual disappearance of the adventitious cells present in the beginning.

"Not unusually there is a gain during the succeeding two weeks that brings the total back to the normal five million erethrocyte count, even though this may have been at, or below, one million in the beginning."

Von Norden says: "The blood atrophies." This is true of the *starvation* period, not of *fasting* proper. Much confusion will be avoided if the student will keep clearly in mind the fact that destructive changes occur only after the exhaustion of the body's reserves. Von Norden, Kellogg and others never tired of detailing the destructive changes that occur in the body during "starvation." Indeed, they were right in their details if they had used the term starvation properly. But they believed that the changes seen in starvation belong, also, to the fasting period. They made no distinction between the two processes. Later, investigators have corrected this old mistake, although few writers on the subject in our encyclopedias and standard works seem to have heard of this fact.

The decreased blood alkalinity due to prolonged fasting is often urged against the fast. It is contended that fasting produces acidosis. Fasting does not produce acidosis and the decreased alkalinity is never great enough, even in the most protracted fasts, to result in any deficiency "disease," unless the frequent cases of impotency are to be regarded as due to a loss of vitamins or mineral salts. The blood rapidly regains its normal alkalinity after feeding is resumed and no damage is done.

Mr. Macfadden said: "It has been said that an acid condition of the blood, fluids and tissues (acidosis) is sometimes brought about by fasting. I cannot concede that this is ever the case, in true fasting. As a matter of fact, all the evidence seems to prove that as Dr. Haig expressed it, 'fasting acts like a dose of alkali.' If there is acidity in the system, fasting will remove it and restore the chemical balance of the system. Therapeutic fasting never created acidity, but on the contrary, removes that state when existing. Of course protracted starvation may do so, but then, who ever advised starvation.

"The medical as well as the general idea is that starvation begins practically immediately when meals are discontinued. The impression is that at once the blood and solid structures of the body begin to break down, that organic destruction has begun. Such is far from the case, as results have proved in scores (thousands) of cases. The vital cells of the organs and glands—those doing the active physical and chemical work of these parts—do not begin to disintegrate until actual starvation begins."

During a fast the body lives on its reserves. What is more, these reserves contain sufficient alkaline reserves to prevent the development of so-called acidosis. Dr Weger says: "Varying degrees of acidosis were often in evidence during fasting. These we consider physiological. Except in very rare instances, the active symptoms are of short duration and easily overcome without interfering with or curtailing the fast." He describes the "symptoms of acidosis during a fast" as "lassitude, headache, leg and back ache, irritability, restlessness, redness of the buccal (mouth) mucous membrane and tongue, sometimes drowsiness, and also a fruity odor to the breath."

These symptoms develop at the beginning of the fast and grow less and less as the fast continues, until they cease altogether. If fasting produces acidosis the evidence should increase as the fast progresses. I believe that all of these symptoms may be explained without regarding them as evidences of acidosis. They result, I believe, from the withdrawal of the accustomed *stimulation*—coffee, tea, cholocate, cocoa, alcohol, tobacco, meat, pepper, spices, salt, etc., etc.—and are identical with these same symptoms when they develop in the man or woman who gives up coffee or tobacco, but who does not cease to eat. I do not think the "fruity odor" of the breath can be explained in this manner. However, in thousands of fasts I have conducted, I have never met with such a phenomenon— the breath in all cases being very foul and much like that of the fever patient or like the bad breath most people have, only much intensified.

Dr. Weger, himself, says: *"Fasting is not and cannot be the cause of acidosis,* for the symptom-complex of acidosis is quite common in full-fed plethoric individuals, in whom the makings of acidosis exist as a result of an over-crowded nutrition. It is true that symptoms of acidosis frequently occur and make patients decidedly uncomfortable during the early stages of the fast. However, these symptoms are due to excessively rapid consumption of the body fat— a catalytic action—and the checking of elimination because of sub-oxidation. In less than ten per cent of such cases do these discomforts last more than three or four days. This indicates to us that the acidosis, as such, was a latent condition that would be excited into activity by any other equally potent provocative. This condition is analogous to a crisis which might occur in the form of an acute disease. The sicker one is made by a fast, the greater the need for it."

In general I agree with these words of Dr. Weger, but I have noted these supposed symptoms of acidosis in cases where there was no rapid breaking down of tissue, and in cases in which physical activity was sufficient to keep up normal oxidation and in which elimination was normal or super-normal. I do regard these symptoms as being part of a crisis and as beneficial in outcome. I have noted repeatedly that the more severe are these symptoms, the more benefit the patient receives from the fast and the sooner do these benefits manifest.

THE SKIN

The exquisite texture and delicate pink color of the skin that develop while fasting attests the rejuvenation the skin undergoes. The clearing up of blotches and blemishes with, even the disappearance of finer lines in the skin, are particularly significant as showing the benefits the skin derives from a period of physiological rest.

That the circulation to the skin is much improved by a period of physiological rest is demonstrated by the way that the blood thoroughly and instantaneously responds to a pinch of the skin. This true "pink of condition" is invariably observed toward the end of the fast and indicates the greatly improved condition of the body. This is to say, the improvement in the skin mirrors the improvement that has taken place within.

THE BONES

There is no evidence of any loss to the bones during a fast. Indeed, as will be shown in another chapter, they may even continue to grow while fasting. When we observe the marrow of the bones, however, we notice a remarkable change. Marrow is stored up food and is readily drawn upon for nourishment when no food is eaten. In *starved* calves, for example, the marrow is reduced to a watery mass. This amount of change does not occur during an ordinary fast.

THE TEETH

Teeth are specialized bones and are subject to the same laws of nutrition as other bones of the body. In certain quarters it is claimed that fasting ruins the teeth. The claim is not true and no one with a knowledge of fasting makes it. No evidence exists that there is any loss to the bones or teeth during a fast. There is an apparent decrease in the amount of organic matter in the teeth of starved rabbits, but the teeth of these animals grow continuously throughout life, and Prof. Morgulis suggests that this decrease may be due simply to a deficiency of building material.

Jackson says: "Like the skeleton, the teeth appear very resistant to inanition. * * * In *total inanition*, or on water alone, the teeth in adults show no appreciable change in weight or structure."

There is simply no truth in the notion that fasting injures the teeth. On the contrary, repeated tests and experiments in the laboratory have shown that the bones and teeth are uninjured by prolonged fasting. I have conducted thousands of fasts and I have never seen any injury accrue to the teeth therefrom. No one makes a trip to the dentist after a fast who would not have gone there had the fast not been taken. Mr. Pearson records that at the end of his fast, "teeth with black cavities became white and clear, all decay seemed to be arrested by the fast, and there was no more tooth-ache."

The only effects upon the teeth which I have observed to occur during a fast are improvements. I have seen teeth that were loose in their sockets become firmly fixed while fasting. I have seen diseased gums heal up while fasting. But I have never, at any time, observed any injurious effects upon the teeth during or after a fast, regardless of the age of the faster and the duration of the fast. This applies only to good teeth. Fasting does sometimes cause fillings to become loose. Although I have always regarded the loosening of fillings in teeth as due to the extraction of the salts of the bad teeth, some of my students have brought up the question: Is the loss of the filling due to an effort of Nature to dislodge a foreign body preparatory to healing the tooth? This question is worthy of study.

THE BRAIN, CORD AND NERVES

The brain and nervous system are supported and lose little or no weight during a fast, while the less important tissues are sacrificed to feed them. They maintain their power and ability to control the functions of the body, as well (and even better) during the most prolonged fast, as when fed the accustomed amounts of "good nourishing food." Relative to the rest of the body, the brain and nervous system increase as the fast continues, due to the fact that little or none of their substances are lost. The spinal cord loses less than 10 per cent in death by starvation—the brain nothing. There are almost no structural changes in the brain and cord even in starvation.

"In general," says Jackson, "the brain appears relatively resistant to the effects of both total and partial inanition. Usually little or no loss in weight or changes in gross or microscopic structure are apparent. In advanced stages of starvation, however, and especially in types of partial inanition (beri beri, pellagra), involving neural or psychic disturbances, there are well-marked degenerative changes in the nerve cells."—*Inanition and Malnutrition*, p. 173.

Here, again, we note a confusing of the effects of actual starvation with those of inadequate diet so that the statement is a bit misleading. We must also emphasize again that losses seen in starvation are not seen in fasting. It is well always to keep the distinction between fasting and starving in mind.

THE KIDNEYS

The losses to the kidneys are insignificant and are usually much less than that of the body as a whole. In the young the kidneys are even more resistant to loss of weight.

THE LIVER

The losses to the liver during a fast are largely water and glycogen. Usually the liver loses more in weight relative to the rest of the body than the other organs, especially in the earlier stages, due to the loss of glycogen and fat.

THE LUNGS

Jackson says: "In uncomplicated cases of *total inanition,* or on water only, the lungs are usually normal in appearance. The loss in weight of the lungs in such cases is usually relatively less than that in the body as a whole, though sometimes equal to, or even relatively greater than, that of the entire body. In the young, the lungs usually appear more resistant to loss in weight."—*Inanition and Malnutrition,* p. 361. That the lungs are greatly benefitted by fasting is shown by their recovery from "disease," even tuberculosis, during a period of abstinence. Shorter fasts are usually required in lung "diseases," than in "disease" of other organs and Carrington thinks this is due to the fact that lung tissue "possesses the inherent power of healing itself in a far shorter time, and more effectually, than any other organ which may be diseased."

THE MUSCLES

It has been shown by investigators that the skeletal muscles may lose 40% of their weight, whereas, the heart muscle loses only 3% by the time death from starvation is reached. The decrease in the size of the muscles extends also to their cells, which similarly decrease in size. Probably there is not an actual lessening of the number of muscle cells in a fast of ordinary duration, but only a consumption of fat, glycogen, and lastly some of the muscle protein and a lessening of the size of the cells. This loss of fat and muscle might occur at any time without damage to health.

In general the skeletal muscles are affected earlier and more intensely than the smooth muscles. There seems to be no actual decrease in the number of muscle fibers, but only a diminution in the size of their cells. The cells are merely reduced in size but remain perfectly sound. In frogs and salmon, fat is stored in the muscles during the eating period, and consumed during the fasting and hibernating period. The decrease in size is due to a loss of fat, not of muscle. Much the same phenomena are often observed in fasting patients.

THE HEART

The heart muscle does not diminish appreciably, deriving its sustenance from the less essential tissues. Its rate of pulsion varies greatly, rising and falling as the needs of the system demand. Studying the respiration rate, Benedict noted various minor fluctuations and arrived at the conclusion that "at least during the first two days of the fast, the pulse rate is much more liable to fluctuations than the respiration rate." That fasting benefits the heart is certain from the results obtained in functional and even in organic heart "disease" during a fast. This arises from three chief causes—namely, (1) it removes the constant *stimulation* of the heart; (2) it takes a heavy load off the heart and permits it to rest; (3) it purifies the blood thus nourishing the heart with better food.

A heart pulsating at the rate of 80 times a minute pulsates 115,200 times in twenty-four hours. Shortly after the fast is instituted, the heart rate decreases and, while it may temporarily go much below 60 pulsations a minute, it ultimately settles at 60 beats a minute and remains there for the duration of the fast. This is 86,400 pulsations in twenty-four hours, or 28,800 fewer pulsations, each day than it was doing before the fast. This represents a decrease of twenty-five per cent of the work of the heart. The saving in work is seen not merely in the reduction of the number of pulsations, but also in the vigor or force of the pulsations. It all sums up to a real vacation—a rest—for the heart. During this rest the heart repairs its damaged structures and replenishes its tissues.

As shown elsewhere, the heart muscle loses only three per cent by the time death occurs from starvation. As in other essential tissues the loss of this small per cent occurs after the exhaustion of the body's nutritive reserves—that is, during the starvation period. This ability of the body to nourish the heart during a prolonged fast is a sure guarantee against damage to the heart resulting from the fast.

Reviewing the chief historical cases of fasting with reference to the pulse beat, Benedict shows that in some cases the pulse remained "normal," and in others it rose or fell. As a result of his review of these cases and of his own series of short experimental fasts, he arrived at no definite conclusions. Carrington says: "That the heart is invariably strengthened and invigorated by fasting is true beyond a doubt. ° * ° I take the stand that fasting is the greatest of all strengtheners of weak hearts—being, in fact, its only rational, physiological cure." He attributes the benefits that accrue to the heart while fasting to increased rest, a purer blood stream and absence of *stimulation.*

The recovery of the heart from serious impairment during a fast (I have had complete and permanent recoveries in what were thought to be incurable organic heart affections), proves that the added rest the fast affords the heart and the general renovation of the body, enable it to repair itself. Dr. Eales says: "Instead of the heart growing weak during a fast it grows stronger every hour as the load it has been carrying is lessened." High blood pressure is invariably lowered and this removes a heavy load from the heart.

On the 15th day of his fast, friends of Dr. Eales brought him the news account of the sudden death of a man in Washington, D. C., while on a fast. The papers attributed the death to the fast, and friends of Dr. Eales warned him of heart failure. Dr. Eales replied to their warnings: "This man's death was not caused by the fast, in fact the fast lengthened his life, for if he had not been fasting he would undoubtedly have died a week or more earlier. He probably resorted to the fast to save his life, but it was too late; his light was too nearly burned out when he started. How many times do we hear of dying after a full meal, when making an after-dinner speech or sitting in their chairs and expiring! That, of course, is regular, but to die when the heart is resting and doing less work than when one is eating, when it is simply worn out and run down from overwork, is always attributed to fasting, if the person is fasting at the time of death."

Of the many thousands who die yearly of heart trouble, probably not more than three or four are fasting at the time of death. In my own practice one death from "heart failure" has occurred during a fast. The patient had been greatly overweight for years, with high blood pressure, nervous troubles, glaucoma, and gave a history of diabetes. Quite naturally the failure of her heart was attributed to the fast and the fact that people in her condition die every day from "heart failure" who have not been fasting, but feeding, escapes notice. Wm. J. Bryan, who never fasted, ate a hearty meal, went to bed for an afternoon nap and never woke up. These things occur daily.

The woman was many pounds overweight at death and there could be no suggestion of starvation in this case. There were ample food reserves left in her body for another forty to fifty days of fasting. I attributed the collapse of the heart in this case to fear. That fear was present was manifest. That the woman had the suggestion of starvation and death dinned into her ears every day of her fast and had the suggestion intensified after the heart became affected is certain. Sudden deaths from fear, shock, etc., are not unknown nor even uncommon.

"How many times," asks Dr. Eales, in discussing the effects of fear in the fast, "have we heard of sad news producing prostration or a fit of sickness; a mother's milk becoming poison during a fit of anger causing sickness to her nursing babe, and in some instances even death?" Again he says: "I find that so long as the mind is free from worry and fear there is not a particle of danger. It is only when the subconscious mind has suggestions of weakness and fear that the body or any of its organs become weak."

THE PANCREAS

Jackson says "that in the early stages of inanition" in young guinea pigs "the pancreas (like the other viscera) appears in general more resistant to loss in weight" and that "the pancreatic losses in the early stages of inanition" are "relatively slight," while in "advanced stages" of inanition the "pancreatic atrophy is extreme, being as a rule relatively greater than that of the entire body." He also says: "upon feeding after inanition, the pancreas recuperates rapidly and is soon restored to normal size and structure." In humans the pancreas becomes small and firm during inanition. Cases are reported in which the pancreas appeared normal after death by starvation. Other cases are reported with considerable pancreatic destruction. Probably there were other causes than starvation at work in these latter cases.

THE SPLEEN

The losses to the spleen during a fast are chiefly water. In starvation resulting in death, the spleen may lose 67 per cent of its total weight.

THE STOMACH

A classical example of the way in which fasting permits the stomach to rejuvenate itself is that of Dr. Tanner. He suffered for years with dyspepsia before his first fast. Indeed, it was this suffering that followed every meal that caused him to refrain from eating in order to miss the distress. So remarkably did his stomach repair itself during its period of rest that he was able, very foolishly, of course, to eat "sufficient food in the first twenty four hours after breaking the fast to gain nine pounds, and thirty-six pounds in eight days, all that I had lost." Although this was a rash procedure, the doctor suffered no apparent ill consequences from it. We cannot approve of such eating following a fast, but cite his example to show what a formerly weakened and dyspeptic stomach can do after a period of fasting.

A stomach rejuvenated through rest returns spontaneously to the normal performance of its function. A weak and dyspeptic stomach resumes normal function after a fast. This alone is sufficient to prove the strengthening results of a rest for the stomach. Both its muscles and its glands are rejuvenated by a period of rest.

It is often objected that fasting permits the stomach to collapse and that it so weakens the stomach that it will no longer be able to digest food. Most stomachs are so weakened by the overwork that results from our national habit of over-eating that the rest that fasting affords is just what most stomachs need most. Fasting provides a rest for the stomach, thus giving it an opportunity to repair itself. Morbid sensibilities are overcome, digestion is improved, a distended and prolapsed stomach shrinks and tends to resume its normal size, ulcers heal, inflammation subsides, gastric catarrh is eliminated and the appetite tends to become normal.

CHEMISTRY CHANGES

The chemical changes which occur in the fasting body are as remarkable as anything that we have described previously. It is quite natural that the fasting body loses some of its substances, but it does not lose all of its elements at the same rate and, what is most re-

—143—

markable, there occurs a redistribution of some of these, due to the urgent need for preserving the integrity of the vital organs. The fasting body does not lose its *inorganic constituents*—minerals—as rapidly as it loses the *organic constituents*—fats, carbohydrates and proteins. It hangs on to these precious minerals while throwing away its excess of acid-forming elements. The more valuable the material the less of it is lost.

The muscles and blood lose relatively much of their mineral constituents, especially is there a decrease in the percentage of sodium, while considerable mineral substances accumulate in the brain, spleen and liver. There is, then a mere shifting of mineral substances from one part of the body to another. While sulphur and phosphorus diminish in the fasting muscles about as rapidly as do the proteins, there is an increase in the amount of calcium in these organs. There occurs an increase in the percentage of potassium in the soft parts of the body taken as a whole, during the fast. These facts show that potassium salts and calcium salts are not lost as rapidly as some of the other of the body's elements. The excess of iron that may be contained in the diet is taken to the cells of the liver and stored by these. It is probable that the iron set free by the breaking down of the red cells is also stored in the liver and spleen, at least it is not excreted in any great amount. The body's iron reserve, in the form of hematogen, is relatively large.

That the body possesses considerable iron reserve, even in pernicious anemia, is shown by the great and rapid blood regeneration and great increase in hemoglobin and red cells during a fast in these cases. During the fast, the iron liberated by the breaking down of tissue is retained in the body and is not thrown away. Considerable iron and proportionately other necessary elements are consumed during the fast, although the body stores much of its iron in the spleen, liver, marrow cells and in the increased number of red blood cells. The reshuffling of protoplasmic substances that occurs during the fast helps to restore normal body chemistry. The body does not merely use up and cast off certain nutrients during the fast; it redistributes certain of its nutrients and attempts to re-establish an equilibrium of its constituents.

Repair of Organs And Tissues During Fasting

CHAPTER VIII

From what has gone before about the body's reserves, its ability to autolyze these reserves and its less important tissues, its ability to shift its materials from one part of the body to another, it should not surprise the intelligent reader to learn that tissues and organs are repaired during a fast; even, that they are often repaired more rapidly than while eating the accustomed amounts of "good nourishing food."

The body has a vast store of reserve foods which are designed for use in emergencies and which may be utilized under such conditions with greater ease and with less tax upon the body than food secured through the laborious process of digestion, for, it is less expensive to the organism to supply the requisite sustenance from its nutritive reserves than to do it by the digestive machinery from raw material. These reserves are available for use in repairing tissue. Repair not only takes place during a fast but it often occurs more rapidly during a fast than when one is eating. Indeed, I have seen wounds and old sores that had long refused to heal, completely and rapidly heal during a fast. I witnessed an operation on a child that had been fasting. The surgeon that performed the operation was puzzled by the unusual rapidity with which the wound healed and remarked to me that he could not explain it. It was no new phenomenon to me and I think that the explanation is very simple. I am sure that the blood-cleansing and tissue rejuvenating work of the fast improves the qualities of the blood and tissues.

Cases of repair of wounds, broken bones and healing of open sores during a fast are too numerous for us to doubt for one instant that even during a fast there is still constructive work going on. Aaron reports that the brain and the bones actually grow during a fast. Dr. Oswald reported a case of a young dog which fell from a high barn loft onto the pavement below and broke two legs and three ribs and apparently injured its lungs. It refused all food except water for twenty days, at the end of which time it took some milk. Not until the twenty-sixth day would it take flesh. The bones knit, the lungs healed and the dog was able to run and bark as lustily as before. Cases of knitting of bones in the absence of food are very common in the animal kingdom and numerous cases are on record as occurring in man. This shows unmistakably that the body utilizes the less important tissues to support the most essential ones. "I saw in human bodies," says Dr. Dewey, "a vast reserve of predigested food, with the brain in possession of power so to absorb as to maintain structural integrity in the absence of food or power to digest it. This eliminated the brain entirely as an organ that needs to be fed from light diet kitchens in times of acute sickness. Only in this self-feeding power of the brain is found the explanation of its functional clearness where bodies have become skeletons."

Aaron found that the bones and brain will grow during a fast. My observations show that the hair growth is slow during a fast and that the beard is much softer than at other times, the body sacrificing the hair in the interest of the more important structures, although fasting frequently stops the falling-out of hair. Pashutin records that in cases of hibernating animals the growth of granulation tissue in wounds goes on during the deepest slumber, even when all functions seem almost to have ceased and the heart may beat as slow as 1 beat in 5 to 8 minutes, the blood circulation being so slow that cuts made in the flesh bleed very slightly.

Fasting planaria live upon themselves, growing smaller meanwhile—this is to say, they draw upon their tissues and convert these, little by little, into food to meet their needs. The higher animals—birds, dogs, men—can do this to a more limited extent, calling first, as before pointed out, upon their reserve stores of fat and glycogen and lastly, upon the actual living substance of glands and muscles and to a lesser extent upon connective tissue. In these higher life forms certain parts are so essential to life that they cannot or must not be liquidated. The heart is little affected even in starvation. The brain cells are not damaged. The bones are not liquidated or hurt. It is only in the starvation period that the muscles waste enough that they are unable to move the parts and the glands waste until they are no longer able to produce their secretions and death results.

If a small oblong piece is cut from the body of a planarian, the piece will throw out an army of new and active cells on both its new frontiers and these, dividing, growing and differentiating, at the expense of the rest, for the piece has no mouth and cannot eat, form themselves into a head and a tail end. At the beginning the new parts are too small for the body, but a remodeling process goes on both in the new parts and in the original fragment. They grow, it shrinks. They both alter their shapes, until finally, what was at first a helpless fragment is a well-proportioned little flat-worm. The building up of new structures and redistribution of nutritive matter seen in this regeneration is common to a greater or lesser degree to all forms of animal life during a fast. We have, in the case of the fragment of a planarian becoming a new worm, the complete construction of a new organism out of food stored in the fragment without receiving fresh supplies from without.

A starfish may grow new tube feet, new arms, or even a new stomach, if it loses its old one. This animal feeds by holding open the hinged valves of a clam or oyster, everting its stomach and performing the preliminary digestion within the shell of its victim. It sometimes has its stomach pinched off in the process and is forced to fast while growing a new one. The sea cucumber frequently dispenses with its digestive apparatus, by casting it out, when forced to exist in stale water. It fasts while growing another digestive apparatus. During the fasting period the water may improve and, as biologists tell us "the trick (of discarding its digestive system) may save its life."

The remarkable changes which insects undergo in their metamorphosis from one form into another are accomplished while fasting. In some states, even where there is no change of form, the softness of their cutting organs prevents feeding. This is seen in the case of caterpillars. Where considerable changes are evolved the period of fasting is prolonged, leading to the existence of a third state, the pupa stage, intermediate between the other two. During these periods of great organizational changes, when old structures are torn down and new structures built up, so that the resulting form is wholly different from and much more complex than the preceding form, no food is consumed. The food reserves stored in the body of the metamorphosing insect and the material contained in the discarded structures are employed as materials out of which to build the new structures.

The growth of whole new organs, and new digestive systems, the building up of new forms of life in metamorphosing insects and the construction of whole new organisms from the stores in a fragment of a worm, all while fasting, are remarkable examples of the internal resources of the living organism, and its power to meet emergencies and to even use these for its own betterment.

The Influence of Fasting on Growth
And Regeneration

CHAPTER IX

In a previous chapter I have discussed the chemistry changes in the body during a fast and have there shown how the body distributes its reserves as need arises. At this point I desire to approach this subject from a slightly different angle. A brief study of *Growth* and *Regeneration* during the fast will help us to see the remarkable power of the body to refine and use the materials it has on hand when deprived of food from without.

Growth is determined by two groups of causes—namely; the internal factor of *Growth Impulse*, and the external factor of *Growth Control*. The nature of the growth force or impulse, which is the real cause of growth, is wholly unknown. It is deeply rooted in the constitution of the organism and we say it is a predetermined, hereditary impulse to grow to a certain maximum under the most favorable conditions. This growth impulse is latent in the germ plasm and may be considered identical with life. The factors that control growth are pretty well known. These are food, water, air, warmth, sun light, or the absence of these. Internally we find, in the ductless glands, a remarkable chemical mechanism for regulating growth.

As before stated the growth capacity, which varies greatly with various species, is determined by heredity. Experiment seems to show that this impulse cannot be increased or completely repressed, although it is subject to considerable limitation. The interruption of nutrition by food deficiency or insufficiency or by inanition interferes with growth, but neither of these wholly suspends it. Judged by the gross weight of the body, growth may seem to be at a standstill, or even seem to be sliding backward. But this is very deceptive. A fasting organism that is losing weight and is consuming its reserves quite rapidly, may still be growing.

Prof. Morgulis says the body "is a mosaic of interrelated parts, each, however, having its own growth history. The growth curve of one portion of the organism may be ascending while that of another has already reached the peak of its growth or indeed is on the downward course. Furthermore, the growth impulse of one may be great and that of another feeble. At times of plenty when there is enough nutriment to furnish building material for every part of the organism, the gross increase in weight is a good measure of the resultant growth; but it obscures the essential fact of the composite nature of the growth phenomenon. Walter's experiments with growing calves and Aaron's work on dogs illustrate this idea. These investigators discovered independently of each other that through chronic under-feeding they could keep their animals at a constant body weight but could not bring about complete standstill of the growing process. The part of the organism which at that phase of the development possesses the strongest growth impulse is potent to attract to itself whatever building material is available, and this not sufficing, will even encroach upon the reserves of other tissues. We witness, therefore, cataplasia or reduction of certain parts of an organism along with a progressive building up, or euplasia, of others. Such a condition has already been shown to exist in the salmon during the spawning season when these animals take no food sometimes for several months, and while all organs are used up, especially the muscles, in furnishing energy to the starving salmon, their gonads grow and develop luxuriantly. The young calves and dogs whose diet was thoroughly adequate in quality but not enough in amount, continued to grow though retaining a constant weight, but the growth was limited only to the skeleton. This increased both in size and mass, and as a result the animal actually grew in stature. Even the muscles were depleted of their stored material to satisfy the growth impulse of the skeleton."

The process of "robbing Peter to pay Paul" seen in these phenomena shows to a remarkable extent the power possessed by the body to distribute its supplies according to need, and thus preserve the integrity of the whole. If the robbing of Peter is not carried too far, no harm comes from it, for the consumed stores are readily and quickly replenished as soon as food is added. Growth seems to be independent of food in the sense that food is not the cause but only the material of growth. Dr. Morgulis finds in the phenomenon of regeneration a most remarkable exemplification of the fact "that the growth impulse of a particular organ may be sufficiently puissant to draw to itself nutriment and to infringe upon the reserves of the less active tissues and cause them to undergo cataplasia."

Properly conducted, fasting actually promotes growth. Thompson and Mendel found that a period of suppressed growth, due to under-feeding is followed by increased growth when better food is given, and that the acceleration of growth following this suppression, is ordinarily accomplished on less food than is consumed during a period of equal growth at normal rate from the same initial weight.

Morgulis says: "It has been repeatedly emphasized that just as soon as an animal, which through acute or any other form of inanition lost weight, is given proper nourishment, it commences to grow at a spectacular rate and in a comparatively brief period regains all it had lost or even increases beyond the original level. The rapid gain in weight is a manifestation of a vigorous process of growth. There is not merely an accumulation of reserve substance, but a true growth in the sense defined previously. There is prolific cell multiplication, great expansion of the cells and a reaccumulation of reserves in the form of intracellular and intercellular deposits of products of their metabolism. Nitrogen is retained with an avidity characteristic of the young growing organism. Frequently, in a short span of time an increase of the body mass is accomplished, which required years of normal growth to bring about. The inanition has produced a rejuvenation of the organism. In the study of histological phenomena accompanying inanition, it has already been learned that except in the advanced stages (in the starvation period) there is scarcely any evidence of tissue degeneration. On the contrary, the cells remain intact though they lose a large portion of their substance. In the keen competition which reigns in the organism subjected to inanition the weaker and less essential parts of the cellular organism are sacrificed first, just as we have seen this to happen to the less essential parts of the entire organism. The more vital parts remain and the vitality of the cells and their vigor is thereby improved. This seems to be the rationale of the invigorating and rejuvenating effects of inanition. Biologically speaking, though the organism acquires no new assets it becomes stronger by ridding itself of liabilities. In the foregoing it has been pointed out that the cell-nucleus ratio changes in such a manner as to increase the preponderance of the nucleus. Morphologically, therefore, the cells composing the entire organism assume a youthful condition. They resemble more the embryonic cell in this respect, and this may account for the expansive growth which they display under the proper nutritive regimen."

Again, he says: "Further experiments performed with the salamander, demonstrated that the growth impulse and not the quantity of food consumed plays the leading role. These experiments substantiated the idea that growth which ensues after a preliminary inanition is not unlike embryonic growth in its intensity. It is well to bear in mind that the reduced size of the cell, or rather the altered cell-nucleus ratio is probably in some way responsible for the vigorous growth process and that the rejuvenescence of the organism is dependent upon this condition. Many years ago, Kagan observed that following 17 days of complete inanition rabbits gained 56 per cent in weight on a diet which could just barely maintain a state of equilibrium in the normal condition."

Regeneration is common to a greater or lesser degree to all plants and animals. If man loses a fingernail, he quickly grows another, but even more remarkable examples of regeneration are seen in many animals, some of them being able to grow a new head, a complete new limb or an eye. In some worms a mere fragment of the body is capable of becoming a complete new worm. Many examples of this have been presented in a prior volume. Prof. Morgulis says: "It is a remarkable fact that the starving organism does not lose its regenerative power. An organism already much emaciated through prolonged inanition will draw upon its scanty reserves in the effort to renew a severed part of its body. The little flat worms, *planaria*, commonly found in stagnant waters, possess an extraordinary regenerative capacity. Morgan has shown that even in advanced stages of inanition, when the planarian has been reduced to a small fraction of its original size, the regenerative impulse is still sufficiently strong to reduce still further the much depleted tissues in rebuilding parts of the body which have been cut off. Of course, during inanition the missing organ does not regenerate as rapidly or as fully as in a well-fed animal. The important thing, however, is that inanition does not deprive the organism of its inherent regenerative impulse."

Dr. Harold W. Parker of the Natural History Museum of London and Dr. Mark Boeseman of Leiden, the Netherlands, studying the huge European shark, the Basking shark, discovered that it sheds its teeth in winter and fasts through the winter months. This shark (*Cetorhinus maximus*) feeds upon marine animals and seems to be the second largest "fish" in the world, achieving a length of nearly thirty feet. In winter they vanish and it had long been thought that they migrate southward. But these biologists reported finding and catching specimens resting on the bottom of the sea, devoid of their gillrakers or teeth. They concluded that they lose their rakers in October and November in northwest European waters and "undergo a resting, non-feeding demersal (submerged) stage" until they grow a new set of teeth and warm weather returns. That they fast for the whole of the duration of the winter is not fully proved, but if they do, it means that they grow a new set of teeth or gill-rakers while fasting. It is logically assumed that they do not eat in the absence of their gill-rakers and it is also noted that there is a great scarcity of their food supplies during the winter months. It may also logically be inferred that if they continued to eat during this period, they would be seen cruising on the surface with the mouth wide open in order to catch their food supply.

Discussing the fact that fasting does not interfere with the regeneration and growth of a new tail in the salamander, whose tail has been cut off, Morgulis tells us that, although the tail grows slower while the animal is fasting than the tails of animals not fasting, "when, after several weeks of starvation (fasting), the salamanders having in the meantime lost one-fourth their original weight, they were fed once more, the regeneration of the tail was immediately improved and in the course of time attained or even exceeded in length the tails which were cut off."

The Rhine salmon take no food from the time they enter the fresh water until their spawning season is over; a period varying from eight to fifteen months. The King Salmon of the Pacific coast, the largest and finest of the salmons, present an even more remarkable case of growth while fasting. They make a long and extremely exhausting journey upstream without food. There is evidence to show that they cease to feed before they begin their migration upstream.

Salmon waste quite rapidly during their migrations, due not only to their vigorous activities, but to the rapid growth of their gonads. It has been estimated by Paton that 5 per cent of the fat and 14 per cent of the proteins of the wasting muscles of male salmon go to build up their rapidly growing testicles; while 12 per cent of the fat and 23 per cent of the protein of the muscles of the female go to build up the rapidly growing ovaries. The rest of the fat and protein that disappear from the muscles are used up in maintenance and work. Despite the rapid wasting of muscles in fasting salmon, Miescher maintains that not a fiber undergoes actual disintegration.

Our interest in these phenomena at this place, is to point out the remarkable manner in which the body regulates its internal economy and distributes its stored supplies to various parts of the body as need arises. This ability to analyze and redistribute and re-synthesize the supplies on hand, is our supreme guarantee that none of the vital tissues shall ever be damaged for lack of food, so long as the body's reserves hold out. The continuance of growth while fasting and the rapid acceleration of growth after the fast, indicate very strongly that the body holds onto and uses to greater advantages those substances or qualities in food which are called vitamins and which are claimed to play such important roles in growth and regeneration of tissue. It may even be true that the body does not lose any of its stored supply of vitamins during the most prolonged fast. The complete lack of evidence to show that it does lose vitamins is as suggestive as is the positive evidence that fasting not only does not stop growth but, actually, accelerates it.

Changes in The Fundamental Functions While Fasting

CHAPTER X

Professor Morgulis says: "Laboratory as well as clinical experience corroborates the rejuvenating effects of inanition. If it is not too prolonged it is distinctly beneficent and may be used in overcoming somnolence and lassitude as well as in improving the fundamental organic functions (circulation, respiration), muscular strength, or the acuity of the senses." These improvements are typical of the improvements which occur, both in structure and function throughout the body when one fasts.

The medical profession and the public have been slow in recognizing the benefits to be derived from judicious fasting. Even today there are few doctors of any and all of the rival schools of "healing" who understand fasting and who are qualified to properly conduct a fast. Few "natural therapists" and almost no medical men are sufficiently acquainted with fasting to properly carry one through it. Practically all of them insist on supplementing the fast and "aiding nature" with their various *stimulating* and suppressive measures. Many of the evils attributed to fasting are due to these measures and are common in patients treated by such methods, but who have not fasted. The other "evils of fasting" are imaginary evils.

PHYSIOLOGICAL REST

An important object secured by the fast is the rest of the organs of the body. The overworking of the physiological functions, which results from over-eating, weakens and impairs them. Fasting reverses this and permits them to recuperate. During the rest thus afforded, these organs are enabled to repair their damaged structures and restore their fagging energies, thus they are prepared for renewed function and are given a new lease on life. A fast is to the organs of the body what a night of restful repose is to the tired laborer.

Digestion and assimilation of food are a tax on the vital powers of the organism and increase the work of the stomach, liver, intestines, heart, lungs, kidneys, glands, etc. The more food eaten the more work these already overworked organs are called upon to perform. How can increasing the work of the organs help the sick? If feeding does not prevent sickness how may overfeeding restore health?

That fasting is a period of physiological rest was emphasized by all the early *Hygienists*—Jennings, Graham, Trall, etc. Thomas Low Nichols says: "in fevers and all inflammatory diseases fasting . . . is a matter of the first importance. As a rule, nature herself points out this remedy. When animals have any malady, they stop eating. Loss of appetite is a symptom of disease, and it points also to the mode of cure. ° ° ° Not only must the stomach have rest, but all the organs of nutrition, and the nerves which produce their action. When we stop food in fevers and inflammations, we diminish the volume of the blood and relieve the action of the heart; and by relieving the system of the labor of digestion and assimilation, we allow the nervous force to expend itself in recuperative action . . . a cold is a sort of fever and there is no better remedy for a cold than abstinence from food." After pointing out that the loss of appetite, seen in all acute diseases and common in chronic disease, is "the voice of nature forbidding us to eat," and lamenting the fact that physicians and nurses disregard this "voice of nature" and force food down the throats of "disgusted patients," Nichols says, "rest for the stomach, the liver, all the organs of the nutritive system, may be the one thing needful. It is the only rest we will not permit . . . In certain states of disease, where the organs of digestion are weakened and disordered, the best beginning of a cure may be total abstinence from all kinds of food. There is no cure like it. If the stomach cannot digest, the best way is to give it a rest. It is the one thing which it needs."—*The Diet Cure,* 1881.

Dewey referred to fasting as the "rest cure," and said that rest "is not to do any of the curing (healing) any more than it heals the broken bone or the wound; it is only going to furnish the condition for cure." Here he was speaking of physiological rest or fasting. Mr. Carrington also insists upon the necessity of physiological rest in disease, but he stresses particularly rest of the digestive system, even prescribing forcing measures that prevent rest of other systems of the body. Both Tilden and Weger emphasized the fact that fasting is a period of physiological rest. Perhaps Walter stressed this fact more than anyone else.

I think it necessary to emphasize the rest that fasting affords to the other organs of the body and not overstress the rest the digestive system receives. Let us take the heart: it is no uncommon thing to have patients come to us whose hearts are pulsating eighty or more times a minute against increased resistance. This is to say, the heart is rapid and the blood pressure is increased. The heart is slowly wearing itself out by this work.

I have seen many diseased hearts that were supposed to be "incurable" fully recover during an extended fast. A few years ago a business executive came to me for care. Repeatedly during the preceding two years he had been refused life insurance because his heart was diseased. One month after a forty days' fast he bought ten thousand dollars worth of life insurance.

The ductless glands, the respiratory system, the nervous system, in fact, the whole organism rests during a fast. The exception is the excretory system. This system does more work, at least through a large part of the fast, in freeing the body of its accumulated toxins. This inner rest, that is, this rest of the internal organs which fasting affords, is what is meant by physiological rest.

Rest! Where is there a rest like fasting? People go away for a rest. They get a change of scenery, a change of food, a change of activity, but they fail to secure the rest they need. If they would but fast a few days they would return to their old duties with renewed zest and increased energy. Nothing can give renewed power of digestion to a worn-out digestive system, nothing affords such rest to over-wrought nerves, to fatigued bowels, or to an over-worked heart and glandular system as a fast—physiological rest.

Most vacationists go away and increase their physical exercise and eat more because of increased appetite and come back worse than before. Physiological rest, decreased physical activity and long hours of recuperating sleep, will do more for these people in a few days, than months spent in the conventional manner.

METABOLISM DURING THE FAST

No definition of metabolism that I have ever seen is entirely satisfactory. Nor has it ever seemed to me that the measurements of the metabolic rate do more than inaccurately measure the katabolic phase of metabolism. Metabolism is the term applied to the changes that foodstuffs undergo in the body in the process of becoming part of the body and being used and discarded after use. The tendency today is to define metabolism in chemical terms and this enables the pharmacologists to talk of the metabolism of drugs. Drugs do undergo chemical changes in the body, but there is no metabolism of drugs. Metabolism is a physiolgical or a biological process and is confined in its activities to those substances that are susceptible of being used by the living organism.

Metabolism logically falls into two separate sets of activities; the first, a building up process—*anabolism;* the second, a tearing down process—*katabolism.* Perhaps we may say that anabolism is that phase of metabolism in which the foods taken in are assimilated and made into cell substance; katabolism is that phase of metabolism during which the assimilated foodstuffs are used and disassimilated.

Metabolism is measured by measuring and analyzing the excretions—the breath, urine, heat, etc. Special emphasis is placed on heat production. These measurements do not measure anabolism. There is nothing in them that differentiates between a normal and an abnormal metabolism. The heat produced by a large tumor or a cancerous growth is measured along with the heat produced by the normal activities of life. The fact is that measurements of development are never included in studies of metabolism.

If we accept the definition that "katabolism is the process by which body material is broken down as a result of oxidation and cleavage," and measure the resulting carbon-dioxide and heat, we certainly have not provided any index to the rate at which the "transformation of food material into body material" is taking place. What does the measure of the amount of heat produced and the carbon-dioxide given off tell us of the rate of bone formation or of brain growth? When it is assumed that "anabolism follows the ingestion of food," and is taken for granted that it is at a standstill when no food is taken, a great mistake is made. The statement is made that when no food is taken, the "anabolic activities may be depressed to such an extent as to make the study (of the metabolism of the fast) essentially one of katabolism." I regard such an assumption as highly incorrect and think that it must be based on ignorance of the phenomena of fasting.

Indeed, it seems to me that katabolism may be reduced more than anabolism during a fast of considerable length. Here, I have no reference to the formation of fat and sugar from protein that seems certain to occur during the fast, but to positive constructive activities, by which tissues are repaired, new tissues built, wounds healed, broken bones reunited, and actual growth of structure takes place. There is the same need for tissue repair in fasting as in periods of eating, and if this does not take place at an unslackened rate, the consequences may be disastrous.

ANABOLISM DURING THE FAST

During fifteen days of fasting the pupa of the honey bee metamorphoses into a full-grown bee, the change undergone amounting to a transformation of one form of life into another and entirely different one, with different organs, different functions and a radically different way of life. Here is anabolism of a very intense kind and many examples of this kind could be cited. The process is less dramatic in the larger animals, but nonetheless real.

It has previously been pointed out that the functioning tissues of the body must be nourished during the fast and that they are nourished off the food stores that abound. As the fasting body feels among its supplies for proteins, carbohydrates, fats, minerals and vitamins and redistributes, utilizes and conserves these, it exercises an ingenuity that seems almost super-human. By thus analyzing (autolyzing) its food reserves and redistributing them according to need, the functioning tissues are supported and this means that an intense anabolism is in process. How else could the heart, for instance, go on pulsating sixty or more times a minute, day and night, throughout a long fast, without wearing itself out, were it not replenished as when eating? How could the respiratory muscles keep up the breathing process throughout a long fast if they were not nourished as certainly as when their owner is eating?

What, then, is the basic difference, save, perhaps, in rate, between the anabolism of the fasting period and that of the eating period? Primarily it is this: While eating, the functioning tissues of the body are daily replenished from fresh supplies of nutriment that are received from without; while fasting, these same tissues are daily replenished from the stored nutritive reserves that are held within.

All of this is so evident to the experienced man that one naturally marvels at the foolish statements that are made by physiologists in dealing with the subject of metabolism in the fast. In the sixth

(1955) edition of their *Physiological Basis of Medical Practice*, Best and Taylor discuss what they call the "Metabolism of Starvation." What they say is of little value, as they lump "findings" together without reference to the stage or the period of inanition and without discriminating between the different results in different animals, nor do they differentiate between *fasting* and *starving*. They say that the gonads lose from 2 to 8 per cent in what they call prolonged starvation, whereas, it is well known that in many animals the gonads increase in size and functioning power during periods of abstinence. In the fasting salmon, the gonads undergo luxuriant growth during the lengthy fast (accompanied with great physical activity) of their mating season, and they produce enormous numbers of ova and spermatozoa.

It is impossible to think that the muscles of the salmon, in almost continuous and vigorous, even violent activity during their long swim up the rivers, are not replenished as certainly as while eating, else would they waste to nothingness before the long journey is completed. The production of milk by the hibernating bear and the fasting gray seal, the laying of eggs by the fasting penguin, and a host of similar phenomena of this nature all show unmistakably that an intense anabolism is in progress throughout the whole length of the fast. The bear maintains a comparatively high body temperature during her long period of hibernation, and secretes milk for her immature young, which weigh at birth, no more than a pound each.

The growth of fasting calves, including growth of bones, the regeneration of lost parts by animals that have lost limbs, stomach, head, etc., while fasting, the radical and rapid constructive changes that take place in the metamorphosis of pupa, the changes in the fasting tadpole, the healing of wounds and broken bones in fasting animals and man—growth of hair and nails—these and many more such phenomena dramatically highlight the anabolic activities that occur during periods of prolonged abstinence.

I must return to the fasting pupa in which we observe a most intense anabolism. Indeed, here is anabolism as it is observed in the embryo. Here is the most active construction proceeding at a rapid rate, producing, as a result, a being so unlike the one that wrapped itself in its cocoon as to lead to the thought that it is a different being altogether. Not only is there autolysis, with the transfer of materials from one part to another, but there is reorganization of the materials on a radically different plan. Something akin to this occurs in the case of the female bear during hibernation. From her own tissues, which are first prepared by autolysis, she supplies the requisite building materials for her unborn young, just as, after the cubs are born, she supplies from the same tissues, the materials out of which she produces milk.

A question obtrudes itself at this point: How are we to regard the autolytic disintegration of fat, bone marrow, glycogen and other stored reserves, their transportation, by the circulation, to functioning tissues of the body, and their incorporation into these tissues? This is to ask: is this total process one of anabolism or one of katabolism? It is my thought that the whole process, beginning with the digestion of reserves and ending with the appropriation by the vital cells of the finished product is one of anabolism. Fat that is oxidized is no longer useful. It has been katabolized and is ready for excretion. Fat that has been autolyzed is still useful and is ready to be conveyed to the cells that are in need of the food substances it provides. It is probable that all fat must first be autolyzed and incorporated into the functioning cells before it can be katabolized.

Autolysis is a prominent feature in all utilization of reserves. The fasting tadpole autolyzes its tail, absorbs and redistributes and finally utilizes the substances in it. The fasting salamander, growing a new tail, autolyzes some of its internal stores to provide materials for the production of the new tail, including bones. The growing of bones and organs of the fasting calf can occur only if the growing parts are supplied with materials from the stored reserves and these are made available by autolysis. An animal suffering with a broken leg fasts while the bone is healing. Materials for this work of repair are supplied from the food reserves of the animal and are made available by autolysis.

A very remarkable example of regeneration, necessitating, as it does, active anabolism is supplied us by those forms of life that, under conditions of surfeit, reproduce parthenogenetically, the male disappearing, and, which, while fasting, reproduce the male and reproduce sexually. All reproductive activity must be classed as anabolic, and when we observe animals, some of them high in the scale of life, reproducing while fasting, some of them reproducing at no other time, we are faced with a most remarkable evidence of the continuation of anabolism during the fast.

If we turn our attention to the vegetable kingdom, we find other evidences of active anabolism during periods of abstinence. If we take a cutting from such plants as the rose bush, the fig tree or the weeping willow, and stick one end of it into the ground, and water it, it will put out roots and leaves and grow into a full-sized plant. In the absence of roots the cutting is incapable of taking up minerals from the soil; in the absence of leaves it cannot take carbon from the air and, by photosynthesis, manufacture carbohydrates. It is forced to rely upon its own internal resources.

Roots and leaves are put out, but the materials out of which these are made come from within. Materials stored in the cutting are utilized in their production and only after these have been produced can the cutting take food from the air and soil. These facts prove that there is circulation in the cutting, that there is a transfer of autolyzed materials from one part of the cutting to another.

Turn in whatever direction we may, in both plant and animal, we find evidence that anabolism is very active during periods of fasting. More remarkable, however, than this, is the obvious fact, as shown by the maintenance of the heart, brain, and nervous system, that there is anabolism even during starvation, this is to say, after the exhaustion of the organism's stored reserves. It would seem that so long as there is any life left and so long as nutrients may be secured from whatever source, the constructive processes of life are never completely suspended. Always the processes of repair and maintenance of tissue are in operation. Activities are reduced, certain functions are temporarily suspended, conservative measures are adopted, but life or living processes are not suspended. If fasting resulted in a suspension of the anabolic process, there would be a steady decline in all of the tissues of the body from the omission of the first meal, until death ended the matter. This is the exact opposite of what we regularly observe during a fast, even a most prolonged fast.

KATABOLISM IN THE FAST

It seems, from what we observe during the early days of the fast, particularly in fat individuals, that there may be a slight increase in katabolic activities immediately upon the beginning of a fast. The rate of weight loss is often great for the first few days, although all of this loss does not represent tissue loss. After a short period, however, the rate of loss slackens and tends to slacken still more as the fast proceeds. We frequently see individuals who lose not more than an ounce to two ounces of weight a day after thirty to thirty-five days of abstinence. That the rate of metabolism is slowed after the end of the first period of the fasting experience as classified by Morgulis, has already been discussed. The reduced intake of oxygen and reduced output of carbon dioxide are but a small part of the evidence of this reduction.

The reduction of katabolism grows out of several precedent and concomitant reductions. There is a reduction of physical and commonly of emotional activity, a reduction of those activities associated with the digestion of food, a reduction (after a time) of endocrine secretion, a reduction of oxygen intake, a reduction of heart activity, a fall in blood pressure, and a slowing up of the complex functional activities of the body. All of this indicates that the tearing down processes of life are greatly reduced.

Except for the predominant role played by autolysis, metabolism in the fasting organism is not radically different from that in the feeding state. The rate of metabolism is changed; the emphasis is on the conservative processes; waste is reduced to a minimum, but no new elements are introduced into the process and no normal elements of metabolism are missing. Life goes on, more or less, in the regular pattern, even if at a slightly (in some cases) slackened tempo, so long as the stored reserves endure. In the hibernating and æstivating animal the tempo of life is greatly reduced; in the fasting Alaskan fur seal bull and in the fasting salmon there is enormous activity. In the fasting patient, put to bed, made comfortable, kept warm and freed of worries and anxieties, the tempo of life fluctuates around a standard that may be about midway between that of the tempo of life of the hibernating bear and that of the fasting fur seal bull.

A phenomenon that is quite uniform in repeated fasts in the same individual is that the rate of loss, from the outset of the fast, is slower in second and third fasts than in the first. If the second fast comes years after the first fast, this fact is not so noticeable, but if it follows within a few weeks or a few months, the slower loss in the second fast is very marked. These observations of the progressive reduction of the rate of loss, as the fast progresses and the slower rate of loss in second and third fasts, have led to the conclusion that the body learns to conserve its resources. The experience gained in one fast is not lost when, at a later time, another fast is undertaken.

Whether the rate of loss in the early days of the fast indicates that katabolism is increased over the pre-fasting level or remains the same, the reduction of the rate of loss, as the fast continues, reveals that katabolism is markedly reduced. Thus it appears, that, instead of anabolism being greatly reduced in the fast and katabolism being increased, as may be thought, the opposite is the case. The greatest reduction is seen in katabolism, not in anabolism. It may be true, that, in some instances at least, there is a slowing down of anabolism, but this is certainly far from the general rule.

With these preliminary remarks out of the way let us turn to more detailed studies, beginning with:

METABOLISM DURING HIBERNATION

In hibernation respiration and circulation are frequently almost suspended; no food is taken, the animal subsisting entirely on fat and other food reserves stored during the Summer and Fall. The animal enters hibernation in a state of fatness; he emerges from hibernation in the Spring in an emaciated condition, although strong and active. In cold-blooded animals in a state of hibernation metabolism is almost at a complete standstill. Indeed, in some of them, as well as in frozen caterpillars, it must be at a complete standstill. Not so the metabolism of warm-blooded animals. These must maintain a minimum of physiological activity and keep up a certain amount of body heat or freeze to death. At the same time, they must maintain metabolism at as low a level as is compatible with continued existence, else their food reserves may be exhausted before the end of winter, at which time they will also die of freezing.

Animals that fast during the mating season are commonly intensively active, both physically and sexually, the fur seal bull taking no sleep throughout the whole of the period. Their great activity necessitates the intake of great quantities of oxygen, the speeding up of heart activity and circulation, with a consequent high rate of metabolism. Due to these factors they use up their reserves at a much faster rate than do hibernating and æstivating animals. But the æstivating and hibernating and the mating animals enter their periods of abstinence with large reserves of food that sustain them through long periods of fasting.

Hibernating and æstivating animals remain quiescent or dormant. Metabolism is at the lowest ebb compatible with continued living existence. The food reserves are used extremely slowly. Heart action is slow, circulation is slow, respiration is slow, all the activities of life are slowed down. Certain activities in these animals do, however, proceed. In the frog, for example, preparations are made for the laying and fertilizating of eggs almost immediately after awakening from the winter sleep. The bear gives birth to her cubs while still asleep and suckles them during this time. She produces milk for them after birth as well as provides food for them before birth. They are born nude so they must depend upon her for warmth after they are born. This would indicate that, despite the intense cold outside her hibernating quaters, she maintains a high degree of temperature inside.

Although the temperature of hibernating mammals falls considerably below their normal temperatures in the active state, there is a point below which it cannot fall without proving fatal to the animal. A ground squirrel which hibernated in a temperature of 35.6° F., had a body temperature exactly the same, although the "normal" temperature is several degrees higher than this.

The low rate of metabolism in the hibernating bat, manifest by slow respiration, slow heart action and sluggish circulation, means a very slow use of nutritive reserves. The same slow circulation, slow heart action and lessened rate of breathing seen in the hibernating bear also mean the same slow consumption of reserves. Exhaustion of reserves before the return of warm weather would result in death from starvation.

Griffin says that "in spite of the low level to which the metabolic processes have fallen, a hibernating bat will awaken in a few minutes if handled or even disturbed by lights and talking. Once awake, the bat is as lively and active as ever. His temperature, circulation, and respiration have returned to normal." Were this activity continued, exhaustion of food stores would rapidly result. He tells us that "after flying around for a few minutes they hang up again and relapse into the torpor of hibernation."

Mr. Griffin tells us that the metabolic rate of an animal in hibernation depends on the temperature of his surroundings: "he will burn more fat at a higher temperature, just as any chemical reaction is speeded up by a rise in temperature." This is not good physiology and I doubt the correctness of his statement. He, himself, shows that the hibernating bat may be awakened and become active, his temperature, circulation and respiration becoming normal in spite of the low temperature of his surroundings. I think we must regard hibernation as a function of life that is vitally controlled and not absolutely determined by the temperature of the surrounding air. The control of metabolism is from within and not from without. There is a purposive conserving of food stores, not a mere passive non-use of these.

We witness, not a mere slowing down of "chemical reactions" by a lowering of temperature, but a reduction of physiological activities by a process somewhat analogous to sleep. By his own showing, these physiological activities are not helpless in the grip of temperature. They are speeded up or slowed down by the bat in the same temperature. Mr. Griffin may be a biologist, but he talks like a chemist. He thinks of the bat in terms of test-tubes, reagent bottles, retorts, etc., and not as a living organism that takes an active part in the control of its behavior.

The bat is not a cold-blooded animal and, even in hibernation, with metabolism reduced to the lowest point compatible with continued life, is able to maintain a body temperature slightly higher than that of its surroundings. It is able to increase or decrease its metabolism in the same temperature. It can be active or dormant in the same temperature. Hibernation seems to be an adjustment to certain environmental conditions—the absence of food supply seems to be more important in inducing this state than the reduction of temperature—rather than a passive yielding to outside influences. The reduction of metabolism is not the result of cold, but the result of the need to conserve food reserves. Oxydation in the animal body, while a chemical process, is a rigidly controlled process. The body does not start to burn and just continue to burn until it is consumed. The body's fat stores do not catch fire on hot days and go up in flames. Even in the hottest weather the fasting animal reduces its metabolic rate and conserves its food reserves. As a matter of fact, non-hibernating animals conserve their food reserves better in hot than in cold weather. This is due to the fact that more heat must be produced in cold weather to maintain normal body temperature. This "chemical reaction" is not speeded up by a rise in temperature; for, internally, there is no rise in temperature, though the surface of the body may feel chilly and the faster may complain of being cold even in hot weather.

It would be interesting to know what is the internal temperature of the bat in hibernation. It is, no doubt, much lower than in the active state. But the question remains to be answered: *Is lowered temperature due to reduced metabolism, or is lowered metabolism due to lowered temperature?*

If the lowering of temperature comes from without and is responsible for the reduction of metabolism, it would seem to be impossible for the bat to arouse itself or be aroused from its state of "torpor" by anything short of an increase of temperature. So long as the temperature of the cave is thirty-three degrees, Fahrenheit, that of the bat should remain nearly as low and "torpor" should persist. It could not fly out of its cave to see if Spring has arrived, or more accurately, perhaps, to see if there is a food supply in evidence. If control is from without, the bat should be helpless until the control —temperature—is changed. Only the coming of warm weather should awaken him. Bats leaving a cave and flying to another when its temperature starts to drop to too low levels shows that the reduction of their metabolism is not a result of lowered temperature. For, if it were, a further lowering of temperature would further decrease metabolism and make it impossible for the bat to awaken and fly in search of a more sheltered abode.

The fact that some species commence their period of hibernation while the temperature is still relatively high and food is still to be had, indicates that the control of metabolism is from within, not from without. The hibernating animal is not helpless in the grip of external conditions.

FASTING METABOLISM IN MAN

Metabolism is lowered from one-fourth to two-fifths during the fast. This falls quite rapidly during the first part of the fast until the true physiological minimum for metabolism is reached. From this point on, until the return of hunger, metabolism is maintained at a fairly uniform level. If food is not consumed when hunger returns there follows, soon, a rapid dropping of metabolism to new low, but pathological levels.

During the first fifteen days of Levanzin's fast there was an appreciable decrease in oxygen consumption and in carbon-dioxide production. During the first seven days of the fast he consumed 352.6 liters of oxygen and produced 260.4 liters of carbon-dioxide. During the second half of the first fifteen day period he consumed 303.2 liters of oxygen and produced 219.5 liters of carbon-dioxide. During the first half of the second fifteen day period he consumed 272.3 liters of oxygen and produced 193.7 liters of carbon-dioxide. During the last half of the second period he consumed 270.3 liters of oxygen and produced 192.9 liters of carbon-dioxide.

In a general way the changes in the metabolism of proteins, fats, etc., run fairly parallel with carbohydrate metabolism. Nitrogen metabolism in the fasting baby supplies a remarkable apparent exception to this. Nitrogen excretion tends to increase from day to day, rather than decrease. The small supply of glycogen possessed by the baby is rapidly oxidized and it is compelled to draw upon its proteins for maintenance. It will be recalled that the growing infant utilizes its proteins primarily for the building up of tissue and that it normally excretes less nitrogen than is consumed.

Dr. Kunde quotes Dr. Carlson who suggests that "the higher metabolism after prolonged fasts may be due to temporary excess activity of such glands as the thyroid and the gonads that seem to have direct effects on the metabolic rate.

"It is well established that fasting induces a marked atrophy of these glands. The recuperation of these glands on the resumption of eating may carry them for a while beyond the level of activity normal for the age of the subject. This would in all probability lead to a higher metabolism."

That this explanation is incorrect is evident from the following considerations:

(1) Fasting does not cause atrophy of the glands. Atrophy takes place in starvation.

(2) There is no reason to believe that atrophied glands will function excessively. They would be more likely to function deficiently.

(3) The increased metabolic rate begins immediately upon the resumption of eating, before the "atrophied" glands have had time to recuperate.

John Arthur Glaze records in the *American Journal of Psychology* that one result of a two weeks' fast which he observed was a marked intensification of the sexual impulse after the fast was over, though it was largely inhibited during the fast. This certainly cannot be due to atrophy of the gonads. It indicates increased gonadal efficiency corresponding to the increased acuteness of the senses of sight, taste, smell, hearing and feeling. We would not attribute better eyesight following a fast to optic atrophy or better hearing to auditory atrophy.

One is constrained to ask, what is the "level of (glandular) activity normal for the age of the subject?" The level of activity presented in the old man and woman of today is a pathological level rather than a physiological or biological norm.

Kunde dwells at length on the increased metabolic rate (oxygen consumption) following a fast and suggests that this may be due to the cell membranes becoming more permeable to food than before the fast. The doctor does not seem to understand the significance of toxin elimination by fasting. Lack of understanding of toxemia and its role in reducing physiological processes leads to much misinterpretation of phenomena.

Kunde continues: "But the fact that there is a tendency for the metabolic rate to return to its former level points to internal coordination processes that are not permanently altered by fasting." But this may point to a speedy reproduction of the pre-fasting "physiological" condition by a return to the former mode of living. Living cannot be left out of the formula. What is meant, for example, by a normal diet? New protoplasm built by a "normal" diet may not be of better quality than that lost during the fast.

RESPIRATION

This is one of the fundamental organic functions which Morgulis states is improved by fasting. The remarkable effects of fasting upon the breathing of asthmatics can be really appreciated only by those who have watched it in many cases.

During the fast the excretion of carbon dioxide decreases. During the first stage of the fast the amount of carbon dioxide produced grows steadily less as the fast progresses, until the fasting level for metabolism is reached. This is due to decreased activity and lowered metabolism, and not to any lessening of the efficiency of the excretory function of the lungs. The breath is exceedingly foul; so much so at times that one can hardly remain in the same room with the patient.

ELIMINATION

Fasting is nature's own method of ridding the body of "diseased" tissues, excess nutriment and accumulations of waste and toxins. Nothing else will increase elimination through every channel of excretion as will fasting. Nothing else affords the organs of elimination the same opportunity to catch up with the work they are behind on and thus bring their work up to date.

At the start of the fast there occurs a temporary increase in elimination over the amounts usually thrown out, after which there follows a very rapid drop to lower levels. The fasting body strikes a new balance of excretion, one which represents a closer approach to the true wastes of the daily activities of life. Much of the larger amounts eliminated daily previous to the fast was due to the daily intake of much more food than the body required. As soon as this surplus is excreted, elimination seeks a lower level.

As the fast progresses, the blood and lymph (lymph makes up from 25 per cent to 35 per cent of the body weight; blood only amounts to about 5 per cent of body weight) becomes purified; pent-up excretions are expelled from the body; the nervous system and all the vital organs rest. As the nervous system secures relief, body and mind become rested and the bodily irritations that have caused the mental irritations and the mental bad conduct cease; indeed, the individual is "made over." Ridding the cells and fluids of accumulated toxins accounts for most of the benefits derived from fasting. The benefits last until the toxins reaccumulate and in most cases, this takes place quite rapidly due to subsequent return to a toxogenic mode of living.

One great source of toxins is decomposing food in the digestive tract. Fasting soon eliminates this completely. The alimentary canal becomes practically free of bacteria. Only a week of fasting is required to result in the complete disappearance of all germs from the stomach. The small intestine becomes sterile. The hibernating bear and other hibernating animals lose all their colon bacilli during hibernation. Typhoid cases that fast through their illness are free of "typhoid bacilli" at the end of the acute stage and are not "dangerous" as "carriers."

ORGANIC HOUSE CLEANING

The vital cells of the body must be nourished during the fast. These are nourished off the food reserves stored in the body and off the less essential tissues, or off the salvable portions of the "diseased" and dead tissues. The body possesses power to refine and use the materials it has on hand during a fast of reasonable length. The popular belief that immediately upon the discontinuance of meals the blood and solid structures of the body begin to break down and that organic destruction sets in, is unfounded as is proved by the results obtained in many thousands of cases of fasting patients. The vital cells of the organs and glands of the body, those cells doing the actual physical and chemical work of these organs, do not begin to disintegrate until actual starvation sets in. We know that it is not until the total of the body's reserves have been consumed that death from starvation sets in and it is only after these are consumed that nature will permit a single vital organ to be damaged. Under favorable conditions of rest and warmth these reserve stores may hold out for weeks and even months.

The faster lives on the same thing when fasting as when eating, the difference being that when eating, he replenishes his nutritive stores each day, while in fasting he gradually consumes them. The faster lives on those portions of his body which represent stored food and not upon the vital or functioning tissues of his body. The vital cells are not injured unless the fast is prolonged beyond the point where all the body's nutritive reserves are consumed and no fasting advocate believes in or practices such a thing.

The fasting body begins to grow smaller, and in order to maintain the integrity of its vital organs, it utilizes all the surplus material it has on hand. Growths, deposits, effusions, dropsical swellings, infiltrations, fat, etc., are absorbed and used to support these organs. With no digestive drudgery on hand, nature employs the long desired leisure for general house cleaning purposes. Accumulations of surplus tissues are overhauled and analyzed; the available component parts are turned over to the department of nutrition, while the refuse is thoroughly and permanently removed.

Emaciation frees the body of excess inert materials in its tissues and proves thereby to be a great boon. One of the first things that nature does in an acute "disease" is to cast off a lot of her surplus weight. She dispenses with the unnecessary burden. The lowering of weight is a natural method of defense. It represents a reduction of the body's nutritive labors, so that these may be fulfilled without exhausting the visceral organs.

There is no known measure that is equal to fasting as a means of accelerating the processes of elimination. When food is withheld, only a short time elapses before the organs of elimination increase their work of throwing off accumulated waste products. Secretions begin a physiological house cleaning.

Carrington and others insist that in fasting accumulated waste and toxins are eliminated first and until these are eliminated none of the really valuable tissues of the body will be destroyed. This is to say, excess food materials in the body and diseased tissues are utilized first in the fast. Carrington, indeed, thinks that "the whole physiology of the fast is contained in" this principle. He says that *"weakness* is due *not* to lack of food, but to the poisons of the disease; *emaciation* is due not to the fact that too little food is supplied the system, but to the fact that disease wastes the body—by poisoning it."

ACTIONS IN RELATION TO POISONS

The nervous system of the faster becomes relatively larger than at other times and its sensibilities become more acute. For this reason, the actions of the body in relation to drugs are more prompt and vigorous when fasting than when feeding. Because this is so, fasting usually compels one to discontinue one's drug habits. This will be discussed more fully in a later chapter. The faster should avoid drugs of all kinds.

The Mind and Special Senses
During a Fast

CHAPTER XI

The mental effects of fasting have been known for ages and have been much discussed by all writers on fasting. A few years ago a group of young men and women at the University of Chicago lived for one week without food. During this period they attended their classes and engaged in their usual sports, following out their usual routine. Their mental alertness was so much greater during the period that their progress in their school work was cited as remarkable. Several repetitions of this experiment, always with the same results, proved that this was not exceptional.

All the purely mental powers of man improve while fasting. The ability to reason is increased. Memory is improved. Attention and association are quickened. The so-called spiritual forces of man—intuition, sympathy, love, etc.—are all increased. All of man's intellectual and emotional qualities are given new life. At no other time can the purely intellectual and æsthetic activities be so successfully pursued as during a fast. Sinclair says: "I went out of doors and lay in the sun all day, reading; and the same for the third and fourth days—intense physical lassitude, but with great clearness of mind. After the fifth day I felt stronger, and walked a good deal, and I also began some writing. No phase of the experience surprised me more than the activity of my mind, I read and wrote more than I had dared to do for years before."

People seem to learn faster when hungry and to rate higher in intelligence tests when hungry than when the stomach is full. This means that, as the old Romans used to say: "a full stomach does not like to think." This well expresses a fact that is known to all mental workers. A full meal leaves them dull, unable to think clearly and continuously and often makes them stupid and sleepy. Mental workers have learned to eat a light breakfast and lunch and have their heavy meal in the evening after the day's work is done. When I was a high school boy, I used to miss a meal entirely when I knew I had an examination ahead. At that time I knew nothing of fasting, but I had learned that I could think better on an empty stomach.

These facts are due to physiological causes. Large amounts of blood and nervous energies have to be sent to the digestive organs to digest a meal. If these energies are not required there, they may be drawn upon by the brain in thinking.

In my experience with fasting, I seldom see any increase in mental powers at the beginning of a fast. This is because we deal with the sick and these people are all inebriates and addicts—food inebriates, coffee and tea inebriates, tobacco and alcohol addicts. As soon as these things are taken from them they suffer a period of depression with headaches and various slight pains. After a few days, that is, when the body has had sufficient time to readjust itself and overcome the depression, the mind brightens up. The special senses also become acute.

Levanzin says: "But if physical strength is not lost during a fast, the mental power and clarity are extraordinarily increased. Memory develops itself in a wonderful way, imagination is at its best." One of the most remarkable things about the fast, one that impresses patients even more than the physical gains made while fasting, is the mental benefit that accrues from a period of abstinence. The clearness of the mind, the ease with which previously difficult problems can be handled, the improvement of memory, etc., all surprise and please the patients. These improvements must be attributed to clearing the body of toxins.

The almost universal testimony of fasters is that their mind becomes clearer and their abilities to think and solve intricate problems are enhanced. They are more alert and their minds seem to open up into new fields. This increase in mental power may not manifest in the first few days of the fast, due to the fact that when patients are taken off their coffee, tea, alcohol, and stimulating viands, there is likely to be a general physical and mental let-down. But after a few days, re-action sets in and they improve both physically and mentally. Experiments on students have shown that short fasts greatly enhance mental powers.

Why should fasting result in an increase in mental abilities? Primarily, I think, because it affords the body an opportunity to throw off its load of toxins, hence the brain is fed by a cleaner blood-stream. Secondarily, I think that the rest of all the functions of life that fasting provides, supplies the brain with more power to think. Who can doubt that modern living tends to dull the mental powers?

Especially our national drug addictions and our almost universal overeating tend to reduce mental abilities.

SPIRITUAL POWERS

A few words about the effects of fasting upon the so-called spiritual powers may be appropriately introduced here. In detailing his experiences during his forty days' fast, taken some years since, Dr. Tanner said: "My mental powers were greatly augmented, to the very great surprise of my medical attendants, who were constantly on watch for mental collapse, which was freely predicted, if I persisted in the experiment until the tenth day. About the middle of my first experiment, I, too, had visions; like Paul of old, I seemed to be intromitted to the third heaven and there saw things which not even the pen of Milton or Shakespeare could portray in all their vivid reality. As a result of my experiment, I came to comprehend why the old prophets and seers so often resorted to fasting as a means of spiritual illumination."

That the mental powers of the faster are elevated instead of decreased by the fast, I have shown, but I pause here to express my opinion about these visions that fasters see. They are, I believe, due to hysteria or auto-hypnosis. They are seen by people who are called psychic which means they are easily swayed by suggestion, particularly auto-suggestion. Fasting tends to increase temporarily this suggestibility and for this reason was and is employed by all mystic religions for purposes of "illumination." Auto-suggestion, during these religious fasts takes the form of frequent and repeated prayers. To add to the religious power of the fast, sexual desires disappear and thoughts of sex cease to obtrude upon the mind. In India the priests connected with the sacred temples are pledged to the strictest chastity. The Hindu high priest is forced to undergo a long period of training and purification and to pass through many severe trials to prove that he has thoroughly conquered his sexual appetites and passions and has them well under control of the higher powers of mind before he is admitted to the priesthood. In these days when the fallacies of psychology and psycho-analysis are on the lips of everyone and when feminine leaders declare chastity and continence to be neither desirable nor practicable and insist that they would be harmful if put into effect, methods of attaining self-control in matters of sex are frowned upon. This feature of fasting may not, therefore, appeal to many who read these lines. Fasting does increase one's control over all one's appetites and passions and this will account in some measure for its use by high priests and others in the religions of old.

INSANITY

Nowhere does the beneficial office of physiological rest in enhancing mental clearness show more clearly than in fasting by the insane. I shall have more to say about this in a future chapter. Here it is necessary only to deal with it briefly. Dr. Dewey tells of an insane woman who was completely restored to sanity by a fast of forty-five days. Dr. Rabagliati tells of similar cases, although he more often employed greatly restricted diets, rather than a complete fast. A small quantity of whey each day was a favorite of his.

The common practice is to feed nervous patients all the "good nourishing food" they can be induced to swallow. If they are deprived of food and their accustomed stimulants, there follows a period of depression and an increased nervous irritability. Feeding and drugging smother these symptoms just as a dose of morphine relieves the addict who is suffering from forced abstinence from his drug, and this leads physician and patient to believe he is improved thereby. Yet, these very measures, so frequently employed to *cure,* are often the cause of nervousness.

If such patients are permitted to fast for a few days, a remarkable change occurs in their mental and nervous symptoms. One example must suffice. A young lady once consulted me. She was so extremely nervous that if her husband only pointed his finger at her and said "boo!" she would become hysterical, laughing and crying alternately for sometime before she would finally regain composure. A little noise in the house or outside at night frightened her. She was placed on a fast. It lasted only a week, but her nervousness was completely overcome in this short time. Nothing frightened her any more and nothing would cause her to become hysterical.

Benedict says: "A characteristic of many delusions is a revulsion towards food and drink, so marked indeed that in many instances all the skill of the trained psychiatrist is required to combat it. In a large proportion of such cases, artificial feeding must be resorted to." He recounts a number of cases from the literature of the subject, none of which will be mentioned here. Let me state, with as much emphasis as I can, that the rejection of food by these patients is, in my opinion, not something to be combatted but to be accepted.

THE MIND AND SPECIAL SENSES DURING A FAST

Instead of forced feeding, they should be permitted to fast. I say this, not alone because I know of the benefits to be derived from fasting, but also because I have seen such cases permited to continue the fast and recover sanity while still fasting. As my observations in this field have necessarily been limited, I have no means of knowing what percentage of them would thus recover. It is my opinion that the revulsion to food is an instinctive move in the right direction as certainly as is the cutting off of the desire for food in acute disease.

Kellogg suggests a "bland diet" "in cases of insane persons who refuse to eat and must be nourished by tube feeding." I helped care for one such case and we permitted him to fast. For forty days he continued to refuse food, then he developed an uncontrollable hunger and would invade the kitchen, if not watched, and get food at all times. The young man made great improvement both mentally and physically and was able to run and also to put up a stiff fight when efforts were made to restrain him in some of his actions. He committed suicide before his recovery was complete, however.

Insanity is frequently overcome while fasting, and practically all cases are improved by the fast. Max Nordau declared: "Pessimism has a physiological basis." It really has what we call a pathological basis and this is removed by fasting. Many cases of paralysis of the throat, legs, arms and other forms of paralysis have yielded to the kindly influence of fasting.

Dr. Kritzer, following the lead of Dr. Henry Lindlahr, warned against fasting in mental, nervous and "psychic diseases." "Beware of an empty stomach in melancholia," he said, "for the patient's constant brooding causes a congestion of blood in the brain, and unless the blood is withdrawn through the process of digestion, the chances of aggravation of the mental symptoms are increased. All persons negatively inclined physically, mentally or psychically—the 'sensitive types'—would fare better on a properly balanced diet rather than fasting, even though for short periods."

We must deplore this mixing of occultism and spiritualism with physiology and dietetics. I once placed on a fast, a psychic woman who had previously been warned that a fast would ruin her. She improved steadily during the fast and went on to good health. I do not hesitate to fast nervous and mental cases and always with good results. Dr. E. R. Moras tells of placing a woman on a diet of strained orange juice who "had been insane for eight months and treated by eminent neurologists." In seven days the girl called for food and in six weeks was normal. She was "psychic." I have found it best, in those cases who have had shock treatment and long periods on "nerve" drugs to employ relatively short fasts, two or more, rather than the long fast.

Dr. Kritzer said: "The ill effect of prolonged fasting upon the nervous system is, however, more pronounced and of longer duration. Indeed, the individual drifts into a negative condition, becomes irritable and extremely sensitive.

"It often requires years of careful living in order to successfully overcome the shock received by the nervous system after an injudicious long fast."

Dr. Kritzer had not been studying fasting; but a mixture of fasting with hot and cold baths, spinal manipulations, massage, electrical treatment, psychotherapy and other such forms of destructive nonsense. Fasting does not produce the effects he attributes to it. The depletion of the nervous system he and others write about, is due to the insane abuse in the form of so-called treatment to which patients are often subjected in most drugless and semi-drugless institutions, and often occur in patients that are fed. "Those who obtain the best results from fasting and proper dieting," to quote Dr. Weger, "are those whose mental state is not shattered by the long continued use of drugs and by psychic shock." He makes this observation with particular reference to cases of epilepsy, but it is true in general. By this is not meant that even these cases do not derive benefit from fasting and proper diet, but merely that the benefit is not so apparent and requires, often, much longer time to make itself manifest.

Lennox and Cobb, of the Harvard University Medical School, experimented with fasting in epilepsy and reported that except in one patient there was little permanent effect on the "seizures." They found that in the majority of the cases the "seizures" were entirely absent or were greatly reduced during the fast, but that these returned with the resumption of eating. As this experience is wholly out of keeping with my own I shall make a few remarks concerning the "essentially negative results of fasting" which they report. Let me say that I have had only two cases in which the fits returned after the fast. I recall one case, however, which was in a sanatorium with which I was connected. This patient had two fasts of about twenty days each. The milk diet was employed after each fast. It was found that if more than six quarts of milk were consumed in one day a "seizure" would result. It was also found that if he was given milk for six days and no food of any kind on the 7th day, he would go for long periods without trouble; but as soon as he took milk on the 7th day he had a "seizure." This case very forcibly illustrates the relation of eating habits to the "disease." Another of my cases that had been having one and two "seizures" a week, did not have one seizure during over three months under my observation after a fast of less than a week. The fast was followed with proper diet and living reform. The fasting cases of Lennox and Cobb lasted from four to twenty-one days, and the longer fasts were certainly long enough to produce great benefit in these cases. They think that if fasting were employed in the early stages of the "disease" the results might be more encouraging. They also say that it would be strange if an "acute therapeutic dieting measure" should give lasting results in a chronic condition like epilepsy.

I would say, however, in view of my own experience, that their lack of knowledge of fasting and especially their lack of knowledge of proper feeding after the fast, is responsible for their partial results. The effects of fasting are profound and lasting, but these may be totally spoiled by injudicious care. Dr. Weger says: "It is conceded by physicians that most epileptic seizures are precipitated by gastrointestinal derangement, gastric hyperacidity and intestinal fermentation, even by a very slight deviation from normal at any period of the digestive cycle. The most frequent source of irritation is the colon." One of my cases noticed pain in the left pelvic region and a knotting of the colon preceding each "seizure." There was a failure of colonic function before each "attack" with a loss of appetite.

If good digestion is so important in these cases, it should be quite obvious that the permanency of the results obtained by fasting must depend largely upon proper feeding and proper general care after the fast. As Dr. Weger says, "It is absurd to look for good results in this class of cases unless some attention is given to the kind and combination of food. If the same kind, quality, and quantity of food is permitted after the fast that the patient was in the habit of taking before the fast, the experiment is doomed to failure."

Fasting and prayer were prominent among the remedies employed by the ancients in epilepsy. Dr. Rabagliati says that the best remedy for epilepsy "consists of a careful restriction of the diet. ° ° ° I have for many years now advised restriction of the acute cases in epilepsy to two meals daily, and sometimes one, and in acute cases have recommended further and greater restriction to a pint or a pint and a half of milk daily for a considerable period of time. ° ° ° Fasting in fact, seems to be of very great efficacy in the treatment of epilepsy."

"ABNORMAL PSYCHISM"

Dr. Henry Lindlahr conjured into being a condition to which he applied the term "abnormal psychism," which he said often resulted in certian types of individuals when they fasted for prolonged periods. I have found no reference to any such mental aberrations in the writing of any other man who has had great experience with the fast, and I have seen nothing resembling it in my own practice. Nonetheless, as conclusions based on Lindlahr's statements about this condition were revived by the authors of *Basic Naturopathy* (a textbook for students of naturopathy), I think it wise to consider his statements. Before going into it more in detail, let me say that I once heard a student ask Dr. Lindlahr if he had ever thought of these examples of "abnormal psychism" as crises. Instead of giving the student a direct and candid answer, he delivered a lengthy talk on the difference between theory and experience. Yet, he did not dissociate his *experience* from his *theory*; or, since it all stems from the darkened seance room, where magic, slight-o-hand, and many mechanical devises are employed to play upon the credulity of the people, had we not better call it superstition, rather than theory?

I am of the opinion that such developments, if they do occur, are due to other causes. They do develop in people who are not fasting. Many fasting patients have lost their abnormal mental conditions while fasting. All who have had extended experience with fasting have seen cases of insanity recover health while on the fast and many others make great improvement while fasting. Knowing that Dr. Hazzard had had many years of experience with fasting I wrote her for her experience with "abnormal psychism" in the fast. She replied in a letter to me dated December 8, 1931, that the notion that fasting produces such conditions is "absolutely wrong" and that,

"Fasting seems to clarify mentality, not to cloud it. Nor will it develop any abnormal mental symptoms."

The nearest approach to such a condition that I have found recorded in fasting literature, is one related by Carrington. He says: "The patient became practically insane from the second to the fifth day of the fast—normal conditions being restored on the fifth day. When once the crisis was passed, no indications of such a condition ever recurred; the mentality became, on the other hand, far clearer than in years—indicating that the condition was transitory and merely a curative crisis; one aspect of the vital upheaval, affecting, by chance, the mentality. In this case, the condition was undoubtedly brought about by the excessive, morbid action of the liver, which was greatly deranged, causing an excessive flow of bile; and to a disordered circulation. This was undoubtedly the cause, since the patient also turned almost green during these days—her complexion becoming normal as the fast progressed."—*Vitality, Fasting and Nutrition,* p. 535.

Lindlahr says: "Next to the hypnotic or mediumistic process, there is nothing that induces 'abnormal psychism' as quickly as fasting. During a prolonged fast, the purely animal functions of digestion, assimilation and elimination are almost completely at a standstill. This depression of the physical functions arouses and increases the psychic functions and may produce in these emotionalism and abnormal activity of the senses of the spiritual-body, the individual thus becoming abnormally clairvoyant, clairaudient, and otherwise, sensitive to conditions on the spiritual planes of life." He adds: "This explains the spiritual exaltation and the visions of 'heavenly' scenes and beings or the fights with demons which are frequently, indeed, uniformly, reported by hermits, ascetics, saints, yogi, fakirs, and dervishes."

Unhesitatingly, I pronounce this mere twaddle. In more than forty years of experience in fasting patients, in all conditions and at all ages of life, I have never seen a single development such as he here describes. I have conducted well over thirty-five thousand fasts, ranging from a few days to ninety days in duration. Men, women, and children, the stolid and the high-strung, the atheist and the religious, the nervous and the mental sufferer and others have been among those who have fasted under my care and none of them has ever become clairvoyant or clairaudient. None of them has become "sensitive" to conditions on any hypothetical "spiritual planes of existence." None of them has had a "heavenly vision," none of them has had any fights with any devils, nor has any of them ever become hypnotically controlled "by 'positive' intelligences either on the physical or on the spiritual plane of being"—hypnotism or mediumism. Lindlahr frankly believed in demonic obsession or possession or, as he also phrased it "spirit control." He says "spirit 'controls' often force their subjects to abstain from food, thus rendering them still more negative and submissive." He thought it "little short of criminal" to "place persons of the negative, sensitive type on prolonged fasts and thus to expose them to the dangers just described."

Theoretically a vegetarian, although reported frequently to indulge in flesh, Lindlahr says that these "negative" and "sensitive" people need "an abundance of the most positive animal and vegetable foods in order to build up and strengthen their physical bodies and their magnetic envelopes, which form the dividing protecting wall between the terrestrial plane and the magnetic field." This mixing of spiritualism and occultism with physiology could but lead him to many false conclusions and many erroneous practices.

Up to the present writing I have had eight cases of mental confusion in my own practice and, as I review these cases, one thing stands out very prominently in all of them; namely, each and every one of the patients was a marked neurotic. Three of them presented histories of previous periods of mental aberration. One of these patients had been thoroughly examined at one of the most famous clinics in America and her husband had been told by the physicians at the clinic, that, due to hardening of the arteries in the brain, she would ultimately become insane. None of these patients has resembled anything described by Dr. Lindlahr and there were no signs that they were being controlled by "spirit beings."

Some years ago a woman was brought in from a distant city who was troubled by what she called "elementals." For several years she had dabbled in occultism and spiritualism and had studied with the swamies and she was convinced that every night these "elementals" were annoying her. She fasted several days and she lost her "elementals" and the symptoms that they were supposed to be inducing in the first two weeks of her fast. Meat eating had not saved her from her "negative" and "sensitive" state; fasting soon brought her out of it. I am convinced that the developments in the aforementioned eight cases were in the nature of crises and that they were in no wise due to fasting and shall set forth my reasons for thinking so. They are:

1. The condition develops extremely rarely, whereas, if the fast were responsible for its development, it would be common.

2. It has not developed in those patients who have had the longest fasts, but in all save two cases, after relatively short fasts. If the fast produces the trouble, the longer fasts should be the ones after which the trouble develops. In one patient the mental symptoms developed after only nine days of fasting. It is well to note that after a subsequent fast of over thirty days, this patient had no such developments.

3. The symptoms never manifest while the fast is in progress, but only after it has been broken, the first symptoms so appearing three days to two weeks after the fast has ended. If the condition results from the fast, it should develop at least part of the time while the patient is fasting.

4. The condition develops only in certain types of individuals, and in these types of cases, such developments are quite common while eating three square meals a day in people who never fast. While I have emphasized the fact that these developments occur, so far as my experience extends, only in pronounced neurotics, they are rare, even in these patients. I have had many neurotics to fast for prolonged periods and receive nothing but benefit. No mental and nervous symptoms have developed during or after the fast in all save the eight we are here considering.

5. In two of my cases the trouble has developed after periods of great physical stress growing out of their diseases and would seem to have been due to the drain placed upon them by their diseases. One of these, a man who developed a severe diarrhea late in the fast that lasted for several days, had slight confusion for three days after his fast was broken, but he never grew irrational. The dysentery constituted a serious drain upon his powers and resources. A second case was unable to take food after the return of hunger. For three days she vomited all food given her. Thereafter she was able to retain food, and after she had begun to eat, she developed mental symptoms that lasted for about three weeks.

6. Certain of these patients who had had such disturbances before fasting have had none since. This is to say, the trouble that

followed breaking the fast was the end of their mental troubles. One woman who had had such periods of confusion before going on the fast, had such a period after the fast was broken, and has had no more such troubles for eighteen years.

7. In one case, at least, the clearing up of the mental symptoms has been accompanied by the disappearance of other symptoms that were of long standing. This woman, a neurotic, psychotic and drug-poisoned patient, became confused three days after the fast was broken (she had had such periods before fasting) and remained so for a period of about seven days. When she became normal, certain subjective head symptoms of which she had complained for over a year were gone and did not recur.

8. Most of these patients are now holding responsible positions and are enjoying good mental health.

There is no means of proving that these people would have had these developments at the times they did had they not fasted, but I think the inference is plain that they would have. In at least four of these cases previous such periods while eating point in this direction. In two other cases in which I have no positive proof of previous such periods, I have some evidence that such periods of mental disturbance had been previously experienced. If we add to this the frequent and great beneficial results that accompany and follow fasting in severe neurotic conditions and in cases of actual insanity, the evidence seems to be complete that the fast is not responsible for these conditions. It may well be said that the chief result of the fast is to retard their development, or even, in many cases, to prevent them altogether.

In considering these developments, it is well for us to keep in mind the ability of the body to nourish and sustain the brain and nervous system and to maintain their functional and structural integrity throughout the most prolonged fast by drawing upon its nutritive reserves, and the actual benefit that is seen to accrue to the nervous system in many cases of paralysis, neuritis, neuralgia, various neuroses and even in insanity, while fasting, even prolonged fasting, all of which should strongly indicate that the brain and nerves are not injured.

THE SPECIAL SENSES

Due, no doubt to wrong life, man's senses are comparatively dulled. In all cases of fasting the senses become more acute. So invariable and distinctive is this that *Hygienists* have long regarded it as more or less certain evidence that the patient is fasting. Professor Morgulis says that "the acuity of the senses is increased by fasting" and that at the end of his thirty-one days abstinence from food "Levanzin could see twice as far as he did at the beginning of the fast."

The acuteness of perception is most marked in fasting cases. Many users of glasses are enabled to discard their glasses and see as well as ever without them. I have had one complete recovery from complete blindness in one eye while fasting. Invariably the eyes become clear and bright.

There are occasional fasters in whom, towards the end of a very prolonged fast, vision grows dim and coordination of their eyes is impaired. They see double, see spots floating before their eyes, and are unable to read. This is a temporary weakness that disappears after the fast is broken. I have never seen any permanent injury follow in these relatively rare cases, but have seen distinct and permanent improvement in vision follow. People who, before the fast were unable to get along without glasses, have been able to discontinue their use after recovering from this temporary weakness.

The sense of touch is invariably sharpened. It is not easy to determine the state of the sense of taste during the fast, but the patient invariably discovers that his sense of taste is more acute and discriminating following the fast than before the fast.

The improvement in the sense of hearing is, commonly, even more marked than that of the other special senses. No doubt part of this improvement in the sense of hearing results from the clearing up of catarrhal conditions in the ears and eustachian tubes. Part of it is the result of the general rise in nervous condition. Although no one makes the claim that all deaf and near-deaf individuals can regain their hearing by fasting, it is, nonetheless, a fact that many deaf people have so regained their hearing. I had one patient who had been completely deaf in one ear for twenty-five years who regained her hearing in thirty days of fasting and was able to hear her watch tick at arm's length with her formerly deaf ear. I had one man who had been completely deaf in the left ear for six years to regain his hearing in this ear on the thirty-sixth day of a fast. It should be understood that spectacular results, such as the recovery of sight by the blind and recovery of hearing by the deaf are not to be expected as a regular result of physiologic rest.

The sense of smell is invariably sharpened, often as a result of the disappearance of nasal catarrh, but even in those cases where there is no catarrh of the nose, the sense of smell becomes very acute. Indeed, its acuteness is often so marked as to be a source of discomfort due to the fact that the faster smells disagreeable odors in his environment that were not detected before the fast. On the other hand he derives added pleasure from smelling agreeable odors.

The following is from a letter from John W. Armstrong which was published in the Yorkshire (England) *Evening Post,* January 16, 1933, and illustrates not merely the heightened acuteness of the sense of smell produced by fasting, but also the strength and endurance an animal may have after fourteen days without food: "Shortly before the war a discussion between Russian professors of medicine and a body of physical culturists resulted in an acid test being made of the respective fitness and sensitivities of well-fed and "starving" (?) bodies. Wolves were chosen for this test, 36 animals being kept in a pit where a stream of fresh running water was diverted to run through and a similar number of the untamed creatures placed in a second pit and fed every day on fresh raw meat and water.

"For 36 hours the unfed wolves were restless and snappy, then, appearing to accept the inevitable, the pack grew quiet and lazy. Until the tenth day they proved the assertions of the Naturopaths that the body never feeds so calmly and easily as when feeding upon its own tissues, by sleeping most of the time. Towards the 14th day they began to grow fierce and super active, having lost all their flesh (the healthy flesh formed of natural food in the wilds in outdoor creatures melts readily and quickly under the internal heat engendered by the process of fasting—thrice as quickly as flesh formed from civilized cooked and prepared food).

"The wolves had reached that stage where fasting is approaching its end and natural hunger is setting in, a stage at which food must be given.

"Released on the 15th day with a herd of deer many miles beyond them and to windward of both packs the unfed pack took scent first, set up the chase and when overtaken by fleet motor-cars, had caught up with their prey and dined off the killed deer, leaving nothing but the bones.

"I leave the reader to judge what this proves, but would add, in passing, the findings of many experienced observers that fasting invariably restores, if conducted long enough, the sense of sight, hearing, smell, taste and touch, and also the gift of speech when lost as in seizures, shock, etc."

I do not agree that fasting will invariably restore sight, hearing, smell, etc., but that it frequently does so is not a matter of doubt. There can be no doubt that all of man's special senses are more or less dulled or weakened by civilized life and by his "disease" and degeneracy. In fasting, without the recorded exception of a single case, the senses are remarkably improved. Indeed, so distinctive a sign is this that we look upon it as evidence that our patient is fasting. I have seen hearing restored on a fast. Catarrhal deafness of long standing, where there are no adhesions in the eustachian tube, is always improved or overcome. Hearing in those who consider their hearing normal becomes so acute that sounds that ordinarily are never heard are noticed often to the extent that the faster is annoyed by them. People who have been deaf for years are enabled to hear the ticking of a watch and low sounds that before was impossible. I have seen the senses of taste and smell, which had long been paralyzed, restored to their normal condition while fasting. The sense of smell becomes so acute that the faster is often annoyed by odors in his daily environment that he never before knew existed. People who have worn glasses for years and who could not read without them are frequently enabled by a fast to discard their glasses and find their sight to be as good as ever. The eyes also become clear and bright. The sense of touch becomes very acute.

The weakening and deadening of man's sense perceptions is due chiefly to depleted energy and the accumulation in the tissues of excess food and retained waste matter. Catarrh of the nose and thickening of the nasal mucosa must always impair the sense of smell. The fast by cleaning out the excesses and wastes and eliminating them from the system and also by permitting nervous recuperation, removes the causes of dulled senses.

Secretions and Excretions

CHAPTER XII

The secretions of the body on the whole are either suspended altogether or greatly reduced during the fast. Secretion is commensurate with need. The body is not wasteful of its supplies, as a brief study of secretion will show.

SALIVA

The saliva is greatly diminished in a fast. Von Noorden says of Succi's experimental fast: "The secretion of saliva diminished in acute starvation even when water was taken ad libitum. Thus, Succi, on the seventh day of his fast, only produced as much saliva by the movements of his jaws in three hours as under ordinary circumstances is secreted in five minutes." Saliva changes during the fast from its normal alkalinity to a neutral or slightly acid state. It again becomes alkaline upon the return of hunger or after eating is resumed.

In some cases the saliva becomes very foul and possesses a very unpleasant taste, sometimes, even causing vomiting. In certain cases it may be thick, tough, transparent, gelatinous, slimy and then gray, yellowish, greenish and even pus-like.

GASTRIC JUICE

The secretion of gastric juice is continuous throughout most of the fast, but in a greatly diminished quantity and is of a weakly acid character. At times its secretion may be accelerated by the usual factors responsible for "psychic secretion."

In cases of gastric hyperacidity, gastric distress continues and may even increase during the first three to four days of the fast. The hypersecretion soon ceases, discomfort wanes and finally ceases entirely, and after a few more days of fasting, eating may be resumed without the previous distress. No other measure will so speedily or so surely end hyperacidity. There are fasting experts of large experience who hold that regularly the secretion of gastric juice ends with the expulsion of the last morsel of food in the stomach and does not recommence until the next meal is taken. On the other hand, I have seen a few cases that regurgitated and expelled gastric juice after the fast had progressed two, three and more weeks.

BILE

The secretion of bile customarily continues during the early days of the fast. Indeed, it may be secreted in increased amounts. In some very foul conditions of the body, the secretion of bile is greatly increased, either during the first few days of the fast, or, at some period of its progress. This is likely to be regurgitated into the stomach where it causes nausea and vomiting. In such cases the bile is invariably evil-smelling and tainted. After a crisis of this kind, the patient's condition is seen to be much improved. The amount of bile secreted is then greatly decreased in amount.

A profuse cholerrhagia (flow of bile) through the bowels or by vomiting, is often seen in fasting. This produces drainage of bile through the bowels, instead of by cholecystotomy (the surgical way of draining the gall-bladder) in these cases and should convince the most skeptical of the superiority of this plan of care.

Normally bile is poured into the intestine only in response to a need for it in the work of digestion. It is poured out as the chyme from the stomach empties into the duodenum. If no food is eaten no bile is poured out. Physiologists are agreed that when an animal is fasting no bile enters the intestine. This is probably also true of a really healthy man; but it is certainly not true of the sick man.

The liver, among other things, is an organ of elimination. The products it takes from the blood are made into bile and poured out as such. When the sick man fasts the liver greatly increases the production of bile and this is poured into the intestine. The quantity and character of bile secreted during a fast as well as its degrees of alkalinity or possible acidity seem to be dependent upon the toxic overload under which the patient is struggling. Habitual hearty eaters, particularly those who consume large quantities of proteins and carbohydrates, produce the most bile and suffer most discomfort as a result.

Observations upon thousands of fasting cases have convinced me that the sooner the "over-production" of bile commences, after the cessation of eating, and the more bile is thrown off, the more rapidly the patient recovers his or her health. The patient is cleaning out. It is doubtful if such bile would have much value as a digestive fluid. In many cases, at least, its alkalinity is greatly reduced and it may even be slightly acid at times. When vomited it ranges in color from almost that of water, having but little bile pigment in it, to very dark. If often has a very offensive odor, not an odor of decay, and is commonly mixed with large amounts of mucus, this latter coming largely from the stomach, no doubt. Such bile must be considered as almost wholly a product of the excretory function of the liver. The secretory function is probably at rest like that of the glands which secrete digestive juices.

This is only one of the evidences of increased elimination during a fast and the cleaning out accomplished by this is of immense value in restoring health to those who have, through abuse or neglect, permitted their health to slip away.

PANCREATIC AND INTESTINAL JUICES

The pancreatic and intestinal juices are reasonably thought to be secreted in reduced quantities. It is known that they are weaker in digestive power than normally, but little else is known concerning them. They are customarily secreted and poured into the intestine in response to the need for them and, when no need exists, little or no juice is secreted. What secretion is present is probably lacking in enzymes.

MILK

It is usual for a female hibernating bear to bring forth her young and secrete sufficient milk to maintain her cubs. The human mother is not so fortunate. Fasting occasions a rapid reduction in milk secretion and for this reason should be resorted to during lactation only when urgently necessary.

SWEAT

The sweat is foul and in rare cases profuse. Under ordinary circumstances sweating can hardly be regarded as an eliminating process, but apparently there is increased elimination through the skin during a fast.

MUCUS

During a fast some patients will throw off an almost incredible amount of thick, tough, transparent, white, gelatinous and slimy expectoration. Later this may become gray, yellowish or greenish and pus-like in quality. The discharge from the nose may also increase at first and then gradually lessen. In chronic bronchitis, asthma, etc., the same gradual cessation of the catarrhal condition and of the cough and expectoration occurs. The discharge from the nasal sinuses gradually ceases as the catarrhal condition ends. In cases of "diseased" and long abused stomachs such matters may be thrown out by the gastric mucosa and vomited. Thus we see how nature adopts every possible avenue of elimination as a means of cleansing the system. In cases of mucous colitis, the amount of long, tenacious, worm-like ropes of mucus that will be passed is astounding. After a time this ceases and the "disease" is ended.

Acid secretions of the vagina, leukorrheal discharges, etc., soon cease and the secretions become normal through fasting. The foul stench that comes from the vagina and womb of the woman suffering from female troubles, or tumor of the womb, soon ceases and the odor becomes normal.

URINE

The volume of urine excreted during a fast, as at other times of life, is determined by the amount of water taken and by the amount of sweating done.

In the early days of the fast, the urine is invariably dark in color and high in specific gravity, strongly acid in reaction with abundance of urea, phosphates and bile pigment. Its odor is foul and strong. It becomes lighter in color and loses its offensive odor as the fast progresses. After the first increase in elimination has passed, specific gravity is lowered, and the quantity of mineral substances decreases. Specific gravity may go as low as 1.010. Its acidity is increased at first, but towards the end of a complete fast the urine may become neutral or even alkaline in reaction.

Dr. Hazzard says: "The hibernating bear never soils his den with urine or ordure, for no waste is formed, consequently none is voided." This is a very marked difference between hibernation and fasting.

Examination of the urine of Succi, made by Apollo and Solard, showed its toxicity to be much increased. Dr. Kellogg draws from the increased elimination of toxins from the body, the strange conclusion that it shows conclusively that fasting is not an efficient means of cleansing the body of poisons. The increased elimination of toxins, shown in the case of Succi, proved to Dr. Kellogg that elimination is checked. True, he thinks the increased urinary toxicity results from absorption from the colon, but there is no reason why there should be more absorption from the colon during a fast than when one is eating, and certainly there is less in the colon to be absorbed. He tells us that fasting produces all the evidences of intestinal auto-intoxication. This is decidedly not true, but on the contrary, fasting is the speediest means of eradicating such intoxication. It has been my observation that intestinal auto-intoxication is found in those who habitually eat, and eat excessively. In discussing intestinal auto-intoxication Kellogg himself traces it chiefly to dietetic errors rather than to fasting.

The increased toxicity of the urine of the fasting person is due to increased elimination and not, as Kellogg reasons, to the fact that "fasting is not, as claimed, an efficient means of cleansing the body of poisons." I presume that to satisfy Kellogg that fasting is an efficient means of increasing elimination we would have to prove that the kidneys wholly cease to excrete toxins. He seems to think that fasting should send the toxins out of the body through some secret channel rather than through the organs of elimination, or else, that by some subtle alchemy, these toxins should be transmuted into angels of mercy and left in the body. The fact that they are eliminated in greater abundance somehow proves to him that elimination is checked by the fast.

Benedict says of the urine during a fast: "Complete fasting during which no water is consumed results in lowering in a marked manner the total amounts of urine voided per day.°°°In general, when water is taken during a fast, the volume of urine approaches more nearly that voided by people under normal conditions. Indeed, when moderate amounts of water are consumed, the volume of urine presents as a rule no noticeable abnormalities.°°°In general, then, during the early stages of a fast, with the exception of the first day, the volume of urine is in large measure determined by the quantity of drinking water consumed. If the amount of ingested water is small, the volume of urine may exceed it several times. When the volume of drinking water is over 1000 cc., the volume of urine is usually not far from that of the water consumed.°°°In all of the samples of urine, whether tested by periods or for the whole day, the reaction was acid. The pressure of other work prevented an accurate determination of acidity. According to Brugsch, however, the acidity, at least in the later stages of a prolonged fast, remains nearly constant from day to day.°°°All the specific gravities observed came well within what would be termed normal limits.°°°In general, the average amount of total solids during the different experiments is not far from 40 grams per day.°°°The only data regarding the ash elimination during fasting with which we are familiar are the quantities in the urine of J. A. On the last day with food the total ash of urine amounted to 23.0

grams; in the five fasting days, the total ash eliminated was 14.7, 6.7, 5.7, 5.0, and 4.5 grams respectively°°°In general, the amount (of organic matter) eliminated ranges somewhere between 30 and 40 grams.°°°The proportion of ash in total solids, as a rule, is greatest on the first day and markedly less on the second day.°°°There is a tendency for the nitrogen excretion to approach constancy on the fourth day.°°°In considering the long experiments, it is noteworthy that the carbon elimination is invariably lowest on the first day, and on the remaining days is relatively constant.°°°The excretion of total creatinine, namely, preformed creatinine plus creatinine formed by heating the creatinine of the urine with acid, remains singularly constant on all days of the fast, even during the 7-day fast, experiment No. 75.°°°While the quantity of preformed creatinine gradually diminishes as the fast progresses, the amount of creatinine, which in normal urine, is extremely small, gradually increases, and on the sixth day of the fast, there is excreted 0.585 grams of creatine.°°° The proportion of creatinine has a distinct tendency to diminish as the fast progresses.°°°During even a short period of inanition, the uric acid output may be greatly reduced.°°°The excretion of sulphur increases on the second day. There is an increase on the third day, and a steady diminution on the succeeding days of the fast.°°° There is, as a rule, a tendency for the phosphoric acid to increase for a few days after fasting begins and then subsequently diminish.°°°The chlorine elimination on the last food day is invariably larger and on the first fasting day there is usually a marked diminution in the amount."

Dr. Eales says: "I have a record of a case where on the twenty-eighth day a large amount of sediment appeared in the urine and the temperature, which had been sub-normal for years, immediately rose to normal after the urine cleared." This case is of interest, not merely as indicating increased elimination of toxins by the fast; but also as showing how the fast brings about a return to normal temperature in cases where sub-normal temperature exists. In this case, at least, it would seem to have returned to normal as a result of the elimination of material which had interfered with heat production or heat conservation. One of my own cases passed a large quantity of sediment in the urine which was flaked and looked like flakes of iron rust. No analysis was made to determine the character of the sediment. Another case had an abscess of one kidney (which had been diagnosed, after being X-rayed, as a kidney stone and for which an operation had been advised) to drain, an eight-ounce glass full of pus passing at one time.

Daily determination of the specific gravity of the urine was made during the fast of Dr. Eales. On the first and second days of the fast his urine had a specific gravity of 1.015. On the third day the specific gravity of the urine was 1.018. It rose to 1.020 on the fourth day and to 1.023 on the fifth day. On the sixth day it dropped to 1.022; was 1.020 on the seventh and eighth days; 1.018 on the ninth and tenth days; 1.020 on the eleventh and twelfth days; 1.022 on the thirteenth; 1.020 on the fourteenth, fifteenth and sixteenth days; 1.019 on the twenty-first day; 1.018 on the twenty-second and twenty-third days; dropped to 1.005 on the twenty-fourth day, due to the consumption of large quantities of water; rose to 1.012 on the twenty-fifth day; back to 1.018 on the twenty-sixth; 1.020 on the twenty-seventh; 1.016 on the twenty-eighth; and 1.018 for the last three days of the fast. During the day of the tenth day of the fast, following an enema and a bath, the specific gravity of the urine fell to 1.010.

Except during the first five days, the doctor consumed habitually during the fast two quarts of distilled water each twenty-four hours. The volume of urine kept up through the whole of the fast, about sixty-five ounces being excreted every twenty-four hours. On the last day of his fast his record shows his urine to have been normal in color and reaction.

Bowel Action During Fasting

CHAPTER XIII

After the digestion of the last meal prior to the fast, the bowels practically cease to function. They take a rest. Dr. Oswald says: "The colon contracts, and the smaller intestines retain all but the most irritating ingesta." Sometimes they will continue to move regularly for the first three or four days of the fast. In rare cases a diarrhea will develop even after fifteen or more days of fasting. Mark Twain describes cases of *starving* shipwrecked men whose bowels had not moved for twenty and thirty days. For this reason most advocates of fasting insist upon the daily use of the enema. I think that the enema is a distinct evil and should not be employed.

Kellogg quotes Von Noorden as saying: "in fasting, the stools were highly putrid and 'similar in appearance to the feces passed when the diet is mainly composed of meat.'" Both these men should have conducted a few hundred fasts and then wrote about the matter. Their mistake is based on the notion that the fasting patient is on a meat diet and should have the stools of a meat eater. It is an assumption, not a fact. Even if we grant the contention that the fasting body's reserves are of a different character to the nutritive supplies of the feasting organism (and they are not) we are still left with the fact that the stools are not made up of these reserves.

The stomach, intestines and colon are given a complete rest by the fast and are enabled to repair damaged structures. Piles, proctitis, colitis, appendicitis, enteritis, enteric fever (typhoid), gastritis, etc., speedily recover under the fast. The alimentary tract becomes practically free of bacteria during a fast. The small intestines become sterile. But a week of fasting is required to result in a complete disappearance of all germs from the stomach. The quickest means of remedying bacterial decomposition in the digestive tract is fasting. Dr. Tilden says: "The fact that the hibernating bear loses its colon bacilli is not acted upon, and a fast recommended when disease results from overeating, bacterial decomposition and toxin poisoning."

Bowel action is necessarily more or less absent during a fast. There may be two or three actions during the course of a comparatively short fast, or no action at all during a most prolonged fast. The use of the enema during the fast, so much advocated in many quarters, is both unnecessary and pernicious, How unnecessary it is will be shown by the following cases.

Dr. Dewey tells of placing a dyspeptic, with feeble body and very low mental state, who had been under the care of physicians for ten years, on one meal a day. He says, (*The Fasting Cure,* p. 196) "The constipated bowels were permitted their own time for action." Further on he adds (page 107): "My patient's bowels gave no hint of their locality until the eighteenth day, when they acted with little effort; on the twenty-fourth day again in a perfect way, and daily thereafter."

It has been said that Dr. Dewey's fasting cases would have recovered more promptly had he employed the enema. But I find no satisfactory evidence that his cases, as a whole, were any longer recovering than the cases of those who employ the enema. Where they do appear to be longer in recovering, I think this may be accounted for more satisfactorily by the fact that in many of his cases he employed certain drugs, especially drugs to deaden sensation (relieve pain), and by the further fact that his limited knowledge of diet and his prejudices against fruit, which he had brought over with him from his medical training, did not give his patients the best after-care. Many of the fasts conducted by Dewey were under fifteen days. His records do not indicate that his fasts lasted longer or that his results were less satisfactory than those of Hazzard who employed the enema more, perhaps, than any other advocate of fasting. His fasts were not unduly long. But I think the best answer to this charge against Dewey's practice is the fact that patients who are placed on a fast today and who are not given the enema recover sooner and more satisfactorily than those who do get enemas. The enervating effect of the enema is indisputable and no one of experience will deny that it is a trying ordeal for most patients to go through. In many cases it leaves an immediate weakness which lasts, often, for hours.

Dr. Eales' bowels moved at least once a day during the first week of his fast; with a slight movement about once a week thereafter. He records movements on the eleventh, and seventeenth days.

He employed one enema a week and had both an enema and a spontaneous movement on the seventeenth day. His bowels began moving within twelve hours after breaking the fast and moved twice a day thereafter.

I cared for a case in my institution in February and March, 1929, in which the patient had a small bowel movement on the second day of an absolute fast, another on the fourth day, a copious movement on the ninth day and medium sized movements on the eleventh and thirteenth days. No enema was employed at any time during the fast, which lasted sixteen days.

I had another case of a young man who had a bowel movement on the second day of his fast, a small movement on the morning of the sixth day and a large movement on the evening of the same day. Again on the ninth day he had a small evacuation and a very copious movement in the evening of the same day. This man had suffered with acne vulgaris for several years and his face was thickly covered with eruptions when he began the fast. There was nothing of these except the discoloration by the end of the tenth day. Later a lady fasted nine days under my direction, and had a good bowel movement on each of the seventh and eighth days.

Two ladies fasted here in the institution at the same time; one for eight days, the other for nine days. In both cases regular bowel action began on the third day after breaking the fast and continued thereafter. Both of these women made rapid progress and did not suffer during or after the fast. There was not at any time any evidence of poisoning in either case.

A patient took enemas contrary to my instructions, for the first three days of the fast, but abandoned them thereafter because of the discomfort and sickness which they produced. On the twenty-third day of the fast she had two spontaneous movements of the bowels—one at 5 A.M., the other at 11 A.M. On the morning of the twenty-fourth day there was another movement.

A lady arrived at my place on January 4, 1932, after having fasted since the morning of December 12, 1931. During the whole of her fast before reaching my place she had had a daily enema. I stopped the use of the enema and her bowels acted spontaneously on January 8th. There were no more bowel actions during the rest of the fast. The fast was broken on January 21, and the bowels acted immediately.

—197—

Another lady whose bowel action had not been good was placed upon a fast as a means of overcoming arthritis. Her bowels moved twice on the fifth day, once on the eighth day and again on the twelfth day of her fast. Another case, that of a man, with a brain tumor, had bowel actions on the fourth and ninth days and two actions on the eighteenth day of his fast. A woman who fasted under my direction in February, 1932, had a bowel movement on each of the fourth, tenth and fifteenth days of her fast. Another woman's bowels acted on the fourth, fifth and seventh days of her fast.

In Dec. 1932 and Jan. 1933 a patient fasted 31 days in my Health School. His bowels moved on the 2nd, 6th, 7th, 13th and 20th days of the fast. Another patient who took a short fast in December, 1932 had a bowel movement on each of the 4th, 8th and 9th days. This patient then took a longer fast in Jan. 1933 with bowel movements on the 1st, 3rd and 9th days, there being a diarrhea on the 9th day. Another case was that of a young lady who had a bowel movement on the 21st day of her fast.

On July 21, 1933, a woman, age 68 began a fast in my Health School. The fast was broken on the evening of the thirteenth day. She had a bowel movement on the first and second days of the fast, on the third and fourth days there were loose stools; there was no movement on the fifth day; on the sixth day there was one movement and a small movement, only one small piece of feces passing, on the seventh day. This woman had orange juice all day on the fourteenth day, six oranges on the fifteenth day and a good bowel movement followed on the morning of the sixteenth day.

On the same day the foregoing woman began her fast another woman, age 37, was placed on a fast. For a period of twelve days or more, this woman had suffered with a persistent diarrhea. The fast lasted for a period of twenty-eight days and the bowels did not move once throughout the whole of her fast after the first day. The fast was uneventful, there were no crises and no signs of poisoning, but a steady improvement in healh.

In April and May of 1948 I had in the Health School a woman from Chicago who fasted ten days and had a bowel movement every day of her fast. This is a rare case, but fasters who have several bowel movements during the course of a fast are very common.

At the end of the year 1949 a woman came to the Health School from San Francisco and fasted thirty-five days. She had eleven bowel movements during the first three weeks of her fast and another movement on the thirty-fourth day.

Contrast these with the case of a young woman, age 25, who was placed on a fast on Feb. 24, 1933 in my Health School and whose bowels moved on the twenty-first day of the fast. In this case there were no crises, none of the symptoms "re-absorption of toxins" is said to cause, but a steady gain in health.

These few cases out of many prove that the bowels will move when there is need for a movement; also they show, as do hundreds of others, that there is no injury from waiting upon the bowels. These cases particularly refute the notion entertained in some quarters that a prolonged fast paralyzes the bowels. This notion finds lodgement in the minds of some who know nothing about fasting, and one usually finds that they do not want to know anything about it. Most of the foregoing cases all fasted before the first edition of this volume was published. Since that time hundreds of similar experiences have been observed here at the Health School.

Prof. Benedict says: "Fasting***affects first the amount and regularity of defecation.***Owing to long retention in the colon, fasting feces become hard, much dried and pilular, and frequently cause considerable uneasiness. Much difficulty is experienced in passing them, and at times they may cause considerable pain with slight hemorrhages. The use of an enema to remove the fecal matter during inanition is quite common. This method was employed throughout the 30-day fast of Succi—reported by Luciani.***Depending upon the amount of food consumed on the day previous, the defecation of the first day of fasting may be quite as regular as on the ordinary days.***The most important factor noted was that feces were frequently retained for a number of days together, during fasting with no apparent attempt on the part of nature to effect a movement."

The hard feces he mentions does sometimes form during a fast, but it is by no means the regular or usual development. On the contrary, it is relatively rare and is usually easily voided. Only in cases of hemorrhoids do they give real trouble. A hard plug of feces stops the anus of the hibernating bear, but he has no difficulty in getting rid of it when he resumes eating in the spring. The feces of the faster is commonly soft, at times loose, only rarely large enough and hard enough to occasion difficulty in passing. In those cases where there is spastic constipation, and in hemorrhoids, the plug does sometimes, although by no means always, become sufficiently hardened as to occasion pain and bleeding in passing. In such cases, it is my practice to employ an enema after the fast is broken, when the patient feels the first urge for stool. No enemas are employed during the fast, even in these cases.

During the first five years of my practice I employed the enema, both in the fast and while my patients were eating, but I particularly employed it in the fast. I had been taught that it was necessary in the fast, that if the enema was not used to wash out the colon, waste matter that had been thrown into this would be re-absorbed and the patient would suffer from auto-intoxication. Two facts caused me, finally, to begin to doubt the wisdom of employing the enema. These were:

1. I found the enema painful when I took it myself and I noticed that most of my patients also found it painful.

2. I found it left me with a feeling of weakness when I took an enema and I found the same thing to be true when my patients were given enemas.

These experiences caused me to do some effective thinking. The first question I asked myself was this: Am I doing right in employing an enervating measure in my care of my patients? I could not get an affirmative answer to this question, no matter how I tried. Then I ran my mind back over my studies of fasting among animals. The question came naturally to mind: If fasting animals, many of which fast for much longer periods than man can ever fast, do not need enemas, why does fasting man require them? I could find no logical reason why man required them while fasting. Then I reviewed the literature of fasting and I discovered that Jennings, Dewey, Tanner and others had not employed the enema. Cautiously, I began to test the no-enema plan. I soon became convinced of its superiority over the enema plan. I found Dr. Claunch rejecting the enema. I discovered that Dr. Page was not an advocate of its use. I had arrived at my conclusion the hard way, only to find that I was not alone.

Dr. Tilden, a frequent and regular user of the enema, admitted that it was enervating. But why should we employ methods of care that further enervate our patients? It is our duty, in caring for our patients, to conserve the energy of each patient in every way possible and not to needlessly dissipate the precious energies of life.

It is our duty at all times to conserve the energies of our patients. All enervating practices should be eliminated from our care of the sick. We may say that no such practices are ever justifiable, except where they are the lesser of two evils and there are rare instances wheie the enema may be the lesser of two evils. Macfadden, himself a great advocate of the use of the enema and of its use in the fast, said: "But enemas are somewhat enervating, and when the patient is already weak, he may find it a drain upon his vitality to take many of these."—*Encyclopedia of Physcal Culture*, Vol. III, p. 1374.

I soon became convinced from tests I made that there is no absorption of toxins from the colon. At that time, thirty-seven years ago, physiologists were still teaching that toxins are absorbed from the colon. Since then, they have changed their minds. The lining membrane of the colon no more absorbs toxins than does the lining membrane of the bladder. If the bladder does not absorb urine which is liquid, how can the lining membrane of the colon absorb feces, which is more or less solid? Answer this question in any way you may, there is one thing of which I am certain and this is, that, no symptoms of auto-intoxication develop during a fast of the longest duration when no enemas are employed.

I am certain of another important matter, namely, that the frequent use of the enema during the fast, as at other times, impairs bowel function, so that after the fast is broken, bowel function is not as efficient as in those patients who have not had enemas. My good friend, Dr. Carlos Arguello, of Nicaragua, put this matter to a test by dividing his patients into two groups and giving one group enemas and the other no enemas during their fasts. After their fasts were broken he kept careful records of the bowel movements of the members of both groups. Those who received no enemas had nearly a third more movement in the same period of time following the breaking of their fasts.

The regular and frequent use of the enema induces several important evils in the colon and its use is not to be recommended at any period of life, certainly not when one is sick and weak and needs to conserve oneself in every way possible. At the beginning of 1925 I ceased using the enema and I am much better satisfied with its non-use in the fast than with its use. My patients also escape the discomforts it induces.

The use of "purgative" drugs and mineral waters during a fast is even worse than the use of the enema. Taken by mouth, as these are, they occasion excited and wasteful action with the secretion of much watery mucus along the whole length of the alimentary canal; whereas, the enema reaches only the colon, except in those many cases of chronic constipation in which there exists insufficiency of the ileocecal valve. In these cases the water and the feces in the colon are frequently sent back, by reverse peristalsis, into the small intestine, and in some cases, the feces and water are carried all the way back to the stomach and from here vomited. The same thing occurs sometimes with the colonic irrigation, which is but an oversized enema, which costs more and cannot be administered by the patient himself.

In these days when we live for our bowel movements and are miserable if they fail to move by the time we are ready to go to work in the morning, the truth about our bowels is hard to get into our heads. We have been well trained by those who have constipation "cures" to sell.

Dr. Tanner, during and after his first fast, had no bowel movement from the 15th of July to the 31st of August, a period of forty-seven days. In commenting upon this fact, Dr. Hazzard declares, "To carry out a fast today in this manner would be deemed a bid for disaster." Why a "bid for disaster?" Both Dr. Tanner and Dr. Dewey repudiated the enema, and to quote Dr. Hazzard, "preferred and insisted upon waiting upon the bowels to act 'naturally' as he (Dewey) termed it." Jennings did not employ the enema, nor did Page. In my own practice I have not employed it for thirty-seven years. I had one patient to go for over fifty days without an evacuation and no disaster befell him.

Levanzin reports of his fast of 31 days that, "during my whole fast I had no defecations. I had a bowel movement just before I started the fast, and the next was thirty-two days afterward, when I broke it." He adds: "I did not try to provoke any, as I did not wish to spoil the scientific results; and so, the bad, bitter and upsetting taste in my mouth was very trying." The implication of this statement is that the use of the enema prevents the bad, bitter taste of the mouth. This is not true, as anyone who has ever fasted and employed enemas can testify. The tongue becomes just as heavily coated, the teeth just as pasty and the taste in the mouth just as foul when enemas are used as when they are not used.

Professor Benedict writes of Levanzin that "when discussing the question of defecation he stated that in some of his long fasts he had defecated only once or twice, often he did this shortly after the beginning of the fast, and then not again until after the fast was over, but after beginning eating he was quite normal."

Dr. Jennings reported cases in which the bowels did not act for weeks. I had one man to fast for thirty-six days in my institution without a bowel movement, the bowels acting for the first time on the third day after the fast was broken. Another man fasted forty-nine days with no bowel action during the time. His bowels also acted on the third day after breaking the fast.

One young lady began a fast under my direction on Dec. 3, 1929, and ended it on Dec. 28th. Her bowels did not act during the whole of this period, acting the first time on Jan. 4, 1930; a period of thirty-three days from one bowel action to the next. This lady suffered with the worst case of psoriasis I have ever seen. Her whole body, face, neck and limbs included, being covered. The skin cleared up rapidly and beautifully during the fast.

Shortly after the foregoing case came to me, a young man suffering with constipation, digestive troubles and "nervousness" began a fast in my institution. He fasted twelve days, during which time his bowels did not act. They acted first on the fifth day after breaking the fast. During these seventeen days without a bowel movement the patient made great improvement.

No harm ever came from waiting upon the bowels. They may be depended on to function if there is a need for action. If no need exists, there can be no gain from forcing them to act. We should learn to distinguish between the forcing and the actual need for bowel action.

It has been noted that dogs and other animals do have bowel actions during a fast. In my own practice I have noticed that the stronger and more vigorous are more likely to have bowel evacuations. The weak, those who suffer with lowered gastro-intestinal tone or with visceroptosis are least likely to have an action of the colon while fasting. In any case no harm results from letting the colon alone and forgetting that it exists.

Dr. Harry Finkle makes the absurd claim that fasting paralyzes the colon. It does nothing of the kind, but improves colonic function in every instance. The enemas, colonic irrigations, purges, etc., almost do what he says the fast does. The great difficulties many men have with fasting arise out of the fact that they have not observed the effects of fasting, but fasting plus a lot of therapeutic measures. They think they are observing the effects of fasting, when they are merely watching the effects of something else. They insist upon treating their fasting patients with all of the harmful cure-alls which chance to be in fashion, and then attribute any evil results to the fast, although such evils are frequent results of these treatments when applied to non-fasters.

Fasting animals, whether hibernating, æstivating, fasting during the mating season, fasting during illness, or fasting because of a lack of something to eat, do not have and do not need enemas. Some of these animals fast for much longer periods than is possible for any man and do not die of nor suffer from the much-feared poisoning by absorption from the colon. I can find no proof that poisons are ever absorbed from the colon; but, assuming that they sometimes are, the absorption of a very small fraction of what was thrown into the colon can certainly produce none of the evils attributed to it. If it could, the whole of the material thrown into the colon would have killed the patient before it was thrown therein.

The Canadian bear enters upon hibernation with a flesh that is repugnant to flesh-eaters. When he comes out of hibernation his flesh is sweet and is considered a great delicacy by the people of the North. Canadian biologists describe the bowels of a bear that had just settled for the winter, and which they opened, after killing the bear, as emitting a stench that was "overpowering," the flesh "nauseating, fishy and unfit for food." By Spring the bear's flesh has undergone a complete and remarkable change, so that it is "the most sought-after of all northern foods." By this time very little residue is found in the digestive tract and "the bowel was odorless and quite sterile. No cultures of any of the usual intestinal flora or bacilli could be obtained."

This complete sterilizing and deodorizing of the intestinal tract together with the sweetening of the flesh of the bear, all without a bowel movement in four to five months, or in some cases longer, will not be easily explained by those who insist upon the urgent need of enemas in the fast. As the hibernating bear never suffers with auto-intoxication during the most prolonged period of hibernation, we are forced to accept the fact that he is not poisoned by any hypothetical re-absorption of waste from the colon.

Fasting and Sex

CHAPTER XIV

The effects of fasting upon the sexual functions are so variable that no generalization is possible. The examples of the salmon and the Alaskan fur seal bull were given in a previous chapter. These are not typical. In dealing with the effects of fasting on the higher invertebrates, Jackson tells us that "the gonads themselves are usually very resistant to starvation, being (like the nervous system) as a rule among the last of the organs to undergo involution. There are, however, evident variations in different species and individuals." —*Inanition and Malnutrition*, p. 28.

The rutting season in animals is almost always a veritable orgy. Both males and females indulge so much and so often during this period as to give the impression that they are trying to compress a year's sexual activity into a few days. Indulgence goes on at frequent intervals both day and night. In the case of the bull who may have to satisfy the demands of two or more cows, this orgy lasts for days. One may expect that a period of such intense activity would be accompanied by voracious eating. The opposite is almost the rule. Sexual activity seems to suspend the desire for food.

Fasting often restores sexual reproduction, bringing back the male, in organisms that, with abundant food supplies, reproduce asexually or parthenogenetically. The restoration of the male in parthenogenetically reproducing forms is but one example of many that fasting may prove beneficial to the sex function.

Surfeit seems to be antagonistic to the highest genetic purposes and fasting becomes necessary as a means of assisting at least, towards a re-establishment of a tolerable degree of domestic (organic) symbiosis. Asexual reproduction in lower forms is associated with surfeit and the introduction of the sexual link in the alternate sexual-asexual reproduction of these forms, is in all cases, dependent on a previous reduction of the nutritive overflow, the overfed asexual units, or "nurses," being incapable of the physiological labor required by sexual reproduction. Alternation of generation is, in fact, the result of changing nutritive conditions. Asexual generation is the expression of excess or antisymbiotic nutritive conditions, while sexual generation is conditioned upon a normal metabolic rate growing out of strenuousness and moderation. Thousands of studies and experiments by biologists show unmistakably that nutritive redundancy is the necessary condition of the overgrowth which makes asexual reproduction possible and interferes with sexual reproduction, while a reduction of the nutritive overflow and a return to legitimate nutrition restores sexual normality.

In hibernation the ovaries and testes undergo certain changes in size, structure and function. The testicles of the frog are largest in August, smallest in the Spring. Nussbaum observed growth in the sex glands of fasting frogs. Male frogs, immediately upon resuming activities in the Spring, this is to say, at the end of hibernation, take on distinguishing seasonal marks, as brighter colors, swollen forefinger, or some unusual feature. The females lay their eggs and the males fertilize them soon after they emerge from hibernation.

While these changes in color and structure and the reproductive activity seen in frogs follow immediately upon the ending of hibernation, with its prolonged period of abstinence from food, they must have been prepared for during the period of fasting. The fact that reproduction follows so closely upon the period of abstinence, even, in the more northerly latitudes, after prolonged fasting, indicates that fasting has no ill effect upon the reproductive function.

No specific changes in the sex glands of the hibernating gopher are found. In the hibernating marmot no sperm cells are produced. Cyclic changes are observed in the interstitial cells of the ovaries and testicles of the hibernating woodchuck which undergo gradual enlargement during this period.

Enforced fasting in non-hibernating animals also produces variable results similar to those seen in hibernation. Where losses and changes occur in the ovaries and testes in fasting they are about the same as those that occur in these structures in hibernation. In general, the testicles lose less rapidly than the body as a whole, the production of sperm cells is greatly diminished or ceases altogether; rapid gains upon resumption of feeding, which often lag behind the general systemic gains, but early restoration of normal function, is the rule. This is the general rule in the ovaries also.

Morgulis, experimenting with the newt *Diemyctylus*, found that the "ripe" female withstands fasting best, because she actually absorbs and utilizes the large reserve of stored food in the nature of eggs and thereby saves her other organs and tissues from wasting. Heidkamp found, in experiments with *Tritoncristatus*, a fresh water salmon, that when the female is denied food the fully developed eggs in her body are the first to be absorbed.

In males the process is a bit different. No spermatozoa are produced during inanition. The spermatozoa already present usually die after a time. Some degeneration occurs in the cells lining the seminiferous tubules, so that, as Urginov discovered, the young born of starved males present distinct signs of degeneration, whereas the young of starved or malnourished females (but sired by normally fed males), as Rudolski has shown, merely show evidences of malnutrition.

Fasting in animals is frequently associated with reproductive activity. In some instances, the male alone fasts, in other instances the female alone fasts and in others both sexes fast. There are even instances in which the young also fast. Commonly, fasts during the mating season or following the birth of the young, are seasons of great physical and sexual activity.

Ordinarily a friendly animal, the fur seal bull, becomes an ugly specimen during the mating season. The bulls stage frequent battles, these usually caused by one male trying to steal a female from the harem of another. These harems sometimes contain from fifty to two hundred females. Physically as well as sexually active, these bulls fast throughout the mating season.

The Emperor Penguin of the Adele Islands is the largest of the seventeen species of penguins known, the males reaching a height of over three feet and a weight of over eighty pounds. The males among these penguins go without food during the two months he sets on the eggs, after which he goes on a long treck to the sea in search of food. It is significant that the young, which cannot be affected by the paternal fast, are still wabbly in their walk, after three months, and mature slowly despite a high protein diet.

In fasting male salmon and certain other animals the testicles greatly enlarge during the seasonal fasting period. The ovaries of fasting female salmon also enlarge. In the frog, as in the salmon, part of its muscles are sacrificed to serve as material in the development of the sex glands. "These are conspicuous examples of dystrophic growth changes during adult inanition, certain portions of the body growing at the expense of others, as occurs generally during chronic inanition in young organisms."

Scientists say that the "mystery of this starvation during reproduction" is all the greater because "maturity is delayed and sexual activity usually decreases during periods of famine." That food scarcity generally occasions a reduction in sexual activity is true enough, but then, so do certain types of overfeeding. It may well be that fasting becomes necessary in certain over-indulgent animals in order to restore sexual potency and reproductive capacity.

Fasting accelerates the normal process of metamorphosis in tadpoles—indeed, the tadpoles of some frogs normally cease to eat at a certain stage in their development, and develop their legs at the expense of their tails. A similar "physiological inanition" is seen at certain stages of the metamorphosis of insects. These present numerous examples of dystrophic growth changes during fasting. Jackson found an increase of 22 per cent in the ovaries of adult albino rats subjected to acute inanition until they had lost 33 per cent in body weight.

Jackson says: "Morgulis, Howe and Hawk found no apparent abnormality in the ovaries of a dog as a result of protracted inanition. Ova were present in all stages of normal development."—*Inanition and Malnutrition*, p. 395.

It has been found that the cells lining the seminiferous tubules in the testicles which give rise to germ cells, preserve their normal character for the longest period of time when no food is taken and undergo degenerative changes only during the starvation period. Even then, parts of these structures remain entirely normal. In the unaffected areas Simonowitch found the seminiferous tubules of starved rabbits and guinea pigs to be filled with living spermatozoa. In fasting dogs Loisel found that spermatogenesis ceases. Grandis found that no spermatozoa are produced in pigeons during inanition, although already formed spermatozoa may continue to grow. He found however that the spermatozoa in the tubules usually die. In some forms the embryo tends to develop at the expense of the maternal organism; in others the eggs or embryo are absorbed by the maternal body and utilized as food.

Both male and female organs are enabled to heal and repair themselves during a fast. Menstruation is often brought on a week or two weeks ahead of the regular time. After this it usually ceases altogether. Disorders of ovulation yield quite rapidly to the kindly influence of fasting.

Sexual desire must vary as much as the previously noted changes. The male goose (gander) loses about one-fourth in body weight during the period just preceding and at the breeding season. There is a concomitant awakening of the sex instinct. This is similar to what is seen in the salmon and the seal. Other animals soon discontinue all sexual activity if forced to go without food.

There seems to have been no actual studies made of the effects of fasting and starvation, as distinct from malnutrition and its many causes, upon the human ovary and testicle. Noting ovarian and testicular changes in all human cachexias certainly is a far cry from the effects of fasting. These studies of "inanition" are not separated from pathology due to many causes.

Carrington found that all the fasters he questioned said that sexual intercourse during a prolonged fast becomes a practical impossibility "after the first few days." As he points out this "impotency" is merely a temporary suspension of the sexual function, for "the function returns, in its full vigor and force, together with hunger." He points out that this lack of sexual vigor is almost invariably present, irrespective of the vigor of the faster, which may be increased, but that sexual vigor returns together with hunger and before any food has been ingested. It is true, as he points out, that many cases of impotency of years' standing, and female sterility, are frequently remedied by fasting.

That fasting, usually, in such instances reduces or abolishes sexual desire and sexual power in men and women is certain. That this is only temporary is equally certain. On the other hand, some fasters, continue to indulge sexually during the fast while nocturnal emissions are occasionally seen in men, even in advanced fasting. I have made no effort to determine the presence or absence of spermatozoa in such instances. That these results are not invariable should be stressed. I have seen impotent men regain potency during a fast and aged and long impotent men have nocturnal emissions. Young and sexually vigorous men often manifest no reduction in sexual vigor. In the winter of 1961-62 I had a forty-two year old woman who had been frigid and sexually quiescent for six years to regain sexual desire after two weeks of fasting. She retained this sexual drive thereafter. Reduced or absent sexual desire and relative sterility may form the rule in fasting men and women, but this is by no means an invariable rule. Mr. Johnson, whose fast will be mentioned later, was neither impotent nor sterile during a forty days' fast I supervised for him. One of my women patients was annoyed as much by sexual desire while fasting as while eating. Another was so annoyed by such desire, we were forced to break the fast. Desire ceased after eating was resumed.

Tolstoy pointed out the close connection between idleness and gluttony on the one hand and unchastity on the other, and recommended fasting as a means of controlling strong sexual passions. This should be understood to mean that fasting is to be employed to aid in removing the surfeit that is responsible for the abnormal sexual desire that is a common result of nutritive redundancy, not that fasting should be employed to suppress normal sexual urges. Fasting should not be looked upon as a means of conquering human nature—it is no ascetic program that *Hygienists* offer the world.

While it seems to be the rule for impotency to develop during a prolonged fast, the sexual powers return with full, even renewed vigor with the resumption of eating, often even with the return of hunger. Sometimes there is a brief delay in their return. One elderly patient of mine, who had been impotent for years, quickly regained virility after a fast of thirty-one days. Another case of impotency of several years duration regained potency after only a short fast.

We have previously pointed out that there are many animals, of which the male salmon and Alaskan fur seal bull are outstanding examples, that fast throughout the whole of the mating season with no impairment of sexual vigor and fecundity. Indeed, fasting often restores sexual reproduction, bringing back the male in organisms that, with abundant food supplies, reproduce asexually or parthenogenetically. Sexual activity among fur seals is confined to the fasting period. The Adelie penguins fast during the breeding period and Prof. J. A. Thomson says many other examples occur among animals. Love seems also to diminish the desire for food in boys and girls.

The fear of permanent sterility in females, from fasting, fostered in laboratory works on this subject, is unfounded. The fact is that we frequently see previously sterile women conceive shortly after a fast, even a lengthy one. One of my patients, unable to conceive for several years, conceived shortly after a fast of forty days' duration. Her baby was normal in every way and presented none of the abnormalities against which we are warned. Another, married ten years with no conception during this time, conceived shortly after a fast of ten days. A third patient conceived at her first intercourse two weeks after a fast of thirty days. This woman had not been previously sterile. A young woman, married for several years and failing to conceive, had a fast of thirty days and conceived soon thereafter. Cases of this kind could be multiplied indefinitely.

Rejuvenescence Through Fasting

CHAPTER XV

Upton Sinclair says: "The great thing about the fast is that it sets you a new standard of health." Old and young alike are renewed and have their whole organism repaired and their functions improved. Fasting supplies opportunities to the body to eliminate accumulated excess weight.

Regeneration of the body is a ceaseless process. The daily renewal of its cells and tissues prevents old age and early death for considerable time, despite the worst abuses which are heaped upon the bodies of most of us. Fasting enables the processes of renewal to out-distance the processes of degeneration and the result is a higher standard of health. Regeneration of the flesh, even the very marrow of the bones, is possible through this method. By it we may actually tear down much of the body and then rebuild it and have a new or renewed one.

When once we have learned that the body is able to rip its structures to pieces and re-use and re-arrange their constituents to match and fit its organs, we are prepared to understand how fasting so quickly brings about a rejuvenation of the body. The texture and tone and feeling and look and utility of your organs and functions will be as fine, after they have gone through the cleansing, refining process of fasting, as are soiled silks or laces after these have gone through the process of cleaning. The rejuvenating effect upon the skin is visible to all who have eyes to see. Lines, wrinkles, blotches, pimples and discolorations disappear, the skin becomes more youthful, acquires a better color and a better texture. The eyes clear up and become brighter. One looks younger. The visible rejuvenation in the skin and eyes is matched by manifest evidences of similar but invisible rejuvenescence throughout the body.

Most of my readers are familiar with the method of propagating certain plants from "cuttings" and from "buds" rather than from seeds. Parts of some plants and of some of the simpler forms of animal life are able to reconstitute the whole plant or animal.

Prof. Child and others have shown that the reconstituted organisms are physiologically younger than the plant or animal from which they were derived. "The degree of rejuvenescence" in such cases "is in general proportionate to the degree of re-organization in the process of reconstruction of the piece into a whole." There is reason to believe, as H. Reinheimer has pointed out, that the virtue of these processes of re-organization and reconstruction lies in a simultaneous reduction of what he thinks is best described as a "nutritive overflow." Reorganization and redistribution as we have already seen, occur in the body of the faster concomitantly and coetaneously with the reduction of surplus nutrition. We know that reduction of a "nutritive overflow" will not account for all the rejuvenating effects observed, for we see these also in the undernourished, mal-nourished and under-weight persons.

Exhaustive experiments by Prof. Morgulis have proved beyond a doubt that fasting rejuvenates. He has also shown that the body does not tear down its tissues nor impair them structurally. The cells are reduced in size but there is little or no destruction of cells except in cases of actual starvation. The nuclei of the cells tend usually to retain their size and lose so little of their bulk that they become relatively larger in proportion to the rest of the cell. Such a cell has the capacity for assimilation and growth which characterizes the cells of embryos and young animals. This accounts for the rapid gains in tissue after a fast. The layman may see these remarkable changes in the skin for this often becomes as fine grained and smooth, almost as that of a child. Drs. Carlson and Kunde, of the department of Physiology of the University of Chicago, showed that a fast of two weeks temporarily restores the tissues of a man of forty to the physiological condition of the tissues of a youth of seventeen.

How long this youthful condition can be maintained these investigators do not know and could not have shown, for they have no knowledge of the causes of the aging process and therefore did not see that these were not returned to after the fast. The fasters simply returned to their accustomed habits of living. Mr. Hoelzel, who took part in this experiment, assures me that neither he nor Dr. Kunde smoked or took alcoholics after the fast, but he thinks that he did overeat. Every faster knows that his body and his energies are renewed by the fast and where he lives properly afterward, he knows that the improvement is lasting. These facts are not new. They were only new to Drs. Carlson and Kunde.

Dr. Kunde says, "It is evident that where the initial weight was reduced by 45 per cent, and subsequently restored by normal diet, approximately one-half of the restored body is made up of new protoplasm. In this there is rejuvenescence." It should be pointed out that much of the 55 per cent of the body that was not lost has undergone rejuvenating changes of great significance.

By repeating the rejuvenating fasts at appropriate intervals, the individual can keep himself younger, year after year, much younger physiologically, than he would otherwise be—in short, stave off old age.

Mr. Hoelzel gives it as his opinion that little rejuvenation can be expected after the age of thirty-five. This is not borne out by the observations of men who have had greatest experience with the fast. Thirty-five years is a fixed chronological point, but in the human organism we deal with a biological entity of very variable physiological status, so that marked distinctions are made between the physiological, the psychological and the chronological ages of a man or woman. Perhaps at thirty-five or thereafter, we could more properly refer to the pathological age of the individual seeking rejuvenation. I would say that, instead of the age of the person being, *per se*, the factor determining the amount of rejuvenation possible, it depends, rather, upon the aggregate amount of irremediable pathological developments present in the individual organism, so that, the possibilities for rejuvenation are different in all men and women of the same chronological ages. Dr. Rabagliatti quoted some one as having said that "old people bear abstinence well, and that they bear over-feeding badly," a fact which he thought was full of hope in the attempt to prolong the lives of old people and in relieving them of their sufferings.

Our flesh is renewed through a renovation of our ways of life. Through fasting we have unloaded the toxic burden and the old flesh and new flesh has been built out of better food, exercise and sunshine with entire abstinence from tobacco, tea, coffee, alcohol, etc. We are renewed and reinvigorated both by a reduction of surfeit and by the excretion of accumulated toxins and their pathologic end-results.

E. Schultz, experimenting with fasting hydra, produced positive proof of the rejuvenating effects of fasting, the animals reverting to an embryonic state. Intensive nourishment results in much poisoning in infusoria and a short fast is needed to restore them to youth. A reduction of surfeit is essential to the most vigorous manifestations of vitality. In higher animals "brief hunger has a beneficial effect." Prof. C. M. Child, of the University of Chicago, took some small flat worms, worms which when fed, grow old, lazy and infirm, and chopped them up into small pieces and each piece grew into a new and *young* worm. He took some of the old worms and fasted them for a long time. They grew smaller and smaller, living off their own internal resources for months. Then, when they had been reduced to a minimum size, he fed them. They started to grow and were just as young in physiological condition as ever they were.

The planarian may continue to shrink until reduced to less than one-hundredth of its original size, to a size even below that at which it hatched from the egg. When this point is reached a supply of food will enable it to grow again. These reduced worms have the proportions of young rather than those of old worms. They look rejuvenated. Prof. Child alternately fed and starved a group of these worms and caused them to live over a period of twelve generations. They showed no signs of progressive aging—whenever they were large they were as old as ordinary worms of the same size; whenever they were small they were as young as ordinary worms. It is stated that if we choose to go to the trouble we could probably keep a single flat-worm alternately going up and down the hill of life and never going beyond a certain age limit for periods that would make Methuselah seem very short-lived.

Professor Child tells us (*Senescence and Rejuvenescence*) *that* with abundant food some species may pass through their whole life history in three or four weeks, but when growth is prevented through loss of food, they may continue active and young for at least three years. "Partial starvation inhibits senescence. The starveling is brought back from an advanced age to the beginning of post-embryonic life; it is almost re-born."

It hardly need be said that in the larger and more complex forms of life the possibilities of rejuvenescence are more narrowly limited than among the lower forms, such as the planaria. Nevertheless, according to Prof. Child, in the organic world, generally, rejuvenescence is as fundamental and important a process as senescence. Prof. Huxley, of England, son of the older Prof. Huxley, took some young planaria, or earth worms, and performed a very interesting and instructive experiment with them. He fed a whole family of these as they ordinarily eat. He isolated one of them and fed it in the same manner, but forced it to undergo at regular intervals, short periods of fasting. It was alternately fasted and fed. The isolated worm was still alive after nineteen generations of his brothers had been born, lived their regular life cycles and passed away. The only difference in the mode of life and the diet of this worm and that of his brother worms was his periodic fasts.

Excess is fatal to healthy action. A reduction of surfeit is essential to the most vigorous manifestations of vitality. Weismann's observations and the results of tissue-culture in the laboratory reveal that there are no limits to vitality. Autogenerated toxins and poisoning from gastro-intestinal putrefaction and fermentation are the chief limiting influences upon life. Surfeit produces and fasting eliminates these. A removal of toxins and surfeit permits tissue regeneration.

An experimenter at the University of Chicago procured some insects of a kind, the normal life of which is only twenty-four hours. He isolated them and placed them where they could not procure food. Instead of starving to death immediately or dying at the end of their normal twenty-four hours' life span, they lived for fifteen days. Fasting enabled them to live for fifteen generations.

Now, these results obtained with the worms and insects only forcefully remind us again that we cannot safely argue from one species to another. Man cannot live for fifteen generations by fasting nor for nineteen generations by periodic short fasts. Nor can he become a minute man by fasting and then, when fed, grow into a new and youthful man as was the case with the worms. But there is a renewal of man's body to a certain extent. His body does become smaller. He does get rid of his surplus tissues, surplus food, accumulated toxins and "diseased" tissues, etc.

Fasting produces no organic deterioration, no pathological changes in the organs of the body. This can occur only after the period of starvation is reached and, even when this occurs, complete recovery generally follows upon the supply of proper nutrition. Active growth and regeneration may go on simultaneously with fasting, as Morgulis and other experimenters have shown. Fasting improves the fundamental organic functions and, up to a certain point, increases muscular strength.

That some of the cells and tissues are consumed in this process is both natural and necessary, but nothing is lost which nature cannot or will not replace when favorable conditions are afforded her. Her reserves are consumed and some of the muscular and glandular tissues are sacrificed to sustain the more vital organs. However, the "germ of the cell" or its own power to renew itself and to build new cells is not destroyed. "The nucleus retains its potentiality to rejuvenate the cell after a period of rest, and it recuperates to function with renewed activity after its environment has been freed of deleterious waste" by the fast.

A great change in cell life and structure takes places during a fast and it is well to continue the fast until this change is complete and nothing but healthy tissue remains. In this way a new body emerges from the process. It is thin, but ready to be re-built upon normal lines. After such an overhauling process, when the body has been largely torn down and thrown away, when the accumulated waste and debris of a life-time have been refined or cast out and, after the chemical readjustment occasioned by the fast, has occurred, the body that is properly cared for is built anew and its youth renewed.

Dr. Carlson found that the increased vigor of the hunger contractions, which appeared in fasting, lasted for some days after a five days' fast. He suggests that this effect may be analogous to the general rejuvenating effect of fasting as seen in animals, and intimates that an occasional period of fasting may exert a beneficial influence in renewing vigor and prolonging life and in increasing one's capacity for work.

Experiments upon human beings and dogs, performed at the Hull Biological Laboratory of the University of Chicago, and reported to the *Journal of Metabolic Research,* showed that a fast of thirty to forty days produces a permanent increase of five to six per cent in the metabolic rate. A decrease in the metabolic rate is one of the phenomena of old age. Fasting by increasing the metabolic rate produces, as one of its effects, *rejuvenation.*

With toxin deposits cleared up; the body purified; the blood rejuvenated; organs renewed; senses improved; digestion and assimilation enhanced; the cells and tissues returned to a more youthful condition; infiltrations, effusions, and growths absorbed; dead and dying tissues removed and new tissues in their places; body chemistry normalized; the body is in very much the same condition as the mattress that has been to the factory for renovation and making over. After the fast has cleared away the accumulations and the devitalized cells, stronger, more vital and healthy tissue is built to take the place of that which was cast away. Regeneration of the body is brought about through the daily renewal of its cells and tissues and fasting hastens this renewal.

On May 18th, 1933, one of the physicians attending Ghandi, during his fast at that time, reported that on that day, the tenth day of his fast, "despite his 64 years, from a physiological point of view, the Indian leader was as healthy as a man of forty."

Gain and Loss of Strength
While Fasting

CHAPTER XVI

"Most men can understand eating to get strong," says Dr. Tilden, "but it takes a long time to educate them to *stop eating* to get strong." As paradoxical as it may seem to those who have had no experience with fasting, there is a frequent, and perhaps always a gain in strength while fasting. Let me begin with a quotation from a thoroughly "orthodox" and "scientific" source. Prof. Benedict, in his report, details a number of experiments upon the strength of Prof. Levanzin during his experimental fast. Then referring to similar tests made by others, he says:

"In the test made by Luciani on Succi in which a dynamometer was used, the strength of the right and left hands showed results seemingly at variance with the popular impression. Thus on the twenty-first day of the fast, Succi was able to register on the dynamometer a stronger grip than when he first began. From the twentieth to the thirtieth day of the fast, however, his strength decreased, being less at the end than in the beginning of the fast. In discussing these results, Luciani points out the fact that Succi believed that he gained strength as the fast progressed. Considering the question of the influence of inanition on the onset of fatigue, Luciani states that the fatigue curve obtained by Succi on the twenty-ninth day was similar to those obtained with an individual under normal conditions."

"On the last days of his fast Succi would ride horseback or ascend the Eiffel Tower of Paris, running up the tremendous staircase that tires the average man to merely ascend it."

Levanzin lost no strength during his thirty-one days' fast as shown by the dynamometric tests. On the last day of the fast, this non-athletic man, used to taking no regular exercise except walking, was able to press up to one hundred and twenty pounds with his left hand. It is somewhat amusing to read that at the end of his fast of thirty-one days in the Carnegie Institute, Levanzin wanted to continue it up to forty days and that Prof. Benedict objected because it would be very expensive and fatiguing to his well-fed men.

Dr. Tanner's strength decreased until after he began to take water, but increased thereafter. He was challenged by a reporter who declared one could not keep up one's strength without eating. The Doctor said: "Here have I been for several years a semi-invalid, suffering from all kinds of diseases, and now I have fasted for two weeks. You are young, healthy, strong and vigorous. I will just take a drink of water and then I will run you a race around this hall and see who can endure the longest." The reporter confidently accepted the challenge and the race began. To the amusement of the audience, who had expected to see the young man easily win, the doctor easily and speedily outran his competitor, who puffed and blowed in his distress.

Mr. Macfadden said: "In several cases treated by myself, and also in a number of cases quoted by Dewey and Carrington, the strength increased from day to day, until the patient was enabled to walk several miles a day toward the close of a long fast, whereas at first he was unable to walk at all!" Again he said: "It is a fact that has been demonstrated again and again that many individuals instead of losing strength by fasting, gain it. In one case a woman was carried to one of our institutions on a stretcher, so weak from malnutrition that she was unable to walk. Her physician had prescribed all kinds of nourishing diets which she had been unable to digest and in spite of food (or because of it—author's note), drugs and nursing she had rapidly grown weaker. She was at once placed on a fast and to her amazement, she, day by day, increased in strength."

In my own practice there is the case of a man who was confined to bed and unable to get out of it, although eating three meals a day. At the end of a week of fasting he was able to get up and walk about the room, although still fasting. There is the case of another man who was so weak he could not walk from one room to another of his home without support. After two weeks of fasting he was able to go down stairs unsupported, go outside and have a sun bath and return upstairs to his bed. After fifty-five days of fasting he was still able to do this. He was much stronger at the end of his fifty-five days without food than when he began the fast.

In 1925, it was announced, from the University of Chicago, that football coaches have found that if they force their players to go without food a short time and then feed them a hearty meal a few hours before the game they are "raring to go, both mentally and physically." Many athletes have found that short fasts during their training periods aid them considerably. The late Harry Wills, Negro heavyweight pugilist, was an outstanding example of this. As an opposite example, habitual gluttony came very near to permanently retiring Babe Ruth from the baseball diamond. Somebody pointed out to him the cause of his troubles and reduced eating restored him to good physical condition, as well as overcame his irrascible temper.

In his *"Why Did Jesus Fast,"* Rev. H. Arndt tells of an Italian fencing master who prepared for contests with a week of fasting and continuous practice and who had never been vanquished. Freddy Welsh, one time light-weight champion of the world, always started his training for important fights with a fast of a week. He found that this shortened considerably the time required to get in condition for the fight. He never had to postpone any fights because of colds, boils, etc., as was often done by Joe Beckett, George Carpentier, and others.

In December 1903, eight athletes under the supervision of Mr. Macfadden entered a seven days' fast and performed feats of great strength and endurance under the watchful eyes of prominent medical men from different parts of New York. These eight men were entered on the list on Saturday night at the beginning of their fast and the same eight athletes presented themselves in the final contest of endurance on the evening of the seventh day of the fast.

Joseph H. Waltering, of New York City, won first prize in the races, winning the 50-yard dash in six and two-fifths seconds, the 220-yard run in twenty-seven and four-fifths seconds, and the mile run in six minutes, fourteen and two-fifths seconds. Gilman Low, of New York City, artist, health-director, athlete, won first prize in strength contests; lifting 900 pounds in a straight hand grip lift and throwing the 56-pound weight thirteen feet six inches. On the sixth day of his fast, Mr. Low lifted with hands alone 500 pounds twenty times in fifteen seconds, and 900 pounds twice in twenty seconds. In the back lift he lifted one ton twelve times in twenty seconds. Following the Saturday night tests in the presence of physicians to whom he desired to demonstrate that there was no deterioration of strength after a week of fasting, he lifted one ton twenty-two times in nineteen seconds.

Mr. Low did not break his fast until the end of the eighth day. Then, at Madison Square Garden, before the astonished gaze of 16,000 people, he established nine world records for strength and endurance, which stood for years before they were broken. These records are:

"1. Raising 950 pounds three times in four seconds.

2. Raising 500 pounds twenty times in fifteen seconds.

3. Throwing 56-pound weight thirteen feet six inches (for height).

4. Leg-lifting — Raising with legs alone 1,000 pounds fifty times in twenty-five seconds.

5. Leg-lifting — Raising with legs alone 1,500 pounds thirty-five times in twenty-five seconds.

6. Raising with legs alone 1,800 pounds eighteen times in eighteen seconds.

7. Back lifting — bringing all the muscles of the back into action raising 2,500 pounds five times in ten seconds.

8. Raising 2,200 pounds twelve times in twelve seconds.

9. Raising 2,200 pounds twenty-nine times in twenty seconds."

These remarkable records were made after eight days of fasting in competition with other men who had been eating regularly, Mr. Low going out of his class to do it. He has set other world records, after fasting at other times. On one occasion in reply to the claim of physicians that should one go without food for a week, one would be so weak one could scarcely walk and a few more days would endanger life, Mr. Low challenged any two of them to handle him in any way suitable to them after he had fasted for fifteen days. He asserted that atfer a fifteen days' fast he underwent a few years previously in Boston, he could have whipped his weight in wildcats.

Prof. Levanzin says: "Those who feel any lack of strength during a fast are to be classed in the same category with those who feel hungry. They are nervous and very impressionable people, and their sufferings are only the baneful effects of their too vivid imagination.

"If you suggest to yourself that you are strong and that you can walk two miles on the thirtieth day of your fast, believe me, you can do it without great difficulty, but if you fix in your weak mind that you are going to faint, and worry, and persist to worry about it, be sure that not a very long time will elapse before you faint really, a victim of your wrong auto-suggestion."

Much to his surprise, Sinclair had none of the weakness during his second fast that he experienced during his first fast. Mrs. Sinclair experienced much weakness during her first fast, but no weakness during her second fast. Macfadden, Carrington and others, record numerous examples of increase of both mental and physical strength during the fast. Everyone who has had experience with fasting has seen similar results. Mr. Carrington used the phenomenon of the increase of energy during a fast as a basis of criticism of the reigning theory of science that energy is derived from food. He also employed it as a basis of interpretation of life. The very title of his book, *Vitality, Fasting and Nutrition,* is significant.

Morgulis says: "Laboratory experience with fasters, as well as long fasting among followers of certain religious sects, prove that no harm can befall the healthy individual who abstains from food." Lacking clinical experience with fasting patients, he says: "Indiscriminate fasting, however, of patients whose strength is already impaired should be discouraged." Prof. Morgulis has never watched a weak patient grow stronger during a fast. He has not seen the day by day improvement in the strength and general condition of such patients. Valuable as his work is, he is not entitled to speak with authority in this field of fasting. "Again," says Dr. Dewey, "let it be borne in mind that recovery from acute disease is attended with a revival of strength in every power that makes life worth living, and that every person not acutely sick who has fasted under my care or who has cut down the waste of brain power by less daily food has found the same revival of power. To this there have been no exceptions."— *The Fasting Cure,* p. 161.

One patient I helped care for a few years ago grew stronger each day during a fast of eighteen days. This man was so weak at the beginning of the fast that he would get down on his hands and knees and crawl up the steps. He told me afterwards that sometimes he thought he would not be able to make it to the top. Before his eighteen days of fasting were up he was able to run up the steps.

It should not be thought, however, that one may fast indefinitely with a continuous increase in strength. On the contrary, when the muscles begin to waste there must come a gradual lessening of strength. In the average case strength should begin to lessen slightly after about the twentieth day. This, however, must vary in keeping with the amount of reserves possessed and the rapidity with which these are consumed. In some cases an increase in strength is registered up to and beyond the thirtieth day.

In the volume on exercise it is pointed out that strength is a combination of muscle (machinery) and nerve force (motive energy). We should add that the purity or impurity of the blood greatly influences both the muscles and the nerves. Fasting brings about the purification of the blood and also conserves nervous energy, so that there is more energy on hand to be used and the condition of nerve and muscle is improved so that they respond more readily to the will. This increase of strength is, therefore, most marked in those who are most toxic and overloaded with excess food. Such an increase cannot continue indefinitely due to the gradual wasting of the muscles. After these have wasted below a certain minimum, while there is no diminution of nervous energy, there will be a decrease in strength.

It is necessary to distinguish between one's actual strength and one's feeling of strength. The man who is accustomed to eating three square meals a day of rich, highly seasoned foods and taking tea and coffee along with these, and using tobacco between meals, will feel miserably weak, languid and shaky when deprived of these. He will feel too weak to sit up, perhaps. This feeling of weakness is due to the withdrawal of energy from the muscles. As the fast progresses, he will feel stronger and more cheerful. Fainting during the fast usually comes, if at all, during these first three or four days.

What we may designate *physical strength* to differentiate it from what we may call *physiological strength*, fluctuates during the fast, being greater one day, lower the next and greater the next or it may increase for a week and then, suddenly, be greatly reduced, only to be increased again a day or so later. One day the faster seems hardly able to lift his head off the pillow; the next day he wants to go to town. Other symptoms fluctuate in much the same manner, with a steady general improvement in them. Much of this apparent weakness seems definitely to be of mental origin, as it is quickly dispelled by a variety of expedients short of breaking the fast. The faster who feels weak will find that he feels much stronger after a few minutes of exercise. The feeling of weakness is due to the withdrawal of energy from the mucles. Exercise causes a great determination of nervous energy to these.

Whatever may be true of the increase of energy during the fast it is not true that there is a continuous increase of strength throughout the length of a long fast. Strength is the ability to express energy and requires the possession of certain mechanisms for the expression. As the fast progresses and the muscles grow smaller, it is inevitable that a time comes when they are less able to manifest energy—that is when muscular strength will diminish.

There are numerous fasting patients in whom there is an unmistakable feeling of weakness even of prostration. Some of them are so weak they cannot raise their heads from the pillow. But it is questionable whether or not the weakness so evident in these patients is real or only apparent. For one thing, it is a common occurrence for them to become suddenly strong as soon as they have taken the first half-glass of orange juice, even before the juice has left the stomach. Where does such a sudden rush of strength come from? If this phenomenon is not to be explained as purely mental, then, the explanation seems to me to lie in the physiological let-down" that fasting occasions.

The apparent increase in strength that follows immediately upon eating is due to the awakening of the body's dormant powers and is not any actual increase in strength. If condiments are taken with the food, as they sometimes are, there is the excitement that is called stimulation. The "weakness" that follows the withdrawal of food is merely the inevitable "let down" that always follows the withdrawal of stimulants. Most people are in the habit of taking stimulating substances with their foods and between meals. The same phenomena are seen when tobacco, alcohol, coffee, morphine, etc., are withheld from the habitual user of these substances. The fact that the greatest let-down is seen in heavy flesh-eaters and the lightest let-down is seen in vegetarians supports this view.

When food and stimulants are withdrawn, there is a general let-down of physical and physiological activities and a cessation of the excited activity that is called stimulation. The slowing up of the heart beat, reduced respiratory rate, lowering of metabolism, etc., mean that the body is resting. It is this physiological let-down that gives one the feeling of weakness. A little activity to speed up the heart, increase respiration and step-up metabolism soon remedies the feeling of weakness.

Long ago Prof. Atwater pointed out that we have neither the means for measuring potential energy as such, nor a unit for expressing such measurements if they were made. We can measure output only. But output is expenditure whereas quiescence is conservation. Trall says: "All persons know how they feel; but all do not apprehend the true sources of their good or bad feelings, and the majority mistake the sense of mere *stimulation* for the condition of actual strength; they do not distinguish between the feeling of strength and vital power; they do not consider that strength or power is only shown in its waste or expenditure, not in its accumulation or possession." —*Hydropathic Encyclopedia*, Vol. I, p. 418.

Carrington pointed out that the immediate feeling of strength and exhiliration that follows upon the taking of the first food after the fast cannot on any possible theory, be derived from the food itself, for the reason that the exhiliration comes immediately, whereas the food cannot possibly give any strength to the organism before it is digested and assimilated. Carrington suggests that the taking of food occasions the rousing up of dormant or latent energy. During the fast, and this is particularly true if the patient has been resting, energy becomes latent. He also points out that much of the exhiliration is mental. I have repeatedly seen patients who were so "weak," they could not raise their heads from the pillow. With the first half glass of fruit juice they were ready to go out and engage in marked activity. In these instances, both the "weakness" and the sudden return of "strength" are so obviously mental that no one who has watched it repeatedly ever doubts it.

Carrington contends that "the vital energies, so far from being lessened, invariably increase, as the fast progresses (no matter what the feelings of weakness may seem to indicate); that the mind is never affected by the fast in any manner whatever, or in any other way than beneficially . . ." Note that he makes a clear distinction between the "feeling of weakness" and an actual lessening of energy. Only by keeping this distinction in mind, can his statement be properly understood. I have seen patients who had fasted for prolonged periods, thirty to forty days and more, manifest most astounding strength and energy.

Carrington points out that the more distinct and uninterrupted gains of energy, while fasting, are seen, and the gain is most marked and steady where the greatest degree of prostration and weakness is observed, and where, if anywhere, we should expect collapse to follow upon the complete withdrawal of food. As he puts it, "In cases which are already weakened by disease, and consequently where the vitality is already at a very low ebb, this increase of energy, consequent upon the withdrawal of food, is always most readily seen and most marked.

"Theoretically, of course, the complete withdrawal of food in such cases, should have the effect of causing the speedy death of the patient, for the reason that the last source (according to science) of bodily energy has been withdrawn. But in actual practice, we find that the very opposite is the fact in the case, and that the patient's strength and energy return and continue to accumulate during the period of fasting."—*Vitality, Fasting and Nutrition*, pp. 260-261.

Gain and Loss of Weight
During Fasting

CHAPTER XVII

A female cat will lose weight and grow skinny while she is nursing her kittens, although she may be well and abundantly fed. She rounds out again by the time she is ready for her next pregnancy. Her very tissues are called upon to supply food for her young. This is very similar to what is seen in fasting. The cat presents no evidence that she is injured in any way by this loss of weight.

When an individual ceases to eat he quite naturally loses weight. Although we usually say that a faster loses about a pound a day, the loss of weight varies greatly, depending on a number of circumstances. Fat subjects lose more rapidly than lean ones. The more physically active one is, the more rapidly one loses weight. The longer the fast progresses, the less rapid is the loss of weight. Losses of five or six pounds a day for the first two or three days are often recorded. But these losses are not losses of flesh. Most of this apparent loss is due to the emptying of the alimentary canal of several pounds of food and feces which is not replaced by more food.

Here is an almost incredible case. Fat people commonly lose weight very rapidly when placed upon a fast. They lose much more than the average pound a day. A very fat woman took a fast of fifty days in the *Health School* in 1952 and lost, in this time, twelve pounds. As she had no way to get food from the outside, had no access to the kitchen and as all the other symptoms indicated that she was fasting, I think I can say that she actually fasted the whole time. She had, before coming to the *Health School*, a very low rate of metabolism. This is the only explanation that I can find for her absurdly low loss of weight in a fast of such length. Her loss through the whole of her fast of an average of a quarter of a pound a day was that of the loss commonly observed in the closing days of an extended fast when metabolism is much reduced.

I took this case up with Mr. Hoelzel in the hope of reaching Dr. Carlson with it, but Hoelzel wrote back saying: "Dr. Carlson would not be likely to be convinced that a fat woman lost only 12 pounds in 50 days of fasting although I believe that this might be possible if her fluid intake was not limited to distilled water." I do not know how hide-bound Dr. Carlson was, but if he was of the type that closes his mind to what may appear to be unusual phenomena, he was poor material out of which to make a scientist. This woman's fluid intake was confined to distilled water.

Luciani found, in his study of Succi, that when mineral water is used, weight can be gained on a fast, due to the storing of water and mineral. I have found, in my extensive experience with fasting, that mineral water is not essential to gaining weight in a fast. It may be done on distilled water.

I discussed this case with both Dr. William L. Esser and Dr. Christopher Gian-Cursio and found that both these men, in extensive experiences with fasting, had cared for similar cases of but little loss during an extended fast. In each of their cases there was low metabolism. I have had several such cases, some of them seeking to reduce weight and they found the experience disappointing. Although none of them were as dramatic as the foregoing case, all of them had a low metabolism.

George S. Keith, M.D., LL.D., F.R.C.P.E., who successfully employed fasting in his care of the sick for many years, says in his *Plea for a Simple Life*: "A healthy man, when he takes no food, loses in weight at first about a pound a day, which is gradually lessened to half a pound if the abstinence is prolonged." In *The Best Thing In the World* Mr. Shaw, recording the developments in his own fast, which he carefully watched, says: "The loss of flesh for many days has been less and less, as compared with the earlier days of the fast . . . The loss of weight grows less and less daily."

It is the history of all fasts that weight is lost more rapidly during the first few days than during the subsequent period. In one fast of thirty days conducted by myself, the loss during the last five days was one-fourth of a pound a day. The patient was moderately active from 9 A.M. to 7 P.M. During Mr. Johnston's thirty days' fast he lost from one-half a pound to two pounds a day. On the thirtieth day of the fast his loss was one-half pound. On the twenty-second and twenty-third days he weighed the same, apparently losing nothing. This however, was due to profuse water drinking. I have seen cases gain weight for two and three days at a time from drinking so much water. At the beginning of his 30 days' fast, Mr. Johnston weighed 154½ lbs. At its completion, his weight was 121½ lbs., his total loss being 23 lbs. During the 20 days of walking from Chicago without food, he lost 37½ lbs., more than in the previous fast of thirty days. It goes without saying that the physically active faster loses more rapidly than the faster who rests most or all of the time.

During the first few days of his fast Sinclair lost fifteen pounds; an indication of the extremely poor state of his tissues. During the next eight days he lost only two pounds, a very unusual thing for this stage of fasting. Levanzin lost 29 pounds during his 31 days' fast in the Carnegie Institute. Major Gotshall says: "For the first eight days of my fast I lost twenty-five pounds." This very unusual loss indicates that his tissues were in very poor condition.

The weight lost by fat patients in the early days of a fast is astounding. I have seen losses of five and six pounds a day for the first few days. A woman who fasted in the *Health School* in January and February of 1950 lost twenty-five pounds in the first two weeks. As before indicated, rapid loss of weight in a fast indicates a poor condition of the tissues. It has been repeatedly noticed that fat individuals who are soft and flabby lose more rapidly than those whose fat is firm and solid. As the fast progresses, the rate of loss decreases in fat patients. Skinny patients commonly lose slowly from the beginning, but one whose tissues are in very poor condition may lose very rapidly at the outset. The difference in the day to day weight loss between fasters who are active and fasters who are kept in bed is surprisingly small. The total difference, over a period of three or more weeks, is considerable.

Mr. Carrington tabulated and published the losses of weight sustained in ten selected patients. In 253 days of fasting these lost 248 pounds, or approximately a pound a day. Such figures supply us with a fairly accurate index to the amount of actual nutritive substance the average person requires each day. By actual nutritive material is meant water-free and waste-free food. The greater part of our foods, as we consume them, is water and indigestible fiber, or bulk. About a pound a day of actual nutritive substance is sufficient to maintain a healthful balance between income and outgo of food.

I present Carrington's table of weight losses from his *Vitality, Fasting and Nutrition:*

Name	Weight at Commencement	Weight at End	Days	Loss of Weight
1. Geo. E. Davis_____	228	174	50	54
2. Mrs. I. Matthews_____	150	123	22	27
3. Rev. N. H. Lohre_____	178	165	10	13
4. Prof. F. W._____	182	158	20	24
5. Mr. J. B._____	165	154	23	11
6. Mrs. J. B._____	135	127	8	8
7. Mr. G. W. Tuthill_____	108½	72½	41	36
8. Mrs. F. J. C._____	136	103	28	33
9. Mrs. T. A._____	117	92	34	25
10. Robert B. _____	135	118	17	17
	1534½	1286½	253	248

It will be noted by a careful study of this chart that the rates of loss varied much in these ten cases. Several factors account for this. Fat patients lose much faster than do thin ones, nervous and emotional patients lose more rapidly than calm and poised individuals, patients that are relaxed and resting lose less weight than those that are tense or active. There is also a correlation between the condition of the patient's tissue and his loss of weight. Fat individuals who are soft and flabby fall away very rapidly. Those fat individuals who are hard and firm lose much slower. There is the added fact that much water drinking tends to keep the weight up by water-logging the tissues, without preventing the usual loss of solid substance. It is also true that the most rapid losses occur in the earliest part of the fast so that on the whole, short fasts show greater average daily losses than do long fasts. Losses are not as great in second, third or fourth fasts as in the first.

On the basis of this table and other data which he considered, Mr. Carrington concluded that: *"The average loss of weight by fasting patients amounts, ceteries paribus, to one pound per diem."* He noted that in some cases there are great variations from this loss and pointed out that the loss is greater at the beginning than at the end of the fast. He says: "A patient loses approximately one and one-half pounds *per diem*, at the very beginning of every fast for one-half pound which is lost toward its close."

As these observations were all made on sick individuals, Mr. Carrington asks the question: How much should the normal man lose? He says: "*more* than a pound a day is obviously too much—denoting obesity; while *less* than half a pound is too little—denoting emaciation." He says that we cannot accept the average loss of weight of a pound a day as the "normal" loss for the reason that: "*All patients who find it necessary to fast absolutely are already in a grossly abnormal condition, and their loss of weight must consequently be considered abnormal also.*" He says that one pound a day must represent the loss of a *diseased* body, and is by no means a normal loss.

Reversing his position that if the normal man fasts, he starves, he takes the position that a loss of a pound a day for a normal man is too great. He mentions a loss of fifteen pounds in a week of fasting by Mr. Macfadden, a loss of nothing at all during a fast of four days by Miss Louise Kops of New York (May 1904) and the gain of three-fourths of a pound by Mr. J. Estapper in a week of fasting. These are exceptional cases and provide no basis for a calculation of the weight a normal person should lose during a fast. From a consideration of various data, however, he reached the conclusion that the fasting normal man should lose an average of *twelve ounces* a day. This, he thinks, represents the actual nutritive needs of the body daily in order to preserve its weight and to replace worn out tissue. Rabagliati arrived at the same conclusion from different data. The reader will understand that food—that is the raw material—is not all nutriment. This does not mean twelve ounces of food, but twelve ounces of nutritive material that the digestive system may extract from the food.

Discussing losses of weight during a short fast, Benedict says: "Losses of body weight in experiments of a few days duration are wholly without significance. With regard to the total cumulative loss as the experiment progresses, it appears that in long experiments of Succi the loss bears in general a direct ratio to the length of the experiment." He recites a fast conducted by Nicholson, using a prisoner for the experiment, in which there was an average daily loss of 1.4 lbs., "the greatest loss appearing during the first part of the experiment."

Observations show that women lose slightly more than men do when fasting. This is thought to be due to the fact that women usually carry more fatty tissue than men. The rate of metabolism in women is lower than in men and we should expect men to lose more rapidly. But it is a well-established fact that the fatter the individual the greater the comparative loss of weight. This is added confirmation of Carrington's conclusion that healthy subjects lose at a slower rate than the sick.

What are lost pounds to those who have recovered from their miseries, so that they may eat in comfort and with pleasure? After they have been restored to good health by a period of physical, mental and physiological rest, they may regain the lost pounds. There is this difference, however; after the fast the patient may put on healthy flesh.

Macleod's *Physiology in Modern Medicine* says that "All of the fat does not disappear from the tissues during starvation. This has led to the concept that a certain amount of fat in a tissue is an essential part of that tissue while the remainder is present as storage material. The essential portion is constant in amount while the storage fat varies with the amount present in the diet, and with the metabolic activity of the tissues." It is the lowering of the metabolic rate that follows the first part of the fast that accounts for the slowing up of the rate of loss.

It is said that a man may lose forty per cent of his normal weight before his life is endangered. We know, however, that many fasting patients lose much more than this without danger or harm. Indeed, Dr. Dewey insists that "when death occurs before the skeleton condition is reached it is always due to old age or some other form of disease or injury and not to starvation." Dr. Hazzard and Mr. Carrington hold the same view and, as will be shown later, there are facts which support this view.

Chossat found that the ultimate proportional losses in different animals experimented on, were almost exactly the same, death occurring when the body had lost two-fifths (40 per cent) of its original weight. Different parts of the body lose weight in different proportions. The chief losses are sustained by the adipose tissues, the muscles and glands. Young organisms are said to die when they have lost twenty per cent of their original weight.

It makes a great difference where one commences to figure the 40% loss that results in death. It must be computed from "normal" weight; not "original" weight. The fast of J. Austin Shaw, of New York, recorded by Dr. Dewey, was of forty-five days duration, during which period he lost but 26¾ lbs. At the beginning of the fast he weighed 199¾ lbs., at the end 173 lbs., being still over-weight. Mr. Propheter, New York, fasted 52 days, losing 43 lbs., from 135½ at the start to 92½ at the end, 40% of his original weight would reduce him to 81.3 lbs. or allow him to lose 11.2 lbs. more, which would have taken three more weeks at the rate he was losing. Young children have, in more than one case, lost more than twenty per cent of their weight before death occurred—see the two cases recorded by Dewey.

Discussing a gain of four pounds during an eight days fast, by a Mrs. Martinson of Stapleton, Staten Island, and a case reported by Dr. Rabagliati of a gain of one and one-half pounds in three weeks, by a patient on less than eight ounces of food a day, about ninety per cent of which was water, Carrington says: "The explanation is in all probability this: In all such cases great density of tissue is present—it is obstipated, as it is called—and when such a person fasts, he or she oxidizes off a part of this too solid tissue, and fills in the interstices with water, which the patient is at liberty to drink during the fast. This is, at least, the explanation which I have been driven to adopt—none other seemingly covered the facts."

J. H. Washburn, of California, was reported to have fasted 43 days in 1870 without losing an ounce of flesh. This, I do not believe. One of the athletes who fasted seven days at Madison Square Garden, in Feb. 1904, actually gained three pounds during the 7 days. The eight athletes were watched during the entire time by paid guards.

Dr. Tanner took no water during the first 16 days of his fast (tissues became dehydrated) and lost weight rapidly. After the sixteenth day he drank considerable amounts of water (tissues rehydrated) and gained four and one-half pounds during the next four days, after which he again commenced to lose weight.

Carrington records that "Miss Louise Kops of New York, lost nothing at all during a four days fast (in May 1904), and in the case of Mr. J. Estapper, Jr., a week's fast resulted in an actual gain of three-fourths of a pound."

The weight of Mr. Estapper was very accurately ascertained, and it is asserted that there was no possible source of error through which a mistake could have been made. The faster was one of the competitors in the seven days' fasting-athletic contest held in Madison

Square Garden during the last week of December, 1903. Measurements and weights were taken with the greatest care, the contestants being under the strictest surveillance during the whole period and were frequently observed and examined by physicians in New York City. Mr. Macfadden, discussing the case in *Physical Culture*, March, 1904, attributed the gain in weight to the retention within his body of a large part of the distilled water, which Mr. Estapper "took in large quantities."

NO DANGER FROM LOSS OF WEIGHT

There is much fear on the part of many, that fasting may result in tuberculosis. They have the idea that to get thin is to lay oneself liable to this "disease." This fear is unfounded and is based on a false view. The thinness in tuberculosis is not the cause of the trouble but the result of its cause. Loss of weight seems to be essential to recovery from acute "disease," and nature makes certain that the acute sufferer loses weight no matter how much food is taken. Indeed, a typhoid fever patient will lose weight and strength more rapidly if fed in the usual manner than if fasting. Due to the fact that the fasting patient recovers more quickly, and even better, during the most prolonged fast, than when fed the accustomed amounts of "good nourishing food," such a patient will lose less weight if he fasts than if he is fed.

The loss of weight during a fast does not represent a loss of vital tissue, but of surplus nutriment, waste, fat, etc. It is just so many pounds of "disease" that one loses. The muscles, for example, decrease in size. But this is due to a decrease in the amount of fat in them and to a decrease in the size of their cells. There is no actual lessening of the number of muscle cells during the ordinary fast.

Tuberculosis quite often develops in the plethoric and "well-fed." Professor Morgulis rightly declares: "as a social phenomenon, malnutrition is not simply a matter of either insufficient or improper nourishment: It is the sinister combination of blighting influences of poverty—overcrowding, under-clothing, unhealthy and unhygienic environment. Here is the fertile soil on which tuberculosis reaps its ghastly harvest."

The weight lost during a fast is rapidly regained, if it is desirable to do so. There is not the slightest danger from loss of weight.

Fasting Does Not Induce
Deficiency "Disease"

CHAPTER XVIII

Deficiency diseases—scurvy, rickets, multiple neuritis (beriberi), pellagra, certain anemias, and similar symptom-complexes—that are due, in great measure to vitamin, mineral and protein deficiencies in the diet or failure to utilize these elements, even though present in the diet, do not result from fasting, even the most prolonged fasts, keeping in mind the definition of fasting employed in this book. So far as I know, I was the first to call attention to the remarkably significant fact that fasting, unlike deficient diets, does not cause deficiency diseases. This I did more than thirty years ago.

Tilden, Weger, Rabagliati, Hay and others have repeatedly shown the value of fasting in anemia; McCullom showed it to be beneficial in rickets; I have employed it with benefit in early pellagra. I am of the opinion that it will prove helpful in multiple neuritis and other deficiency diseases.

In experiments with animals fed on mineral free diets, it was found that they became weak, dull, listless, had fits and died. They reached a point where they refused to eat. Forced feeding was resorted to. It was found that the animals that were forced to eat the mineral-free diet, after their instincts had put out a stop sign, died quicker than animals not fed at all. In experiments of this nature it was found that the nervous system suffered most. A dog so fed showed sudden fits of madness, became weak and uncertain of his movements, trembled and showed signs of nervousness, and grew weaker and weaker until he could hardly crawl.

Years ago Dr. Foster's experiments proved that pigeons and dogs develop symptoms of auto-intoxication and die sooner when fed on foods artificially deprived of their minerals, than when given no food at all. Dogs fed on demineralized food died in twenty-six to thirty days; whereas dogs completely deprived of all food lived for forty to sixty days. One will starve to death with just as much certainty and much more speedily, if one attempts to live upon foods containing only one or two elements of nutrition, as if one were totally abstaining from food. A diet of white flour and water, or white sugar and water, will result in death much sooner than a diet of water only. If no food is eaten the body feeds upon its own food reserves, but it has no provision for meeting the exigencies created by prolonged subsistence on one-sided diets.

If no food is taken the body feeds upon its stored reserves and its less vital tissues. If necessary, until the skeleton condition is reached, it is able to maintain a balance between its elements and will not develop, beyond emaciation, any of the "deficiency diseases." Indeed, judicious fasting is distinctly beneficial in such "diseases." But nature has made no adequate provision for properly nourishing a body that is fed indefinitely upon half-foods. The body does not contain within itself the elements needed to compensate, for more than a brief time, for the deficiency created by denatured foods. Indeed, as pointed out elsewhere, one may starve to death much quicker on some diets, than one will if totally abstaining from food. One will die quicker on a diet of white flour than from fasting, and the more flour one consumes, the more severe will be one's suffering and the sooner will one die. Such foods draw so heavily on certain of the body's reserve elements that these are soon exhausted and body chemistry becomes badly unbalanced.

In innutrition and undernutrition we have a failure to balance the physiological expenditures of the organism. The diet is either inadequate as a whole, or else it is lacking in some essential components. This results in malnutrition. In this condition, there is an unbalanced demand upon the stored reserves of the body caused by the presence of most of the body's needs in the food eaten, with a deficiency of some of its needs. There is, as a consequence, a basic difference between the processes of metabolism under the two sets of conditions. Contrary phenomena occur when the body is fasting. The body easily controls the use and loss of its reserves, using some of them comparatively rapidly, while conserving, hoarding and redistributing others. In this manner chemical balance is maintained and no "deficiency disease" is produced and no organ is crippled. In total fasting, the body's reserves are drawn upon in a balanced manner, or else, those elements that are most abundant are used most rapidly, so that balance is preserved or is restored, as a consequence.

Prof. Morgulis says that "our observation that the chronically underfed dog became debilitated in a measure not commonly noted in animals which undergo a straight fast is also borne out by the more extensive study of this matter by Benedict, Miles, Roth and Smith." This bears out my contention that fasting does not produce the same deplorable results in the body that underfeeding or unbalanced feeding does. Fasting tends to maintain and even to restore chemical balance; whereas, the unbalanced or inadequate diet tends to unbalance the body's chemistry.

Scurvy, typhus, spotted fever, influenza and diarrhea are reported to develop in famine districts. Following in the wake of famine and persisting long afterwards, rickets, diarrhea, various skin eruptions and purulent inflammation of the eyes are found in nearly all children. The famine of 1848 in Ireland left a large number of blind women and men behind. The number of blind increased from 13,812 in 1848 to 45,947 in 1851. It is such experiences as these that have served to prejudice thousands against fasting. They have not known that the most prolonged fasting never produces such results. Fasting never produces blindness, deafness, idiocy, insanity, eye "diseases," rickets, bowel disorders, etc., that follow in the wake of famine. So long as no food is consumed the organism seems to be able to supply from its stored reserves the elements needed to sustain the vital organs and their functions and to supply these elements in correct proportions. These evils are out-growths, not of complete abstinence from food, but of a very one-sided or unbalanced diet. We meet with them in the absence of famine, right here in America, as a result of such diets. Purulent inflammation of the eyes and various skin eruptions are frequent out-growths of carbohydrate excess. Sore eyes, "simple" or "purulent," develop almost wholly in children who eat lots of sugar, syrup, white bread, etc., and who do not get fresh fruits and vegetables. Not even an inadequate diet of fruits and green vegetables ever produces such conditions.

Jackson points out that the teeth are "especially susceptible to rickets and scurvy" and that in both animals and man, there are slight changes in chemical composition, especially in chronic (incomplete) inanition. In the young, such inanition may delay the process of dentition, but persistent growth and development of the teeth (as of the skeleton) occur in young rabbits held at a constant body weight by underfeeding.

"The effects of partial inanition have been studied in rickets and in scurvy. In both human and animal *rickets* there is delayed and abnormal dentition. Both enamel and dentine may be defective and imperfectly calcified."

Without additional quotations about the effects of deficient diets (partial inanition) upon the teeth in rickets and in scurvy, let us point out that dentists who have studied the effects of inadequate and deficient diets upon the teeth and do not know that fasting does not produce the same results as such diets are likely to conclude that fasting injures the teeth. Indeed, there is a tendency in all who study the effects of dietary inadequacies and deficiencies to run away from fasting; for, they reason, "if a defective diet produces such undesirable results, no food at all should produce much worse results." They are blissfully unaware that fasting not only does not produce any of the so-called deficiency "diseases," but that it is actually beneficial in everyone of them.

Jackson says that: "In *scurvy*, the gums are markedly congested and swollen in about 80 per cent of adult human cases, * * * The alveolar bone and peridental membrane undergoes necrosis, with consequent loosening of the teeth, and ulcerations or pyorrhea may occur." In pyorrhea we see inflammation and ulceration of the gums, pus formation, loosening of the teeth, necrosis of the jaw, and even falling out of the teeth. In numerous cases of pyorrhea that we have cared for, the gum inflammation has subsided, the ulcers have healed, pus formation has ceased and the loosened teeth have become firmly fixed in their sockets, and all of this has occurred while the patient was fasting. The effects of fasting must not be confused with the effects of a white-flour-lard-pie-pasteurized-milk-mashed-potato-diet. Not only do such conditions not develop during even a prolonged fast, but they are improved and many of their symptoms completely removed by a fast. This remarkable evidence of the value of fasting is explained by the fact that there is a disproportionate loss of the various constituent elements of the body during the fast and a redistribution of some of these, which results in a near approach to normal body chemistry.

It is quite probable that it is much easier for the body to secure and utilize its mineral reserves during a fast than on a one-sided diet. Several years ago, Prof. Forster, of Munchen, who made experiments on fasting animals and animals fed on mineral-free diets and found that animals fed on mineral-free diets died quicker than animals not fed at all, explained that if no food is eaten the body is nourished on itself and, consequently, a supply of mineral is obtained from the broken down tissues, but if the body is nourished on foods freed of their organic salts, there is no demand made upon the tissues for albumen and carbohydrates and so no minerals are derived from broken down tissue.

The body possesses a reserve from which, in emergency, it may, for a time, draw the required minerals, vitamins and other elements. Animals fed on demineralized foods are compelled to expend their reserves in two directions — (1) in the regular processes of life; and (2) in balancing up the mineral-poor foods they are consuming — while animals deprived of all foods (fasting) are forced to expend their reserves only in carrying on the ordinary (though somewhat reduced) processes of life. The reserves of the fasting animal last much longer and the body's chemical balance is also maintained.

We know, of course, that the body fed on a denatured diet is capable of extracting minerals from its own tissues, but its mineral reserve is never great enough to meet the constant demands made upon it by a mineral-free diet. The mineral-free diet exhausts these reserves very rapidly. During a fast no such demand is made upon the body's mineral reserves. The body's vitamin and complettin reserves, supposed to be stored in the liver and a few other internal organs, are also exhausted much more quickly on a deficient diet than on a fast.

Experiments with deficient diets must be carried out over sufficiently long periods of time to exhaust the body's possibilities of self-help before the effects of the diet can be seen. Its own reserves must first be exhausted before the deficiency will begin to be manifest. However, when a nitrogen-free diet is given the body, it is forced to draw upon its own stores for material. We know that under these circumstances the most important elements are vigorously retained by the body and an intensive nitrogen hunger is induced. The ability to utilize nitrogen is actually improved.

During fasting the same retention of the most important constituents of the body's stored material takes place even more efficiently than when on an inadequate diet. For, while the fast compels the body to draw upon its reserves, the denatured or unbalanced diets draw excessively upon certain of these stores and compel their more rapid utilization. Indeed, the more of the elements supplied by the diet are given, the greater is the demand made upon the stored material not supplied by the diet. It is largely for this reason that death can be produced quicker by a diet of white flour, or white sugar, or meat soup, etc., than by starvation. During the fast the body can regulate the expenditure of its stored materials in its own best interest and can conserve these in such a manner as to make them hold out longest. On a denatured diet, the demand for stored material is such that this regulation is impossible. The stored reserves are soon exhausted by those elements contained in the diet and become as denatured or inadequate or unbalanced or deficient as the diet itself.

There is more malnutrition due to overfeeding with an embargo on assimilation than to underfeeding. More often there is a loss of power to assimilate special elements than an absence of them in the diet. Animal experimentation has shown that when animals are fed mineral-free diets their nervous systems suffer most of all. Nervousness, weak and uncertain movements and fits of madness develop as a result of such diets. On the other hand, the nervous system suffers least of all (almost none at all) in animals that are given no food of any kind, except water, until they die of starvation. This marked difference between the effects of fasting, even of starvation, and the effects of deficient diets may be seen in man if we contrast a case of beri-beri (multiple neuritis) or of pellagra with a man who has fasted forty, fifty or sixty days. Nothing could more clearly demonstrate the terrible drain upon the body's reserves caused by the deficient diet than such a contrast.

In beri-beri, for example, paresis, especially in the lower extremities, paresthesia (diminished feeling), hyperesthesia (excess feeling), tenderness of the nerve trunks and loss of deep reflexes are the chief nervous symptoms present. In its advanced stage, pellagra also presents symptoms referable to widespread changes in the brain and cord. The fasting patient, after a most prolonged fast, not only does not present these or other nervous symptoms, but has lost all or nearly all of the nervous symptoms he may have had at the beginning of the fast. Almost all the effects of fasting, with the exception of the loss of weight and sometimes a temporary loss of strength, are exactly opposite to the effects of the deficient or denatured diet.

Pashutin says that he has found in his experiments on dogs, that "when mineral salts are purposely withheld from the animal's food for long periods, other food from which all mineral salts have been removed being given, the animal will use the mineral salts in the body over and over, none being excreted or passed in the urine, as occurs when the animal has a plentiful supply of mineral salts in its food." This is only partially true. Whether the animal is fasting or on a mineral-free diet, it seeks to retain its minerals as long as possible. There is, however, a day by day loss of more or less of these, so that in the case of the mineral-free diet, minerals must sooner or later be added to the diet or serious trouble results. The mineral exhaustion of the organism occurs much more rapidly, as previously shown, on a denatured diet than on a fast.

Dr. Kellogg offers, among his many objections to fasting, this one: "The body is also continually losing vitamins which are essential for the promotion of the processes of repair and the maintenance of the various vital functions. The daily supply of vitamins is as necessary as the daily supply of air and water. Vitamins cannot be produced by the animal body. They are an exclusive product of plant life. The liver hoards a small store of vitamins sufficient to serve in emergency, but the supply is not sufficient to last indefinitely, and, as shown by the experience of sailors who contract scurvy and those who become the victims of beri-beri through living upon polished rice, the vitamin store of the liver soon becomes exhausted and the body then falls into serious disorder. Fasting deprives the body of vitamins and this involves the risk of serious injury for which no adequate compensation is offered. The total loss of all vitamins must certainly involve greater damage than the loss of one only, yet the absence of but one of the three known vitamins for even a short period produces noticeable injury. Certainly the body can be in no way benefitted by the deprivation of food iron, food lime, and other food salts, and of the precious vitamins, the activators of the vital process."

We have no means of knowing how much of a reserve store of vitamins the body possesses, nor do we know where all of these reserves are stored; still less do we know about how much of these vitamins are lost from the body during a fast. All of this is as unknown to Kellogg and to the writer as to the reader, but we may be sure of one thing:—namely, these stores are sufficient to outlast the most prolonged fast. We know that scurvy and beri-beri never develop on a fast. We know that rickets is positively benefitted by fasting. Kellogg overlooks an important difference between fasting and a polished rice diet—namely, that, whereas, in both, the body is deprived of its daily supply of vitamins, fasting makes little if any demand upon its vitamin reserves, while the polished rice diet rapidly consumes these. If he could show that fasting, even the most prolonged fasting, ever produces "deficiency disease," then his objection would have some weight. As it is, the facts of experience must silence the voice of his theory.

It is well to recall that animal flesh does contain vitamins, certain portions of the animal containing higher concentrations of the various vitamins than other portions. The carnivorous animal secures all of his vitamins from the flesh, bones and blood of his prey. He tends to eat those organs that contain the highest vitamin and mineral concentrations. The vitamins stored in the tissues of the body are released, as weight is lost (this is to say, as the tissues are liquidated), and are made available for use in carrying on the essential nutritive processes of life.

Vitamin deficient diets compel the body to consume its vitamin stores; but we do not know that the body is forced to consume these stores in living off its own internal resources. We cannot say positively that these reserve stores do not contain the vitamins necessary to their utilization. We only know that pathological conditions attributed to avitaminosis do not develop as a result of prolonged fasting. Since there are no such injuries, they do not require adequate compensation. Fasting does not produce deep-seated and hidden injuries that make themselves felt at a later date. There is no harmful destruction of important or vital tissues from fasting. Weger says: "Even though vitamins are in a small degree consumed by fasting, we consider this factor quite negligible compared with the refinement of body chemistry and the overwhelming influence for general good that takes place. After a fast the tissues are more receptive and readily assimilate as well as utilize vitamins that are necessary elements contained in vital or base-forming foods."—*Defense of Rational Fasting.*

Death in the Fast

CHAPTER XIX

Opponents never tire of telling us of the "large number of deaths" that have occurred "as a result of fasting." They read the story of the death of a faster in some sensational newspaper and, without knowing anything of the circumstances of the death, repeat the story over and over. If we were to publish the story of every death of patients while being treated with poisons by the physicians, they would rise up in their organized might and denounce us for insinuating that they are a group of murderers.

It is the general custom for the Press to herald far and wide every death during a fast, and attribute the death to starvation. The many thousands who fast and live, who fast and recover health, are not mentioned. Horrified relatives and enterprising newspaper writers are sure to see that the world receives full information about any case of death during a fast. Cases of death are often attributed to "starvation," where death was due to other causes. We quite naturally expect that where thousands of cases are concerned, there will be an occasional death, whether patients fast or feast. But we may be certain that if we had some means of recording the experiences of a thousand individuals for a period of twenty years or more, while fasting and while eating, more deaths would occur among those taking three meals a day than among those who fast while sick.

A few years ago Theodore Neuffer of Goldsboro, Pa., was reported to have died after only 18 days without food. As a newborn baby can go longer than that without food, it is possible that Neuffer died of causes other than starvation. He was 84 years old and it was said that because of his age he couldn't stand the strain. As numerous people of his age and older have "stood the strain" of much longer fasts with benefit, it is still probable that his death was not due to starvation.

Dewey established the fact that it is physiologically impossible to starve to death before the skeleton condition is reached (by this is meant the mere weight of the skeleton and viscera). This fact has not been fully understood by many of the advocates of fasting, still less by its opponents. Opponents of fasting point to cases of death occurring long before the skeleton condition is reached, while there is still considerable flesh, even fat on the body, sometimes, indeed, within a few days after starting the fast, and declare that these instances disprove Dewey's contention. Physiologists, on the other hand, estimate that "strong adults die when they lose two-fifths of the body weight."

It must be noted that instances of such deaths in fasting are extremely rare. Instances of prolonged fasting by people of all ages and in all possible physical conditions, are very common. Such deaths are, as will be seen, exceptions rather than the rule, and are to be accounted for in some other way than on the assumption that they resulted from starvation. For example, there is the testimony of Miss Marie Davenport Vickers (*The Mazdaznan* Feb., 1906, p. 28) who fasted forty-two days to good health from April 19, to June 1, 1904. She tells us that on two former occasions, before she knew anything of fasting, other than having seen it mentioned in the Bible, she was forced to go without food for some days, owing to lack of funds with which to purchase it. She says: "and I did almost starve to death." I was once called to see a woman on the fourteenth day of a fast she had undertaken at home. She was a large, fat woman, with high blood pressure, heart disease, diabetes, etc. I did not like the general aspect of the case and advised that she break her fast. She refused and in another day began to vomit. Three days later, she fainted while coming from the bath room. This frightened her. She never overcame her fright. Perhaps she would have done so, had a meddlesome and "know-it-all" daughter not kept up her fear-engendering suggestions day and night. I have always been convinced that the chief cause of death in this case was fear. It certainly was not starvation, for at death she weighed nearly two hundred pounds. In Herter's *Lectures On Chemical Pathology* he tells us that death from inanition is not a possibility till the body has lost at least a third of its normal weight.

Sick people are dying all the time. People seldom turn to fasting until they are desperate. It is inevitable that among such a desperately ill class of people a few deaths will occur. A physician who discovered a new "cure" for illness and was permitted to use it only upon cases that had been given up by all other doctors, would be looked upon as a great physician if he effected only an occasional *cure.* It is an indisputable fact that of the thousands who go upon a fast to enable them to recover from their ills, most of them have suffered for years and have given "regular" and "irregular" physicians unlimited opportunity to effect their recovery.

In thousands of fasts ranging from a few days to sixty and even ninety days, no deaths have occurred that could be attributed to the fast. In every case, where an autopsy has been made, this has revealed an organic "disease" which would have resulted in death, with or without food. Dr. Dewey properly maintained, that if one's vitality is so nearly exhausted, or if a vital organ is so badly damaged, that death is near at hand, the result is absolutely certain, eating or fasting. Most people turn to fasting as a last resort, instead of the first resort. They turn to it after their bodies have been wrecked and ruined by years of wrong living, drugging and surgical operations. Under such circumstances we naturally expect that an occasional patient will die even while fasting. Honesty and fairness will not attribute death, under these conditions, to the fast.

We should bear in mind that of the thousands of patients treated in the regular way and regularly fed "plenty of good nourishing food," a large percentage die. How absurd, then, to blame fasting for the exceedingly small number of cases that have died while fasting when, too late, they turned to this method of *healing.* Dr. S. Lief, of England, says in the June 1929 issue of *Health For All:* "During eighteen years' experience in the treatment of thousands of cases, we have not known a single case where death took place as a result of fasting."

Dewey not only emphasized the fact that it is physiologically impossible to starve to death before the skeleton condition is reached, but he also emphasized the fact that nature will always demand food long before this stage is reached, providing it is a remediable case. That people have died before the skeleton stage is reached is true, but in such instances death has been due to causes other than starvation. Too many people turn to fasting as a last resort; whereas, it should be the first resort. If, standing with one foot in the grave and the other on a banana peel, they attempt a fast as a last desperate attempt to save life, and they die while fasting, the fast should not be blamed for the death. Fasting is a natural, vital process, and no such process is injurious unless it is wrongly used or over-used.

Writing in *Physical Culture,* Sept. 1912, Dr. Linda Burfield Hazzard says: "when severe and distressing manifestations arise during the period of abstinence from food, it is virtually certain that defects in organism lie within. Post-mortem examination of bodies of patients who have died while the fast was in progress give proof beyond confutation to this all important point, and in these cases it was further demonstrated that death would have occurred fasting or feeding." In a letter to Mr. R. B. Pearson, dated Nov. 18, 1919, Dr. Hazzard writes, "In sixteen years actual active practice" she had "fasted nearly 2500 cases with eighteen deaths, in every case of *death a post mortem never failed to reveal organic defects* which made death the inevitable outcome, fasting or feeding." Then she adds: "I have never turned a patient away."

Dr. Dewey says (*The No Breakfast Plan and Fasting Cure,* p. 31); "As the months and years went on, it so happened that all my fatalities were of a character as not to involve in the least suggestions of starvation, while the recoveries were a series of demonstrations as clear as anything in mathematics, of evolving strength of all the muscles, of all the senses and faculties as the disease declined.° ° ° For years I saw patients grow in the strength of health without the slightest clue to the mystery, until I chanced to open a new edition of Yeo's Physiology at the page where I found this table of estimated losses that occur in death after starvation.° ° ° And light came as if the sun had suddenly appeared in the zenith at midnight. Instantly I saw in human bodies a vast reserve of pre-digested food.° ° ° I now knew that there could be no death from starvation until the body was reduced to the skeleton condition.° ° ° I could now know that to die of starvation is a matter not of days, but of weeks and months; certainly a period far beyond the average time of recovery from acute disease."

"Death during a fast cannot occur," says Dr. Hazzard, "unless there is organic disease, and not then unless the organ or organs affected are in such degenerated state as not to permit of repair; and it is conclusively demonstrated that in a scientifically directed fast, although death in the condition cited cannot be averted, yet because of organic labor lessened, life is prolonged for days or weeks, and distress and pain, if present, are much alleviated."

Tilden says: "It is safe to say that when anyone dies while going without food it is due to the fact that he died from the disease before the fast could be extended long enough for it to be thrown off, or from fright, or from lack of proper nursing, being allowed to freeze to death. It is a mistake to associate in mind the two terms 'fasting' and 'starving' as one and the same. It requires great skill to fast a patient properly. Any fool can starve a patient to death." There are conditions in the bodies of many patients which lead to death inevitably. If one so afflicted dies while fasting, everyone is only too willing to place the blame for death upon the fast. Dr. Hazzard says that in her experience "death during a fast never has occurred when merely functional disorder was present, nor did it ever result for the sole reason that food was withheld."

True starvation begins only when the body has been reduced to the skeleton and the viscera. Dr. Dewey declares: "When death occurs before the skeleton condition is reached it is always due to old age or some form of disease or injury and not to starvation." The organism deprived of income, must draw upon its capital to meet the expenses of living. Life endures as long as the reserve capital lasts. He records the case of a frail, spare boy of four years, whose stomach was so disorganized by a drink of a solution of caustic potash that not even a swallow of water could be retained. He died on the 75th day of his fast, with the mind clear to the last hour, and with apparently nothing of the body left but bones, ligaments, and a thin skin, and yet the brain had lost neither weight nor functional clearness. "In another city a similar accident happened to a child of about the same age, in whom it took three months for the brain to exhaust entirely the available body-food." If such a prolonged period is required for a small boy to starve to death, death from inanition is certainly a remote possibility in the average adult who carries a much larger reserve of food. It should not be overlooked that the length of time any individual can live without food is determined by the amount of reserve food stored in his or her body. The fat person can go wtihout food much longer than the thin person.

The average patient need have no fear of starving before he recovers from his trouble. I have fasted patients for as much as twenty days who were "skin and bones" at the outset of the fast. In no instance has such a patient been injured by the fast. If fear and worry are absent, if the faster is warm and not forced to exert himself, he may go without food for a long period not only without damage to his body, but with actual benefit.

The *American Encyclopedia* quotes Chossat and Brown-Sequard as saying: "In man, as in animals, the immediate cause of death from starvation is a decline in the animal temperature. Death is accelerated by cold, and delayed by the presence of moisture in the atmosphere." Pashutin mentions the case of a man whose temperature remained normal throughout a 50 days' fast and says: "However, we know from the experiments upon animals that only when the total of the body reserves is consumed, the body temperature decreases markedly."

It is suggested that the "true mode of death" from starvation is from want of heat, due, no doubt, to a lack of combustible material at the end. Chossat found in starving animals, that when death seemed imminent, restoration could be effected by the application of artificial heat. The *American Encyclopedia* recounts that M. Chossat "deprived a number of animals (birds and small mammals) of all sustenance and carefully observed the phenomena that followed, and his experiments throw much light upon the subject of starvation. The temperature in all the animals was maintained at nearly the normal standard until the last day of life, when it began rapidly to fall. The animals previously restless now became quiet, as if stupefied; they fell over on their side unable to stand, the breathing became slower and slower, the pupils dilated, the insensibility grew more profound, and death took place either quietly or attended with convulsions. If when these phenomena were fully developed, external warmth was applied, the animals revived, their muscular force returned, they moved or flew about the room and took greedily to the food that was presented to them. If now they were again left to themselves they speedily perished; but if the external temperature were maintained until the food taken was digested (and from the feeble condition of their digestive organs this often took many hours) they recovered. The immediate cause of death seemed to be cold rather than starvation."

Carrington gives 76° Farenheit as the lowest temperature at which life has survived in human beings, although we know that some warm-blooded animals (hibernating) have survived a body temperature as low as 2° Centigrade. Despite the fact that one maintains normal body temperature on a fast, or even has a rise in temperature, there is a feeling of chilliness in a moderate temperature in which one ordinarily feels comfortable. This is due to decreased cutaneous circulation.

Fasting does not cause death. Starvation results in death, and any death that occurs during a fast must be credited to other causes. Several theories have been offered to account for death from starvation; for, it is known that death is not due to exhaustion of stored food, since fat and other stores may persist in appreciable amounts, but none of them are adequate. The following are the most prominent theories that have been offered to account for death: (1) impoverishment of the blood, resulting from loss of solids; (2) fall of temperature (obviously not applicable to cold-blooded animals); (3) inability of organs to utilize remaining reserve stores (inability not explained); (4) asphyxia resulting from paralysis of respiratory center by accumulation of toxic materials; (5) auto-intoxication, produced by toxins, resulting from disordered metabolism of malnourished tissues; (6) it is suggested that death is due to infection due to lowered resistance; (7) also to disorders of the ductless glands. As all of these conditions are present in varying degree it has been suggested that the immediate cause of death may vary according to circumstances.

The loss of weight in total inanition, in animals, resulting in death, runs from 30 to 65 per cent; averaging about 40 per cent; but varies with the age of the animal, the temperature and activity as well as with different kinds of animals. Certain arthropoda can sustain a loss of ninety per cent of body weight before life ends. In many cases of fasting in man, death has not resulted until after a loss of 60 to 70 per cent of body weight.

Morgulis found that the collie, a high strung nervous dog, dies after a loss of only 30 per cent of body weight, whereas other animals recovered health after a weight loss of 60 per cent, which suggests that mental and nervous peculiarities need to be taken into account in the conduct of a fast. We see many striking examples of this principle in fasting nervous people. We never permit them to go without food long enough to result in death but many of them do not stand fasting as well as the non-nervous types.

Starvation can come only after the body is reduced to the skeleton condition, death resulting then more as a result of cold than anything else. This means that no one will ever starve to death as a result of fasting in "disease." If death occurs at all during the fast it would not occur in the time required to recover from practically all "diseased" states.

Pashutin records the case of a girl who drank sulphuric acid and ruined her digestive tract. He says, "some liquid food was given for four months but not believed absorbed as it was eliminated too rapidly and no chlorides in urine at all. Last 16 days no food at all." In this case the body temperature did not begin to decline until the last 8 days of life. Many fasts of long duration are on record. Mr. Macfadden recorded one of ninety days; nine of the Cork hunger strikers fasted for ninety-four days; thousands have fasted up to forty days and longer. Many fasts have gone to fifty, sixty and seventy days and longer, McSwiney died on the seventy-eighth day of his fast. While this hunger-strike was on, I heard Dr. Lindlahr tell of a fast of seventy days which he conducted. Dr. Dewey records one of three months. In none of these cases has there ever developed deficiency "diseases" nor has death ever been due to so-called acidosis. It would seem that a deficiency "disease" can only develop when the body is being filled with denatured foods. Its vast store of reserves seems to be well-balanced. It is known that the blood has almost unlimited power for resisting analkalinity (acidosis), for it will die before turning acid.

More remarkable proof that death in *Hygienic* fasts is due to irremediable organic troubles, and not to starvation, is the fact that it has been found that in every case where death occurred, there still remained considerable subcutaneous fat, and this is always entirely absent in death by starvation. The heart has been found to be normal in all cases, except where normal development had never occurred, while in real starvation, the heart is always markedly atrophied and contracted. The blood has always been found to be practically normal in volume with no real anemia, while in starvation there is a marked decrease in the relative blood volume with a marked anemia. In death during *Hygienic* fasts the pancreas has been found to be either not affected at all, or but slightly; in starvation this organ is almost entirely absent.

Here, let me emphasize the fact that the destructive and degenerative conditions found in animals, which have been used in laboratory experiments in inanition, are due to starvation and not to fasting. The line of demarkation between fasting and starving is distinct and unmistakable, although few, if any laboratory investigators have ever recognized it. We know that it is only when the total of the body's reserves has been utilized that death from starvation can occur, and it is only then that nature will permit any vital organ to be damaged. The autopsy, in every case of death while fasting, shows that there was some serious organic "disease" which made death inevitable, whether the patient fasted or ate "plenty of good nourishing food." Indeed, it may be affirmed, with a reasonable degree of certainty, that death would have come sooner in practically every instance except for the fast.

Sinclair says: "It is perfectly true that men have died of starvation in three or four days; but the starvation existed in their minds— It was fright that killed them. *** As an example of the part that mental disturbances may play in the fast, I will cite the case of a woman friend who started out to fast for a complication of chronic ailments. She was rather stout, and did not mind it at all—was going cheerfully about her daily tasks; but her husband heard about it and came home to tell her what a fool she was making of herself; and in a few hours she was in a state of complete collapse. No doubt if there had been a physician in the neighborhood, there would have been another tale of a 'victim of a shallow and unscrupulous sensationalist.' Fortunately, however, business called the husband away again, and the next day the woman was all right, and completed an eight days fast with the best results. Bear this in mind, so that if you wake up some morning and find your temperature sub-normal and your pulse at forty, and your arms too weak to lift you, and if your friends get 'round you and tell you that you look like a mummy out of a sarcophagus of the seventh dynasty—you may be able to smile at them good naturedly and tell them that you will never again eat until you are hungry."

Fear of the fast should certainly be avoided. I do not doubt that well-meaning, misguided relatives and friends of fasters have caused the death of more than one by their cultivation of fear in the fasting individual. One hesitates to say that a loving son or daughter kills his or her mother or father, yet the evidence certainly points this way in more than one case. We should encourage and cooperate with the faster and not frighten him to death.

Objections to the Fast

CHAPTER XX

A number of supposedly scientific objections to the fast are offered from various sources but not from any source that is entitled, from actual and broad experience with the fast, to speak with authority. I have not met with a single objection to fasting that was not based upon a lack of knowledge of fasting or upon a mere half-truth. Evils sometimes attributed to fasting are accountable for by other causes. There are many attempting to conduct patients through long fasts who do not know how to do so. Fasting is simple and, when properly done, always beneficial. Those who condemn fasting should first understand it and should have had sufficient experience with it to enable them to know what they are talking about. I read a statement by a prominent medical columnist that often fasting will bring on an "attack" of illness due to too much insulin in the blood, the insulin being secreted by the patient's own pancreas. I wonder how he found this out. As he never places patients on fasts, what can he know of fasting? I fast cases of hyper-insulism with benefit.

In preceding pages many of the commonest objections have been met and disposed of in discussing various parts of our subject, so that but few objections remain for us to discuss at this place.

The old opponents of fasting were open and frank in their attacks upon it. They declared that it weakened the heart, caused the stomach to atrophy, caused adhesions in the stomach, caused the gastric juice to turn upon and digest the stomach and made similar unfounded objections to its use. It was contended by them that a fast of six days would cause the heart to collapse and the patient would die. These old opponents denied that any benefits could come through fasting, but that it constituted a great and immediate danger. Time and experience proved all of these objections to be unfounded and we hear no more of them. Even in cases of death from starvation, nothing has been found to justify the old notion that if we do not eat the gastric juice will "eat up the stomach." The heart does not collapse, even in the longest fast, and this objection has been removed from the encyclopedias.

The present day opponent of fasting is a different type of man and offers a different type of objection to its use. The present attack upon fasting is underhanded. The attacker comes in the guise of a friend. It is now the practice to admit that fasting is often beneficial and then to attempt to kill it by talking learnedly of its imaginary dangers and saying nothing of its benefits. Warnings about the dangers of fasting come from those who know least about it and who have had no experience with it.

Men like McCollum, who have had no experience in caring for patients and who have a wholly wrong conception of the essential nature of so-called "disease" and are unable to rightly interpret symptoms, offer theoretical objections to fasting which grow out of their failure to rightly interpret the developments during a fast. We are gravely warned of the dangers of decomposition of the digestive juices, particularly the bile, during the fast, and are told that the coating of the tongue is proof of this. They tell us also that there is an excess of decomposition products in the urine during a fast. The fact is that there can be no more decomposition products entering the body from the digestive tract when this is empty than enter it when it is full of decomposing food. There is a gradual decrease in the amount of such products in the urine as the fast progresses, until finally, they cease altogether to appear in the urine. The sluggishness of the intestines during the fast may result in a temporary increase in the amount of such products during the early days of the fast, but even this can be so only in a few patients. The digestive juices are all antiseptic and resist decomposition. Bile is antiseptic and aids in keeping the intestine and colon aseptic. It does not decompose readily. It is frequently regurgitated into the stomach and vomited so that there is no posssibility of its decomposing and poisoning the body. The supposed evidences of bile decomposition grow less and less as the fast progresses until finally they completely disappear.

Dr. J. H. Kellogg was long one of the chief foes of fasting. He compiled a number of objections, most of which have been met in preceding pages. There are frequent references to the benefits of fasting in his *New Dietetics* and also much discussion of the damages produced by fasting. He says: "It is certainly irrational to suppose that great benefit can come from prolonged and painful resistance of a natural instinct with which the body is endowed by Nature for its protection by securing the prompt and regular meeting of its essential requirements. Hunger is a sensation through which nature serves notice upon the consciousness that the energy resourecs of the body are running low and need to be reinforced; in other words, that food is needed. Thirst is a sensation which notifies intelligence of the need of water. On purely *a priori* grounds it would seem to be highly unreasonable that man should use his intelligence to thwart this means of automatic defense of the body against injury.

"Argument could be offered in favor of water fasting as well as of food fasting. Indeed, why should not one restrain himself from gratifying the sense of air hunger which prompts constant rhythmic action of the lungs? Air hunger, water hunger, and ordinary hunger are simply nature's demands for supplies of different kinds of foods which the body needs for its protection and the maintenance of its functions."

This objection to fasting reveals that Dr. Kellogg knows nothing at all about fasting and the claims of those who advocate fasting. We all agree fully with the above statements. Nobody advocates continued abstinence from food in the face of hunger. Dr. Kellogg overlooks the essential fact that the instinct that fails to call for food or that produces repugnance to food or that causes the stomach to vomit food or the intestines and colon to hurriedly expel it in a diarrhea, is equally as reliable as the one that calls for food. This man who pleads for the reign of instinct in eating, advocates a carbohydrate diet—"abundant carbohydrate feeding"—in fevers, where there is lacking both the desire for food and the ability to digest it. He feeds despite the most obvious protests of instinct. His insistence upon sugar in some form, even in the most violent stages of "disease," is due, in great measure, to his fear of germs; which, he says "will not grow or at least are not virulent and active in producing toxins in the presence of sugar."

Kellogg says: "Statkewitsch studied the effects of fasting in a large number of animals—cats, dogs, rabbits, pigeons, frogs, lizards, and other animals—and found that after prolonged fasting the cells of the heart, liver, muscles, kidneys, pancreas and other glands were the seat of degenerative processes. These processes were most marked in the muscles and the glands." His objections to fasting are largely based on the damages produced in the starvation period. All the evils attributed to fasting, which are enumerated in the works of laboratory experimenters, are the results of starvation. This is to say, these results are found in animals that have died of starvation, the destructive changes all having occurred after the exhaustion of the body's reserves. Laboratory experimenters are in the habit of thinking that starvation sets in with the omission of the first meal, whereas, starvation does not begin until after the return of hunger. Many of Kellogg's assertions with regard to the effects of fasting are directly contradicted by numerous capable laboratory investigators. Those who fail to differentiate between fasting and starving and who are unaware of the important fact that actual vital tissue damage belongs to the starvation period make many absurd statements about fasting. Kellogg speaks of five days without food as a period of starvation. To him fasting and starving are synonymous.

Although opposed to fasting, Kellogg makes the following admissions of benefits received from it:

1. "Surplus body fat may be disposed of."

2. "Any accumulation of surplus or 'floating' nitrogen or waste which may be present will rapidly disappear during a fast."

3. "Fasting creates an appetite by producing an imperious demand for food, and perhaps at the same time increases the ability of the tissues to assimilate food. This effect of fasting may be an advantage in certain cases, particularly when it is desirable to produce a rapid gain in flesh by subsequent overfeeding."

4. "There is some evidence that a prolonged fast may in some instances produce a sort of rejuvenescence in some of the tissues." (He denies that there is any evidence that this is so in man. He can deny this only by shutting his eyes to the wealth of evidence that exists).

5. "The observation has been made that after a prolonged fast, when the body has been built up by proper feeding, there is apparently present an unusual degree of vigor and an enhanced sense of well-being." He tries to escape the implications of this admission by adding: "It is to be noted, however, that a similar observation is often made following recovery from typhoid fever, or some other acute wasting disease in which the patient has been greatly reduced. It is to be further noted, also, that notwithstanding

this apparent rejuvenation accompanying convalescence from fever, the life expectancy of such persons is only one-half of the average person of the same age. Hence, there is ground for believing that notwithstanding the apparent improvement resulting from the fast as well as from the fever, a certain constitutional damage is done, the effects of which become apparent later."

In typhoid and other acute ills, there are present powerful toxins which induce damages. There are also, in most cases, the powerful drugs of the physician as well as the forced feeding. Damages resulting to the body in such a state which show up later, are not properly attributed to the wasting of the body, while the toxins and the drugs are ignored. Dr. Kellogg should show that the life expectancy of typhoid cases is cut in half where no drugs, serums and food are employed. He should also show that fasting cuts short one's life expectancy. He says that "many persons have passed through the ordeal of a long fast and have survived, and in some instances there has been evidence of a notable improvement in health following the fast."

The two chief objections to the fast are: (1) it produces "acidosis" or decreases the alkalinity of the blood; and (2) it weakens the patient, and lessens his chances of recovery while rendering him more liable to other "diseases."

Fasting not only does not reduce resistance to "disease," but, on the contrary, increases resistance. Resistance is the product of pure blood and an abundant nerve force. Fasting, because it increases elimination and conserves nervous energy, adds to these qualities. I have known fasters to be subjected to all kinds of unfavorable influences, but I have yet to see any "disease" develop as a result. I know that "disease" recovers much more rapidly in fasters than in those who eat. The following words of Geo. S. Weger, M.D., agree perfectly with my own experience with fasting:

"In all my personal experience with fasting, I have yet to see a case of tuberculosis develop as a result of it. On the other hand, I have seen many patients recover from tuberculosis who made their first improvements after a fast followed by moderate feeding."

"Real vital resistance is very rarely lowered by fasting. Temporary muscular weakness should not be classed as lowered vitality. Indeed, I have seen many cases of infection of different kinds recover completely on a fast. Take for example an advanced case of sinusitis after five or six painful operations—frontal, ethmoidal and antrum—with surgical drainage and irrigation two or three times a week, continued over a period of two to five years, with no relief or amelioration of symptoms. After almost unendurable suffering, such patients are, as a rule, thin, and physically and mentally depressed. When they make complete recoveries after a prolonged fast, as the great majority of them do, is this not sufficient proof that fasting somehow or other raises the power of the organism to overcome infection, rather than that fasting renders them more susceptible? What is true of sinusitis is equally true of other infections, even those so situated anatomically that they cannot be surgically drained and must therefore be absorbed."—*In Defense of Rational Fasting.*

We have long insisted that fasting increases resistance to *infections.* This claim has usually been met by the counter claim that resistance is lowered by fasting. Mr. Pearson tells us that after his complete fast, mosquito bites caused no itching and no swelling, and that no amount of exposure would cause a cold. It is almost impossible to have a cold in the last days of a prolonged fast and immediately thereafter. Animal experimenters have shown that *resistance* is increased in some animals, decreased in others (pigeons, for example), and unaffected in others. These results cannot be of great aid to us in studying the effects of fasting upon resistance in man. Morgulis tells us that "A subject still very imperfectly known, but one which merits a most careful investigation, is the increase in resistance to infection revealed by organisms which are recovering from inanition. Roger and Jause report such an increased tolerance towards bacilli coli in rabbits which had undergone a preliminary fast of five to seven days. The inoculation with bacterial culture took place three to eleven days after the fast was broken. In each case the control rabbits succumbed to the infection, while all the rabbits which had previously fasted survived the inoculation. These experiments, however, need verification."

The rejuvenating effects of fasting upon the blood have been noted in a previous chapter. It was there shown that fasting does not produce hypoalkalinity. Dr. Weger says concerning the effects of the fast in improving the blood condition: "We quite agree that considerable iron and proportionately other necessary elements may be consumed during a prolonged fast. However, the needful materials in the body are not lost to the same extent that the unusable waste is lost. It should not be forgotten, as previously stated, that the human body has within itself the power to use and refine the materials it has on hand during a reasonable fasting period.

"The writer has witnessed in a case of anemia, actual rejuvenation of the blood during a twelve-day absolute fast, during which time the red blood cells increased from 1,500,000 to 3,200,000, hemoglobin increased from fifty per cent to eighty-five per cent, and the white cells reduced from 37,000 to 14,000.

"This is but one instance of many that have impressed the value of fasting where to some practitioners it might have been contraindicated. If the body, because of its crowded nutrition, cannot assimilate vitamin bearing food, it can be brought into condition to do this by a purifying fast."—*In Defense of Rational Fasting.*

Another objection offered to fasting is purely theoretical and is based on the reigning theories in biochemistry. That these theories are correct has not been shown and there are serious objections to them. At any rate, the developments we should expect if these objections are valid, do not show up during the fast. The objection is this: "All the energy of our bodies comes from either fat or glucose. In order to produce energy all other foods must be changed into fat or glucose, one or the other. But here is the important fact; when blood-sugar or glucose is burned alone, by itself, energy is produced with maximum efficiency. But when fat is burned alone, it is burned incompletely, and yields as by-products acetone and harmful acids, which accumulate more and more as long as fat continues to be burned without sugar. This is what happens when a person attempts to 'fast,' that is, tries to go without food."

If this objection is valid, it would certainly be impossible for us ever to observe gains in strength and energy in fasting patients. Either this objection is wrong, or else all who have seen gains in strength in fasters have been seeing the same kind of things seen by the drunk watching "pink elephants" on the wall.

We refute this objection, not alone on the grounds of experience, but also upon theoretical grounds. First, there is no rapid exhaustion of the body's sugar reserve as this objection implies, when a fast is undergone; second, the fasting body produces a daily supply of glycogen from its stored reserves. The physiologists, Zoethout and Tuttle, say "during starvation (fasting) the blood sugar falls but little below the normal level (although it is being constantly consumed) and the liver still contains some glycogen; this is due to glyconeogenesis."—*Textbook of Physiology. Glyconeogenesis* is the term applied to the formation of sugar in the animal body out of materials other than carbohydrates. Amino acids, after these have been de-aminized, may be transformed into sugar. This is to say that the portion of the amino acid that is left after the amines have been split off may be transformed into sugar. Glycerol, formed by the digestion of fat, may also be converted into glycogen. Apparently the fatty acids—palmitic, stearic, butyric, etc.—cannot be made into sugar.

What, then, becomes of those acetone bodies about which we hear so much? That they do show up in the fast is not denied. But we have a different explanation of them. One of the surest signs that the fast is nearing its end is the disappearance of acetone from the breath, urine and excreta. The presence of acetone is part of the ketosis that fasting is said, in some quarters, to produce.

Ketosis is the presence in the blood of certain end-products of fat-metabolism, known as ketones. There are three ketones—acetone, aceto-acetic and beta-oxybutyric acids. The presence of these bodies in the blood is said to produce acidosis and damage the body. The damages that these ketones produce are never described and those who have had most experience with fasting have never seen them. It would be interesting to see a catalogue of the evils that flow from the presence of these bodies. Dr. Gian-Cursio, who says he has never seen any evidence of harm from the presence of these bodies, and who thinks of them as evidences of normal adjustment to the fasting state, says that "their absence would be cause for alarm."

These same bodies are present in certain stages of diabetes and from this fact, it is reasoned that they are harmful. It is the rule that when there is ketosis, the blood is slightly alkaline so that the acidosis that is imagined is not actually present. It is even denied that diabetic ketosis is the same as fasting ketosis. We are certain of one thing; namely, that the diabetic faster is able to oxydize sugar. Benjamin Harrow, Ph.D., professor of chemistry, City College, College of the City of New York, says: "The fact that in starvation and diabetes, acetone bodies accumulate in an appreciable degree has led to the view that they are abnormal metabolic products. This view must be revised, for the evidence is accumulating that these substances are indeed normal metabolic products." Thus the more advanced physiologists and bio-chemists do not regard the older theory as any longer tenable.

It is claimed that the sick must eat to "keep up their strength," that food cures "disease," and that it increases resistance to "disease." If food *cures* the sick, how did they become sick? If feeding increases resistance to "disease," how do the well-fed fall ill? If fasting lowers resistance, how do so many fasters recover health? If food builds strength, how do the well-fed grow weak? If fasting, *per se,* robs the faster of his strength, how do so many fasters grow stronger? If food is essential to recovery, how do fasting patients ever recover? Why do not all fasting patients die? Why do they have more comfortable and less protracted illnesses and shorter convalescences? Why do they recover without complications and sequels? If people who are taxed to death by excess food become sick, how will more feeding help them? Why does feeding make them worse? Why does temperature run up and discomfort grow more pronounced after eating? What are the diseases that are caused by fasting? Will somebody please give us a catalogue of them? Dr. Shew declared that abstinence does not cause disease, that even the person who dies from starvation dies from *debility* rather than from disease.

During the last illness of the actor, Joseph Jefferson, Dr. Chas. E. Page made the following memorandum from the published accounts of his illness:

April 16th: "Has not retained nourishment."
April 20th: "The patient is better."
April 20th: "Retained nourishment."
April 21st: "More restless: condition less favorable."

According to the published accounts, Mr. Jefferson, who was said to have had pneumonia and who was said to have suffered with gastritis for several months before developing pneumonia, had no desire for food. He was fed in spite of the lack of desire for food and no possibility of digesting and assimilating it. His illness followed an "attack of indigestion from an indiscretion in diet on a visit to a friend." Forced feeding, alcohol and heart *stimulants* finished him off and it was announced that his "age was against him." Was it age or feeding and drugging that killed him?

A patient in a sanatorium with which I was connected some years ago was too weak to walk up the steps at the time he entered the institution. He was placed upon a fast and did not taste food of any kind for eighteen days. Before this time was up he was able to run up the steps. If food gives strength why was he so weak while eating and why did he gain strength when he ceased to eat? I had one patient who was too weak to walk up the steps at the beginning of a fast, but was forced to crawl up the steps. After a week of fasting, he was able to walk up the same steps. Food is not nutrition. Overeating with continued wasting of the body is an every day experience of life. Reduced eating with gain in weight and health is becoming a more common experience as people learn that gluttonous indulgence is not conducive to health of body and clearness of mind. The most important element in nutrition is the living, active body that utilizes the food, and not the dead, passive food that is utilized. When the body is not in a condition to carry on the processes of nutrition, it is worse than idle waste to feed it. Such a patient should fast.

Whatever may be the source of vital energy, it is certain that no food can supply any of this energy until after it has been digested, absorbed and assimilated. It requires much vital power to digest, absorb and assimilate food, or to maintain it in a state against decomposition, hence it is worse than folly to urge food upon the patient in cases of debility of the stomach or of the whole body, or when there is no natural demand for food. For, beyond a natural call for food, there is no power to make profitable use of it.

Those who have had the least experience with fasting are the ones who offer the greatest number of objections to it. For example, J. Haskel Kritzer, M.D., makes the ridiculous statement that "in prolonged fasting, the teeth often decay—forming cavities." The fact is that in the most prolonged fasts the teeth do not decay and do not develop cavities. As it was shown in a previous chapter that fasting does not injure the teeth, it will not be necessary to devote more attention to this subject at this place.

One writer objected that there can be no such thing as a fast as the body consumes its own tissues during periods of abstinence from food, but this "objection" is not to fasting—which is to abstain from food. He contended that the "fasting" body does eat, but he forgets the meaning of the word eat. This same objector, an advocate of much flesh eating, tells vegetarians that they cannot logically fast, for in so doing they are living on a meat diet. He goes so far as to say that the faster is on a largely fat diet and that this is the poorest possible kind of diet. This objection is based on the assumption that the faster consumes his tissues during the fast, rather than his stored food reserves. The fact is overlooked that these stored reserves are identical with the materials with which his tissues are nourished while eating. The difference is that the eater is daily replenishing his reserves, while the faster is not. Wear and waste with repair and replenishment are continuous and almost simultaneous processes in all living structures.

The inconsistency of these objections is apparent in two particulars: 1. there is the demand for plenty of flesh in the diet and the condemnation of fasting because the faster is "on an exclusive flesh diet;" and 2. there is the assertion that flesh alone can adequately supply certain needs of the body coupled with the condemnation of fasting because the "flesh diet" of the faster is inadequate. The fact is that, during even the most prolonged fast, the blood is maintained in all due richness from the storage tissues.

I have considered the colon and the enema during the fast, at the proper places, but must here disprove an unusual objection to fasting, which involves these matters. Kellogg says: "The colon has another function than that of removing food residues. A highly important and essential part of its function is the removal of the body wastes which are excreted by the liver in the bile and also extracted from the blood by the intestine itself; in other words, the colon is an excretory organ as well as a garbage disposal plant. This excretory function has been quite overlooked by the exploiters of the fasting method. They have thought only of the food residues." Again he reveals a lamentable ignorance of the literature of fasting. It is because of this excretory function that he mentions, that the enema and other means of forcing bowel action are so much in favor. For most of those who employ fasting, forget, like Dr. Kellogg, that the colon is an excretory organ—its chief function they believe with Kellogg, is to secrete toxins into the blood.

Dr. Kritzer says: "As the bowel action is materially lessened during a fast, there is a great possibility for intestinal reabsorption, not only of accumulated fecal matter; but also of the tissue that is being used by the system as a food substitute. Hence, daily enemizing of the bowels is beneficial." He advocates Celery-King tea and Caraway seed tea as the prefered "less drastic means of emptying the bowels." I, long ago, showed the fallacy of this notion, in my *Regeneration of Life*. There is no need for the enema or the drugs during a fast. The bowels will always act during a fast, if there is real and not mere theoretical need for action. There is nothing in fasting to prevent the colon from exercising its excretory function and it does continue to carry on this function. It does not perform any "Hindu tricks" and both secrete and excrete at the same time. We need have no fear of intestinal reabsorption.

Since the first edition of this work was issued, Mr. Frederick Hoelzel, of Chicago, published a brochure on *Fasting, Water and Salt*, in which, though approving of fasting, he puts forth the contention that it always produces a condition of "hidden edema," a term used to designate a slight excess of salt and water in the tissues. He says: "I have not known of any case of fasting, even when for only five days, where some post-fasting edema was not present. I have also noted edema developing in rats after fasting or protein restriction. A 'wet diet' (with plenty of water), in my opinion, only seems to produce edema more easily in rats than a dry diet because rats eat more freely of a wet diet (made up largely of vegetables) and thus also obtain more salts, etc. There seems to be no exception to the rule that edema will develop after starvation or sufficient protein restriction in humans or rats, excepting that there naturally are expected differences in time and degree of edema production."

I have seen several cases of edema of the feet and ankles following prolonged fasting, but these are rare occurrences. However, Mr. Hoelzel discusses "hidden edema" for which there is no accurate test and of the existence of which we cannot always be sure. The "pitting test," whereby the skin on the legs over the shin-bone, is depressed by the fingers, can reveal edema only after it is no longer hidden. The intra-dermal salt solution (called the McClure-Aldrich test), which consists of injecting a little salt water into the skin and noting how long it takes for the blister to disappear, is claimed to be an improvement over the pitting test, but even this fails to reveal slight edema.

Hoelzel thinks that a more accurate and more valuable test of hidden edema than the pitting test and McClure-Aldrich test is the presence of the following symptoms: "Swollen feet and enlarged ankles; a puffy, bloated face; hypersensitiveness to drafts or to shaving; skin that cuts, chaps or bruises easily; a shiny skin, including a shiny nose; frequent colds; some types of headache; a continuous sense of fatigue and lack of ambition; mental depression; abnormal blushing and shyness; cases of obesity in which the fat is not firm; and some troubles associated with menstruation and pregnancy," or what have you? He asks: "how many can say that they are not troubled with any of these common ailments? Or that their troubles at least are not due to some degree of salt-water retention?" Hidden edema would seem to be almost universal without fasting, while the above symptoms are removed by the fast.

He further says that "fasting is not even necessary to predispose one to the development of edema as it develops after simple protein restriction, when this has been sufficiently prolonged. Moreover table-salt is not necessary as many natural and unsalted foods (some vegetables and some types of meat) contain enough natural or mineral salts or unoxidizable crystals to produce edema after sufficient protein restriction. It is now known that carbohydrates can contribute to edema, apparently by being retained as glucose instead of being changed to glycogen." One certainly does not get an excess of salts nor of carbohydrates while fasting, nor is an excess of water consumed if the demands of instinct, rather than of theory, are obeyed. It is the rule that the sodium-chloride-produced edema is eliminated during the fast. As the protein restriction during the fast is no greater than the restriction of other substances (except water and air) the body succeeds in establishing and maintaining a balance.

Mr. Hoelzel's experience with fasting has been extremely limited and his method is not one of which we can approve. He became a technician in gross anatomy at the College of Medicine of the University of Illinois in 1916, but carried on most of his experiments with fasting in the Department of Physiology in the University of Chicago, where he was granted the courtesy of the use of the laboratory from time to time by Prof. A. J. Carlson, to carry on his independent experimentation. He tells of fasting fifteen days in the University of Chicago in 1917 and following this with six days of fasting during which time he took cotton fibre soaked in lemon juice to which common salt was added. He used about one-third of an ounce of salt a day. With this as "food" he gained over two pounds a day in weight, storing fifteen pounds or more of salt water in the six days of "fasting." He says: "I stopped after six days because the edema had become obvious in my legs and I was becoming sluggish generally." He recounts another gain of twelve pounds in twenty-four hours after eating two moderate sized meals which contained salt food (ham and cabbage) and a weight increase of two pounds daily after a nine days fast when only salt (10 gms. daily) was taken in addition to sufficient water to satisfy thirst.

This is not an objection to fasting, nor does it prove that fasting produces hidden edema. It is an objection to salt-using and excess water-drinking. The use of salt and salted foods and the consequent drinking of lots of fluid, water-logs the tissues of all who practice it —fasting or feeding. I know of no one (except Ghandi) who advises the use of salt while fasting. Without salt-using and excess water-drinking, no gains in weight, such as Mr. Hoelzel describes, ever take place. Excess water drinking in the absence of salt never registers more than slight temporary gains. The rapid post-fasting gains he describes do not occur in properly fed cases. The most rapid gains I have seen have been produced by the milk diet, but here again it was a mere water-logging of the tissues from excess fluid intake. Cases fed on fruits, vegetables, and moderate quantities of proteins and carbohydrates do not present the difficulties he describes nor do their tissues fill with excess water. On the other hand, additional protein alone is not always enough to overcome malnutritional edema. It may even aggravate the condition. Simple fasting, of whatever duration, is not open to any of the objections raised by Mr. Hoelzel.

The writer has cared for marked cases of malnutritional edema and has used fasting in these cases with the most gratifying results. One such case had a fast of forty days with results that were all any one could ask for. Every good thing can be misused and abused. Fasting is as much subject to abuse and misuse as any other thing that man uses. Just as he can and frequently does abuse diet, exercise, sunshine, sex, etc., so he can and often does abuse fasting. Indeed, fasting is often abused by those who know little about it and by those who know all about it and know it all wrong. But the abuse of a thing is no argument against its valid use. One does not cease to drink pure water when thirsty, merely because somebody was drowned in the lake.

It has been objected that the faster is a cannibal—an autophage, in fact. This is exactly the same as to say that a woman on a reducing diet, who is also consuming her surpluses, is a cannibal. The faster does not live upon himself, but upon his stored reserves. Is the man a cannibal when he converts the glycogen stored in his liver into sugar and uses this? Does not *autophagy* belong to the starvation period rather than to the fast proper? Certainly the rejuvenating effects of fasting are not due to any gnawing at the faster's vitals.

At the risk of some repetition, permit me here to list a few things that fasting does not do.

Fasting does not cause the stomach to "shrink up"—atrophy.

Fasting does not cause the walls of the stomach to grow together—adhere.

Fasting does not cause the digestive fluids of the stomach to turn upon it and digest the stomach.

Fasting does not paralyze the bowels.

Fasting does not impoverish the blood nor produce anemia.

Fasting does not produce acidosis.

Fasting does not cause the heart to weaken nor to collapse.

Fasting does not produce malnutritional edema.

Fasting does not cause deficiency disease.

Fasting does not produce tuberculosis nor predispose to its development.

Fasting does not reduce *resistance* to "disease."

Fasting does not injure the teeth.

Fasting does not injure the nervous system.

Fasting does not weaken the vital powers.

Fasting does not injure any of the vital organs.

Fasting does not injure the body's glands.

Fasting does not cause abnormal psychism.

Does Fasting Cure Disease?

CHAPTER XXI

If "disease" is remedial effort does fasting *cure* "disease?" If there are no *cures* for "disease," if "disease" does not need to be *cured*, is fasting a *cure?* To us there are not twenty thousand "diseases," but many local states growing out of a common systemic derangement. We do not seek to *cure* "disease," but to remove the causes of impairment and to afford the sick organism every natural or hygienic advantage that will facilitate its own spontaneous return to biological and physiological normality.

Does nature *cure* vomiting, or does she use vomiting as a means of ejecting unwanted materials from the stomach? Does the body *cure* coughing, or is coughing a vital act by which irritants and obstructions are expelled from the respiratory tract? Does diarrhea need to be *cured*, or is diarrhea a process by which obnoxious materials are rushed out of the digestive tract? Does nature *cure* inflammation, or is inflammation a reparative and defensive process by which broken bones are knit, lascerated flesh is healed and foreign bodies are removed from the flesh? Is there a need to *cure* fever, or is fever part of the body's own healing activities? Does not coughing automatically and spontaneously cease when there is no longer any need for it? Does not diarrhea cease when it has freed the digestive tract of all offensive materials? Does not inflammation subside when the bone has knit or the wound healed? What is there to *cure* about the various processes of the body that are collectively labeled disease?

Is it not obvious that if fasting suppressed vomiting, diarrhea, coughing, inflammation, fever, and the other symptoms that make up disease, it would be as evil as drugging? To call fasting "the fasting cure," the "hunger cure" or the "abstinence cure," as many have done, is to place it in a false light, unless, of course, we understand by cure what it originally meant—*care*. Fasting is part of the rational care of the sick body, it does not *cure* disease, as the word *cure* is now commonly used.

We are frequently accused of regarding fasting as a *cure-all*, despite our oft reiterated statement that it is not a *cure* at all. Using the term *cure* in its presently accepted sense, we say that fasting does not *cure* anything. But the charge against us continues to be circulated. This charge grows out of the fact that we employ the fast in all forms of impaired health. Our principle that the forces and processes of life accomplish all healing work, after the causes of impairment and damage have been removed, is not noticed by any of our critics. Indeed, they have shown a singular incapacity for understanding this simple principle. They fasten upon some one of our most commonly used methods of care, the one they think they can use with greatest advantage against us, and ride it for all it is worth.

If we use fasting in nearly all cases, we employ food in exactly all of them. If we employ fasting in nearly all cases we employ exercise in as many. We use sunbathing in nearly all cases, but we never regard it as a *cure,* much less do we regard it as a *cure-all.* Physical and mental rest are employed in every case, but not as a *cure* as this word is commonly misused. Before we employ rest, fasting, exercise, diet, sunshine, or any other means of care, we seek for the causes of the patient's impaired health and seek to eradicate these. Removal of the cause is primary. Why can our critics never understand this simple fact?

There are many men in the various schools of so-called healing who admit the great value of fasting in a variety of diseases, but they say: "The absurdity of the fasting care of the sick is its indiscriminate use in a great variety of diseases." The *Hygienic* answer to this objection is that, if its use is indiscriminate, undoubtedly that indiscriminate use is absurd. But, we add, this observation is as true of any other mode of care and treatment that has been used and is now used by the various healing professions. In the days of venesection, was not bleeding used indiscriminately in almost all diseases? During the recent world war, was not blood transfusion, in one form or another, employed indiscriminately in a wide variety of diseases and traumatic conditions? Have not alcohol, quinine, mercury, tobacco, antimony and a number of other drugs been used indiscriminately in a wide variety of diseases? Are not the sulfonamides, penicillin, streptomycin, and the other "antibiotics" being used indiscriminately, in a wide variety of diseases? Has not the removal of "foci of infection" fad been as indiscriminately applied to a thousand-and-one diseases?

The hydropaths employed their water applications, the chiropractors their spinal adjustments, the osteopaths their manipulations to almost all diseases as indiscriminately as any drug was ever applied. All the schools of so-called healing have been and are guilty of the very indiscriminate use of their therapeutic measures that they charge against the use of fasting. No physician ever purged the bowels of his patients with greater regularity or with less discrimination than the chiropractors have punched the spinal columns of their patients.

When we consider that fasting is not employed to *cure* disease, as are the various therapeutic measures, its wide use loses its appearance of indiscriminate use. More than this, when we consider that *Hygienists* do not recognize the existence of a great number of diseases, it will be realized that they cannot apply it indiscriminately. Take the following so-called different diseases—pleuritis, enteritis, pericarditis, peritonitis, arachnitis, cystitis, metritis, appendicitis, ovaritis, colitis, proctitis, prostatitis, gastritis, menengitis, tonsilitis, rhinitis, etc.—they are only one *disease*—inflammation—in different locations. A different name is imposed on each in order to indicate which organ or tissue is inflamed, but there is no difference in the process of inflammation and there is no difference in its cause. We have many names for disease, according to the location of the inflammation, or functional failure, or atrophy, but we have only one disease. Disease is a unit—*forms* or *modes* of manifestation are many. A so-called disease is a name applied to a symptom-complex and the symptom-complex is clustered about the organ most involved.

The *Hygienic System* is not a system of treating and *curing* "disease" and "disorder." It does not recognize the existence of hundreds, or thousands, of "diseases," but regards all of these many so-called "diseases" as varying expressions of the same thing. *Hygienic* methods are methods of caring for the body. By these we seek to place the body under the most favorable conditions for the prosecution of its own healing activities. Rest and sleep, exercise and cleanliness, water and sunshine—we also employ these in all forms of impaired health. But we do not regard them as *cure-alls* or *cures* at all. There are no "diseased" conditions in which fresh air is not helpful, but it is no *cure*-all, in fact, it is no *cure* at all. There are no "diseased" conditions in which rest is not helpful, but rest is no *panacea*. Why, then, accuse us of regarding fasting as a *cure-all* because it (with rest, sunshine, fresh air, exercise, sleep, quiet, etc.) is found useful in all so-called "diseases?"

Fasting is primarily a rest of the organism. There is no condition of "disease" in which rest of the vital organs is not of benefit to the whole organism. Rest gives all of the organs an opportunity to repair their damaged structures. Rest affords to organs that have been lashed into impotency by overstimulation, an opportunity to recuperate their substances and forces. Fasting is not a process of elimination, but it does permit a marked increase in the elimination of toxins and waste from the body, not alone from the fluids, but also from the tissues of the body. It does permit the organs of elimination to bring their work up to date—to balance their books, as it were. There is no state of impaired health in which this increased elimination is not of distinct value. Fasting means a temporary cessation of the inflow of nutritive substance. This gives the surfeited organism an opportunity to consume its surplus. The removal of a burdensome redundancy always results in increased vigor and improved function.

When fermentative and putrefactive toxins are pouring in from the digestive tract in excess of the body's ability to neutralize and eliminate them and the toxic overflow has been partly stored in the less vital tissues, fasting speedily ends the intake of decomposition-toxins and thus gives the organism an opportunity to catch up with its work of excretion. Not only are the toxins that circulate in the lymph removed, but the toxins deposited in the tissues are removed and excreted. Fasting does not remove the toxins. This is done by the excretory functions of the body. Fasting only affords them the opportunity to perfect their work.

Just as fasting causes the body to consume its excess of fat and use this to nourish its vital tissues, so it causes the body to break down by autolysis, growths, or tumors and use the nutritive substances in these to nourish its vital tissues. In like manner dropsical swellings, edematous swellings, and deposits are absorbed and the usable portions salvaged for use in nourishing the vital tissues. Withholding food from the body for an extended period creates an intense nitrogen hunger and a demand for other nutritive elements. Assimilation is rejuvenated so that frequently the chronically underweight man can gain weight after the fast, who, previous to the fast, could gain in no way. The general increase in functional vigor and the detoxication that take place during the fast contribute greatly to this result.

Due to the disproportionate use of the body's reserves during a fast, to a heavy loss of some elements and a storing of others, fasting results in a chemical normalization which nothing else occasions. Cellular and tissue rejuvenation also occur during a fast. The rejuvenation effected during a fast is of a character and extent not effected by any other method or process in existence.

Fasting does not do anything. It really stops the doing. In thus stopping certain activities, it permits, even enforces certain tissue changes and chemical readjustments in the body which result in increased vigor and improved health. There are no conditions of functional and structural impairment in which these changes are not desirable. To sum up, fasting, by affording the organs of the body a rest, by withholding raw materials and by stopping the inflow of decomposition-poisons from the alvine canal, permits the repair and recuperation of the organs of the body, the consumption of a burdensome nutritive excess, the removal of circulating and deposited toxins, the normalization of blood chemistry, cellular and tissue rejuvenation, the absorption of deposits, exudates, effusions and growths, and improves the body's powers of digestion and assimilation. If there are any "diseased" conditions in which some or all of these results are not desirable, I have not seen them, nor even any description of them. Then, although fasting *cures* nothing and is no panacea, it is useful in all "diseased" conditions.

Fasting is not a *cure;* it will not *cure* any "disease." Rightly conducted, it is a sure, quick, safe way to unload a toxic overload, but healing is a physiological process that succeeds if the toxins have been eliminated and life has been righted. Fasting, followed by rational eating, has proved very satisfactory in helping thousands to re-establish health and strength, but it is not a *cure.* "Cure is an evolution in reverse," said Dr. Dewey. A period of abstinence, or of very light eating, with rest in bed, and the giving up of enervating habits, mental and physical, will allow nature to eliminate the accumulated toxins; after which, if enervating habits are given up, and rational living habits adopted, good health will evolve and will be maintained so long as the individual continues to live correctly.

The real remedy consists of correcting the errors of life that have brought on and perpetuated the toxemia. These errors are not all errors in eating. Personal habits other than dietetic—worry, excesses, dissipations—have as much to do with producing sickness as wrong eating.

When toxemia has been eliminated, or when "disease" is said to be *cured,* this means that an abnormal physiological state has been restored to normal. But the patient may have been reduced down to a dangerous point and he is not in a normal physiological state. Hence, fasting *per se* does not remedy—it does not restore a normal physiological state. It is often necessary to abstain from food until one is far below a normal state in order to give the organism an opportunity to absorb deposits and correct perverted states. For example, fasting will cause a more rapid absorption of dropsical fluid, which has accumulated in the tissues, than any other known measure. A fibroid tumor may be caused to cease growing, its size may be greatly reduced, or it may be completely absorbed by a fast; while the fast is in progress the organism can readjust itself and normalize its secretions and excretions—bring these to a state of equilibrium. This done, the patient may consider himself *cured,* but he is not. He has only commenced to *get well.*

We do not claim that fasting *cures* disease, but simply that it enables the organism to heal itself. What, then, does fasting do?

1. It gives the vital organs a complete rest.

2. It stops the intake of foods that decompose in the intestines and further poison the body.

3. It empties the digestive tract and disposes of putrefactive bacteria.

4. It gives the organs of elimination an opportunity to catch up with their work and promotes elimination.

5. It re-establishes normal physiological chemistry and normal secretions.

6. It promotes the breaking down and absorption of exudates, effusions, deposits, "diseased" tissues, and abnormal growths.

7. It restores a youthful condition of the cells and tissues and rejuvenates the body.

8. It permits the conservation and re-canalization of energy.

9. It increases the powers of digestion and assimilation.

10. It clears and strengthens the mind.

11. It improves function throughout the body.

Each of these statements has been fully proved in the pages of this book.

When we say that fasting is neither a *cure-all* nor a *cure* at all, we do not thereby intend to limit its scope or its field of usefulness. Indeed, the more we learn about this element of nature's hygiene, the more useful we find it to be. As it is used as a rest and is employed where there is great need of a physiological housecleaning, it is effective in all states of disease, even in deficiency diseases, where it is commonly thought that more of certain food factors are essential, the fast has proved to be very helpful. Thus, what may appear, on the surface, to be an indiscriminate resort to the fast, turns out, upon analysis, to be no more indiscriminate than the employment of water or food or exercise in the same great variety of conditions. When we once grasp the fact that fasting is not employed as a *cure* and that it is not something that is good in certain so-called specific diseases, but may not be good in other so-called specific diseases, we understand that its use in all the conditions of impaired health is not an indiscriminate use.

The Rationale of Fasting

CHAPTER XXII

We undertake a fast for an ultimate good and we have a right to demand that the end for which we fast shall justify this means of achieving it. The man or woman faced with the decision—to fast or not to fast—has a right to ask: What is there in it for me? What shall be my reward, my gain, if I deny myself the pleasures of the palate for a period? Before we undergo a fast, we have a right to ask: Why shall I fast? We have, also, a right to ask that, as a permanent possession, something worthwhile shall come out of it. That man and animals do fast, even for long periods, is a highly interesting fact, but this is not, in itself, sufficient reason for fasting. Fasting is futile if it shall not prove productive of great benefit.

In previous chapters four important facts about fasting have been fully established, as follow:

1. Fasting, as a period of physiological rest, affords the tissues and organs of the body an opportunity to repair, renew and replenish themselves. Damaged organs are repaired, worn out and diseased cells are discarded and cast out.

2. Fasting, as a period of physiological rest, affords an opportunity for recuperation of depleted energy.

3. Fasting, because it compels the body to rely upon its internal resources, forces the tearing down (by autolysis) of growths, effusions, infiltrations, deposits, accumulations and excesses. These are thoroughly overhauled, their usable constituents are employed in nourishing the vital tissues, their unusable portions are excreted.

4. Fasting, by the foregoing and related processes, enables the body to regenerate itself to a marked degree. It becomes younger in physiological condition. Its functions are improved, its structures repaired, and its fitness to live increased.

Two replies may be made to those investigators who stress the ephemerality of the cellular regeneration that results while fasting. The first of these was made by Dr. Christopher Gian-Cursio. He says: "it does not take more than a transitory regeneration to remove a structural abnormality and to increase functional efficiency. Even

THE RATIONALE OF FASTING

where the structural impairment cannot be completely removed, there is, nevertheless, great functional betterment through compensation. The activity that removes the toxic influence may be transitory, but the removal of that toxin is permanent." The other reply is that these investigators, in making their experiments, have guaranteed the transitory character of the regeneration that results, by the post-fasting feeding and other care that have been given to their subjects. Always have they sent their "washed sows" back to "their wallowing in the mire." Nothing should be expected to produce permanent regeneration if, after the regeneration has been achieved, the renovated organism returns to the habits of living that accounted for the prior degeneration. Unfortunately, biologists who have observed the structure and function of cells during and after fasting, fail to recognize the part played by unbiological and unphysiological habits of mind and body in inducing pathological changes in the cells and tissues.

Fasting may be regarded as a temporary expedient, but it must, at the same time, be seen as a fundamental and radical process that is older than any other mode of caring for the sick organism, for it was employed by animals long before man was introduced upon the earth. But it is not to be thought that fasting should be instituted only in serious states of illness, that we should continue to eat so long as any digestive power remains. On the contrary, missing a few meals at the beginning of trouble is often enough to prevent the development of serious trouble. When there is but slight functional impairment, as indicated by a coated tongue, bad breath, a bad taste in the mouth, headache, dullness of the mind, a general feeling of malaise, and similar *insignificant* symptoms, a brief fast will enable the body to excrete the systemic toxemia that is responsible for these symptoms before the more formidable stages of disease evolve.

Using the phrase "hunger cure," Dr. Walter said that "a large experience" has shown "that a moderate hunger-cure is exceedingly beneficial in the great majority of diseases. Indeed, in many of them the capacity to appropriate food is entirely destroyed, the very thought of it becoming repugnant to the individual." It was his view that fasting "liberates vitality (energy) to be used in the process of purification," and that this energy would "otherwise be used in the process of appropriating new materials" or, we might add, in excreting materials that cannot be used. That this liberation of energy does take place seems to be certain. In other words, energy not employed in the work of digesting three or more meals a day is available for employment in other and, immediately, more urgent work. This liberation of energy or its recanalization is of utmost importance.

We cannot and do not claim for the fast any power to *cure* disease. We have said repeatedly that fasting does not do anything, that it is a cessation of doing. It is a longer or shorter period of physiological rest. We claim only that the body can do for itself, during this period of rest, what it is not able to do in periods of surfeit and full activity. It is not a "hunger cure," as it was called by German *Nature Curists* and by many early *Hygienists*, for it is not a *cure*, nor is the faster hungry. If he continued hungry throughout the period of a fast, it would not be possible to get him to fast very long and repetitions of the fast would be all but impossible.

NATURE'S PREPARATION FOR A FAST

Writing of a case that passed under his care, Dr. Jennings explains the rationale of fasting, thus: "The child has taken no nourishment for a number of days and may take none for many days to come; if it should live; yet there is nothing to be feared on this account. Take a healthy child from food while its vital machinery is in full operation, and it will use up its own building material and fall to ruin in two or three weeks; but in this case the system has been prepared for a long suspension of the nutritive function. There is now little action of the system generally, and consequently there is but little wear and tear of machinery; and like the dormouse, it might *subsist for months on its own internal resources,* if that were necessary, and everything else favored. *The bowels too have been quiet for a number of days, and they might remain as they are for weeks and months to come without damage,* if this were essential to the prolongation of life. The muscles of voluntary motion are at rest and cost *nothing for their maintenance,* save a slight expenditure of safe-keeping forces to hold them in readiness for action at any future time if their services be needed. So of all other parts and departments; the most perfect economy is everywhere exercised in the appropriation and use of the vital energies. It is an 'extreme case' and calls for extreme measures; but they are all conducted under a perfect law, which adapts with the most punctilious minuteness the means to the end."—*Philosophy of Human Life*, pp. 159-160 (Italics mine, Author).

THEY THAT WORK MUST EAT

The body's reserve stores are designed for use in just such emergencies and may be utilized in such circumstances with greater ease and with less tax upon the body than food secured through the laborious process of digestion. As Jennings explained:

"There is one particular in relation to the lymphatic system of vessels, that deserves special notice and remembrance. In some forms of impaired health, when the nutritive apparatus is disabled, either from defects in its own structure, that require suspension of its action for recuperative purposes, or because the only organic forces that can be used to sustain its action, are, for the time, either exhausted or employed more advantageously in other duties, the lymphatic vessels interpose their kind offices to supply the deficiency by taking up the adipose and fleshy substances wherever they can find them, or any matters that they can work up into nourishment, and throwing it into the general circulation to be distributed among the weary and hungry laborers according to their several necessities— for they that work must eat. Indeed, this expedient is often resorted to in severe cases of illness, particularly in those of protracted general debility; *for it is less expensive to the vital economy to furnish the requisite sustenance in this way, than to do it by the nutritive machinery from raw material.* This wise provision for sustaining life under critical circumstances, should allay all fears and anxieties on the score of eating when there is a lack of appetite; for when there is a demand for nourishment, and the nutritive machinery is in working order, and the necessary forces can be consistently spared to operate it, there always will be appetite, and just in proportion to the necessities of the system for nourishment; for real genuine appetite is simply and only nature's appeal for something with which to supply a want, and if she makes no call, it is either because there is no want to be supplied, or she is not in a condition to meet it, and in either case it would be useless to urge food upon the stomach, either in repugnance to obvious indication, or after having provoked an unnatural appetite.

"In an extreme case, when it is expedient to make dependence on the lymphatic system for nutrimental aid for a long period, until all the material suitable for supply through that medium is exhausted, and starvation becomes the alternative to digestion and assimilation, if it is a remediable case, the nutritive system will be clothed with power sufficient to make a call for food, and on its reception, commence operations; it may be in a very slight degree for a while, and at intervals of some hours, just sufficient to sustain the essential organs in working condition, and may need extreme care in feeding, in quality and quantity lest feeble vitality should be smothered and destroyed. But, if under these circumstances, with proper treatment in other respects, no effort is put forth by the nutritive organs to stay utter extinction of life, it may be regarded as inevitably a fatal case; for neither the incitement nor power to effort in this direction can be increased by artificial means."—*Philosophy of Human Life*, pp. 57-59 (Italics, mine. Author).

The process of nourishing the weary and hungry laborers of the body is not as simple as Jennings describes it, but it must be understood that nothing was known of the process of autolysis at the time he wrote. It will be recalled that Graham also described the process in much the same way as did Jennings. Indeed, as the two men were friends and more than once discussed such matters, it may be that they arrived at a common understanding of how the nourishment of the vital tissues was accomplished during periods of abstinence. In its general outline, however, Jennings' explanation of the way in which the body makes use of fasting in order to better achieve certain ends is correct.

Sylvester Graham explained that when more food is used by the body than is daily supplied, "it is a general law of the vital economy" that "the decomposing absorbents always first lay hold of and remove those substances which are of least use to the economy; and hence, all morbid accumulations, such as wens, tumors, abscesses, etc., are rapidly diminished and often wholly removed under severe and protracted abstinence and fasting." Fasting, by creating a nutritional scarcity, forces the body to surrender superfluities and to eliminate encumberances, which it cannot achieve in a state of surfeit. The surrender of surplus material is compatible with increasing powers and with processes of physiological and, even, biological readjustment.

Recording another case, Jennings declares: "There has been no nourishment taken into the stomach for a number of days, and none will be taken for a number of days to come, for it would be a waste of power to compel the nutritive apparatus to work up raw

material under present circumstances, if this could be done."—
Philosophy of Human Life, p. 166. This principle is susceptible
of a wide application. Its workings are particularly apparent in the
fast. The fasting body is very careful to hoard its materials, but
rapidly absorbs and either eliminates or utilizes the materials contained in growths, deposits, effusions, swellings, etc.

ELIMINATION

The proper management of so-called disease is analogous to
the drainage of marshy land in agriculture. More water is getting
into the ground than is flowing out and, to remedy this situation,
drainage must be established so that water flows out as fast or faster
for a time, than it is flowing in. In disease, more toxins are finding
their way into the fluids and tissues of the body than are flowing out.
Drainage must be increased to the end that the tissues and fluids
may again become sweet and clean. If we can check the inflow of
toxins at the same time that we increase their outflow, so much the
better. Fortunately, both of these things can be done.

It is instructive to note that the specific gravity of the urine
during a fast, and particularly during the earlier stages of the fast,
is frequently as high as 1.030 instead of the 1.010 that is considered
normal. It is noteworthy that, as the fast progresses, the specific
gravity of the urine gradually falls, until, ultimately, it reaches the
1.010 level. Does it mean anything that coincident with the drop in
specific gravity there is also a lightening of the color of the urine,
which, at first may be almost inky black; a clearing up of the tongue,
which commonly becomes heavily coated; a gradual lessening of the
foul taste in the mouth, until the taste becomes sweet and pleasant;
and, in those cases where there was a tendency for the temperature
to drop below normal, a rising of temperature, often to its normal
level? Coincident with these changes, there is a return to normal
of the body's secretions, a clearing up of symptoms, often a healing
of ulcers, wounds, etc., that have long refused to heal, and return of
a feeling of wellbeing such as the patient has not experienced for
years prior to the fast.

If the patient suffering with subnormal temperature goes on
a fast and the temperature rises, in a few instances the temperature
even rising above normal, certainly something has taken place, as
a result of fasting, that removes the detriment to heat production.
If, after the fast is broken and normal eating has been resumed

—281—

the gain is found to be lasting, we may be sure that the body has accomplished some good for itself during this period of physiological rest that it was unable to do while burdened with food.

Burdened with food! The popular idea that man is immediately and utterly dependent upon food, which he supplies every few hours and will starve if he misses a few meals, is false. Food is a basic need of every living organism, but food may become so burdensome that a period of abstinence is demanded, and will prove to be highly beneficial.

In some quarters it is held that when food is taken excretion is suppressed, this is to say that the body cannot both digest and eliminate at the same time. That there is value in this view seems certain, but we must not take it as a statement of absolute truth, for it is essential to life that excretion go on at all times. It may be reduced, it cannot be suspended. The statement that "assimilation arrests elimination" is a catchy one, but not exactly true. The energies of the organism are at all times divided between assimilation and elimination, but there are times and conditions when one demands more attention than the other: times when excretion is most important and assimilation can and is reduced to a bare minimum. Herein lies one of the great benefits of the fast. By suspending the intake of food, thus eliminating the expenditure of energy in digesting and circulating and assimilating the regular food supply, the energies of life may be directed more completely to the work of excretion.

It cannot be doubted that there is a constant effort to maintain the normal condition of the fluids of the body by an unending elimination of body waste and of all else that finds its way into the body and cannot be utilized as food. Hence, it must go on, even while digesting food. It can be only in a very limited sense that "assimilation arrests elimination." In all living bodies, said Graham, there is an economy of disassimilation and excretion co-equal to that of nutrition.

Dr. Joel Shew explained that "the principle on which the hunger cure acts is one on which all physiologists are agreed, and one which is readily explained and understood. We know that, in animal bodies, the law of nature is for the effete and worn-out and least vitalized matter first to be cast off. We see this upon the cuticle, nails, hair, and in the snake casting off its old skin. Now, in wasting or famishing from want of food, this process of elimination goes on in a much more rapid manner than ordinarily, and the vital force which would otherwise be expended in digesting the food eaten acts now in expelling from the vital domain whatever morbific matters it may contain. This, then, is a beautiful idea in regard to the hunger cure—that whenever a meal of food is omitted, the body purifies itself this much from disease, and it becomes apparent in the subsequent amendment, both as regards bodily feeling and strength. It is proved also in the fact that, during the prevalence of epidemics those who have been obliged to live almost in a state of starvation, have been free from attacks, while the well-fed have been cut off in numbers by the merciless disease."

Dr. Oswald says: "A germ disease, as virulent as syphilis, and long considered too persistent for any but palliative methods of treatment (by mercury, etc.), was radically cured by the fasting cures, prescribed in the Arabian hospitals of Egypt, at the time of the French occupation. Avicena already alludes to the efficacy of that specific, which he seems to have employed with similar success against smallpox, and Dr. Robert Barthlow, a stickler for the faith in drugs, admits that 'it certainly is an eminently rational expedient to relieve the organism of a virus by a continuous and gradual process of molecular destruction and a renewal of the anatomical parts.' Such is the hunger-cure of syphilis, an Oriental method of treating that disease. Very satisfactory results have been attained by this means." The point here is that the body tears down the defective parts and eliminates them during the fast, and then builds anew after the fast. With no digestive drudgery on hand, as Dr. Oswald expressed it, nature employs the long desired leisure for general house cleaning purposes. The accumulations of superfluous tissues are over-hauled and analyzed; the available component parts are turned over to the department of nutrition, while the refuse is thoroughly and permanently removed. That this is true will become very apparent as we progress with our study of fasting.

"The organism, stinted in its supply of vital reserves," says Dr. Oswald, "soon begins to curtail its current expenditure. The movements of the respiratory powers decrease;—and before long the retrenchment of the assimilative function reacts on the intestinal organs. The colon contracts and the smaller intestines retain all but the most irritating ingesta."

COMPENSATION

The principle previously presented, that the energy customarily expended in the digestion and assimilation of food may, when no food is eaten, be employed through other channels in the increased work of elimination, is accepted by Mr. Carrington and Mr. Macfadden in this country and Dr. E. Liek and Otto Rosenbach in Germany. Dr. Liek says, "By saving the force required for the process of digestion, the body saves strength and mobilizes forces for other purposes, such as the healing of wounds, combating the microrganisms of disease, etc." Rosenbach has written much in the German language upon fasting.

While fasting bars any direct or measurable income to the system from nourishment, it does not incur any expenditure in digestion. The large sum of energy thus saved is available for use through other channels; that is, in carrying on other, and for the moment, more important functions and processes.

Disease, especially acute disease, is labor, action, struggle—it is often violent action. It uses up energy. It often leaves the patient exhausted at the end of his severe effort. It may so completely exhaust him as to end his life. Disease frequently means a much greater expenditure of energy than the activities of health require, hence the urgent need for conservation of energy in every possible way. Loss of appetite, cessation of digestion, suppression of the digestive secretions, suspension of the muscular contractions of the stomach and of the peristaltic motions of the intestine, inaction of the bowels, skin, liver, kidneys, general debility, prostration, etc., are conservative measures. Energy not expended through these channels is available for more urgent work elsewhere.

The urgent demand for increased effort, which the presence of toxins occasions, is the reason for the increased, even violent effort. But violent effort in one direction means reduced effort in other directions. Fasting by the acutely ill is definitely a compensatory measure and its urgency is in direct proportion to the severity of the symptoms. There is still digestive power in a cold, in pneumonia there is none. By this is meant that the more ill the patient, the greater is the need for fasting. Curious as this may appear at first thought, the return of health and hunger come together.

"Nothing is remedial," said Trall, "except conditions which economize the vital expenditures." Physiological rest (fasting) is the surest way of economizing vital expenditures. Walter pointed out that "the patient often grows stronger through the process of fasting and always better."

Some years ago I laid down the principle that: power cannot be expended with equal and increased intensity in all directions at the same time. I pointed out that increased activities in one part of the body require concomittant and coetaneous diminution of activities in other parts. Power saved through one channel is always available for use through other channels. All forms of power obey this principle. A convenient example is the diminished force with which the water runs in your bath tub, if some one turns on the water in the kitchen. Cut off the water in the kitchen and the force of the flow is immediately increased in the bath tub.

Dr. Jennings understood that the withdrawal of energy from the digestive organs, in "disease," was for the purpose of employing the energy ordinarily expended through these channels, in the work of elimination and repair. Mr. Macfadden said: "We do not perhaps realize to what extent the processes of metabolism draw upon the body energies. It requires an enormous amount of energy to digest, convert, and push through thirty feet of tubing, several pounds of food material, and to carry the normal and excess assimilated food elements through every blood vessel in the body, over and over again. If this energy is not utilized for that purpose, it is free to be utilized in other directions, and in all cases of disease it is in the main actually used for purposes of cure. Many people keep themselves tired and exhausted by using up the energies of the body in continual digestive processes."

There is another and equally important reason why the gross overeating which is so prevalent causes people to be tired. The intestinal toxemia, resulting from excessive food, poisons the tissues and cells throughout the whole body. Sluggishness, laziness, and chronic fatigue are some of the results of this poisoning. The fagging energies of the body revive to a remarkable extent, when eating is discontinued for a few days, due to the conservation of energy and to cutting off the source of toxins.

Dr. Walter also recognizes these facts and says in *Life's Great Law*, p. 209: "No process of treatment ever invented fulfills so many indications for restoration of health as does fasting. It is nature's own primal process, her first requirement in nearly all cases. As a means of promoting circulation, improving nutrition, facilitating excretion, recuperating vital power, and restoring vital vigor, it has no competitor*** In chronic diseases fasting is hardly less important than in acute cases. Obstruction of the vital organs, and especially of the process of nutrition, is the rule. Giving rest to the organs is of utmost importance, in order to improve nutrition, and restore vigor The secondary effect is the exact opposite of the primary.

"Extremes of practice, are, however, to be avoided. Men are always prone to indulge forcing processes. A fast for a few days or at most a week, will often be comforting and valuable; but to compel the organism to live for a month without food is an unnecessary violence. But in acute diseases the fasting may continue for weeks, because nature cannot appropriate the food; we only object to arbitrary fasts for long periods. Fasting is not a cure-all; it may do evil as well as good; but it should always be employed in connection with rest of the general system." Walter's fear of the long fast, in chronic "disease" need not engage our attention at this place, beyond saying that such a process is not essentially violent and that, while the short fast is preferable in some cases, the long fast is alone productive of results in others.

The Length of the Fast

CHAPTER XXIII

It is possible to carry a fast too far. It is possible to break it prematurely. In the first case the patient is damaged, in the second he fails to receive the legitimately expected results. A controversy has long been waged between the advocates of the short fast and the advocates of the fast to completion. The advocates of the short fast depict what they believe to be harm resulting from the long fast. While it is true that the short fast is more popular with most patients, I have yet to see these fancied damages result from a long fast.

For many years Carrington defended the long fast. I can do no better than quote him at this point. He says: "I must contend, and that strenuously, that the breaking of the fast prematurely is one of the most foolish and dangerous experiments that can possibly be made. The prevalent idea is that a fast should be undertaken and persisted in for a certain definite period, which can be fixed upon before the fast is begun, and that the fast can be broken, and even broken with advantage, at the expiration of this period . . . who is there to decide? Were it thus possible to determine *a priori*, the length of time the fast might be protracted, without harm resulting, or with benefit to the fasting patient, this system of treatment would be as blindly experimental, and as whimsical, as the orthodox medical treatment of today—whereas it is nothing of the kind. Nature would institute no such senseless code, no 'law in which there is no law' . . . I wish to impress the following statement upon the minds of my readers, since it is one of the most important facts contained in this entire book; and the failure to appreciate it is, I believe, the cause of almost all the misunderstanding concerning the fasting cure*** . . . *Nature will always indicate when the fast should be broken*".—*Vitality, Fasting and Nutrition*, pp. 543-544.

He adds that "there can never be any mistake by those who are accustomed to watching fasting cases, as to when to terminate the fast. Nature will always indicate when the fast should be broken by a series of symptoms which can never be misunderstood and which she here displays most obviously—to all those whose judgement is not perverted by preconceived ideas, and who possess a sound knowledge of the phenomena and philosophy of fasting."—*Vitality, Fasting and Nutrition*, p. 544. He says that "the return of natural hunger is the great point to note, and the most important indication that the fast is ended, and the system is able and willing to digest and assimilate nutriment, in the form of either solid or liquid food. The spontaneous and precisely coincidental cleaning of the tongue, of the breath, and the other and lesser phenomena which may be observed toward the termination of the 'finish fast,' all indicate that Nature and Nature alone, is the authority to be considered as to when the fast should be broken."

A "finish fast" does not always mean a long fast. It does not mean a fast until all of the body's food reserves are exhausted. It is a curious fact that hunger will return in three days, even where there are abundant reserves on hand, if three days are all that are required for the patient to get well; whereas, it will not return for five weeks or longer, even where there are fewer reserves on hand, providing this time is required for the body to eliminate its accumulated toxins. Fortunately, in most cases it will be perfectly safe for the patient to fast until hunger returns. I have been repeatedly asked by anxious patients: "Are you sure that my hunger will return? Does this always occur?" My answer is: You need have no worry about this matter. You may rest assured that your hunger will return and it will do so in all its youthful intensity and zest.

I have had cases in which hunger returned before the tongue cleared up. I interpret this to mean that the body's reserves have been exhausted before the work of elimination could be completed. I have had a few cases in which the tongue cleared up before the return of hunger. I think that in these cases the body was cleansed before the reserves were exhausted and the body did not begin to demand food until the reserves were exhausted. Both of these types of cases are very rare.

Carrington says: "However long the fast may continue, no danger whatever from starvation need be feared, *since hunger will always return before the danger point is reached.* Thus, so long as hunger is absent, it is a plain indication that no food is required . . . I cannot too strongly impress this point upon my readers—that natural hunger, and that alone should indicate the terminus of the fast . . . That this signal is invariably given at the proper time, and in the proper way, and that absolutely no danger from starvation need be apprehended until the signal has been given, is absolutely true . . . The artificial breaking of the fast; the taking of food in the absence of real hunger, for the reason that the ignorant attendant thinks the patient has 'fasted long enough,' is an abomination, and an outrage upon the system which cannot be too strongly depricated."—*Vitality, Fasting and Nutrition*, pp. 546-547.

His view is that this sudden, artificial check to the healing and cleansing processes that go on during the fast is detrimental to the vital machinery. Dr. Lindlahr once likened this arbitrary control of the processes of healing to the work of renovating a house. The workers come in and tear all the paper off the wall and throw it out into the middle of the floor. They tear away much else and pile it in the middle of the floor. They then go away and cease their work. The condition of the house is worse than before they began to work. While this analogy is not strictly true, due to the fact that the body does not throw its waste into the middle of the floor, it has some relation to facts. In my own experience I have seen the following developments when fasts were broken prematurely, which I interpret to mean that nature was not ready for the fast to be broken:

1. The body often refuses food (by vomiting) before the return of hunger.

2. When the fast is prematurely ended, the tongue tends to remain coated.

3. In many cases no desire for food and no relish of food develops for prolonged periods following premature breaking of the fast.

4. Failure of complete recovery from the state of impaired health that occasioned the fast is common.

5. The patient often does not gain weight thereafter.

Carrington points out that there are cases of paralysis and other diseases in which daily improvement is seen during the fast, but the moment the fast is broken (prematurely) the improvement ceases, so that the organic benefit corresponds to the actual time fasted. Thus, if thirty days of fasting are required for full results and the patient fasts but twenty, he gets but two-thirds of the desired results, for the last days of a fast are often most productive of results.

Many patients make the mistake of breaking their fast prematurely. They decide that they have but two or three more days to fast and that these few days will make but little difference. They reason that, since they will derive so little benefit from two or three more days of fasting, they may as well break it at once and not fast the extra few days. Yet, these few extra days may be the difference between success and failure; or, perhaps more accurately, between complete success and a disappointing partial success.

There is a popular belief that the work of purification can be finished with a diet and, in many cases, this is true, providing the patient is willing to greatly restrict himself for a sufficiently long period of time; but it is the rule that the patient who will not carry the fast to completion will also refuse to control himself and stay with the requisite dietary restrictions sufficiently long to accomplish the desired end. Because it is easier to fast than to restrict one's eating, one is more likely to abandon a restricted diet. It should be known that there are no "seven day cleansing diets."

Carrington says: "We have now seen that it is impossible to tell *a priori*, when to break a fast. No arbitrary time limit can be set, no definite date fixed upon before hand and asserted that it would be the most advantageous for the patient were the fast broken on that day. Nature will always dictate when the fast is to be broken, if we but interpret her right. The return of natural hunger is the great point to note, and the most important indication that the fast is ended, and the system is able and willing to digest and assimilate nourishment, in the form of either solid or liquid—food. The spontaneous and precisely coincidental cleaning of the tongue, of the breath, and of other lesser phenomena which may be observed toward the termination of a 'finish fast,' all indicate that Nature and Nature alone, is the authority to be consulted as to when the fast should be broken; and inversely proves conclusively that fasting is Nature's cure . . ."—*Vitality, Fasting and Nutrition*, pp. 556-557.

I agree fully with Carrington that there is no means of determining in advance how long any patient needs to fast. No arbitrary limit should be set to the fast, except in those instances where the patient has but a limited time to devote to fasting. No definite time can be fixed in advance when the fast should be terminated. The body itself will always signify when the fast should be ended. Theoretically, this is all correct; but we deal with all types of patients, with all types of mentalities and of all degrees of economic wellbeing and with many and varied responsibilities. We are compelled, therefore, to break fasts when in our better judgement, they should not be broken, to break them far in advance of the time nature would indicate they should be broken. Levanzin says: "It is always inadvisable to break a fast before natural hunger appears; and as a rule, there is no reason why you should."

A few more words should be said about the return of hunger. We have many patients saying they are hungry when they are not. They mistake many different sensations, chiefly morbid sensations, for hunger. After a short wait, the supposed hunger passes, whereas, the genuine article persists until food is taken. It is necessary to differentiate between real hunger and the many sensations that are commonly mistaken for hunger.

Individuals undergoing a fast on their own and without supervision, have been known to push their fasts into the starvation period, refusing to eat after the return of hunger, merely because the tongue was not clear. This is a mistake and has proved fatal in more than one case. We may always avoid a mistake of this nature if we keep always in mind the fact that the return of hunger is the central indication that the fast should be broken.

Mr. Carrington writes of a race between the successful elimination of toxins and the amount of flesh upon the body, and hunger not returning before the starvation period or even death occurring, because there is not sufficient flesh upon the body to feed the vital organs while the work of elimination is being completed. I have never seen anything of this nature. I have seen cases in which hunger has returned and the tongue was still heavily coated. I have seen the tongue clear up days in advance of the return of hunger. I have said, as a result of such experiences, that if the tongue is clear and hunger has not returned, it means that the body has been cleared before the reserves have been exhausted; while, if hunger returns and the tongue is still coated, it means that the reserves have been exhausted before the body is fully clean. I have seen a few cases in which the tongue never coated throughout the whole of a long fast. I am sure, also, that if the patient's reserves are carefully conserved by mental, physical and sensory rest, there is much less likelihood of his reserves being exhausted in advance of the completion of the work of elimination.

The man experienced in the employment of the fast does not start out to have his client break all records in fasting; but he does start the fast with definite objectives in view. He wishes to reduce weight, reduce blood pressure, relieve the organism of accumulated waste and of food excess, to rest the vital organs, and relieve the nervous system of irritations. If possible, he wants the fast always to continue until these objectives are accomplished. We should not expect a few days of fasting to completely reverse pathological processes that have been decades in developing, or to enable the body to completely remove the pathological accumulations of years. Too many people go on a fast and, from ignorance of their own or that of their advisors, give up before they have achieved the desired results. These people may often be heard to say: "I *tried* fasting and it did me no good."

There are patients who do not need a complete fast, and those who should not have a complete fast, as well as those who do not get well without a complete fast. No hard and fast rule can be set down to guide us here. Each case will have to be handled according to its own needs and according to the general condition of the patient. Ordinarily the fast should continue until the desired results are achieved; yet there are cases, as will be seen later, where this is not feasible. In *acute "disease,"* one is always safe in continuing the fast as long as the acute symptoms continue and for as long thereafter as nature does not call for food. But in chronic "disease" one may not always fast to completion. If a chronic sufferer has begun a fast and it is giving him no difficulties there can be no reason for discontinuing it until the results desired are obtained, or until nature indicates that it should be broken. But it is not wise to arbitrarily set a goal of thirty days or more, as many fasters have done, and make a stunt of the fast. Where a long fast is required, nature herself can be depended upon to indicate when it should be broken. In many cases it is probably better to resort to a series of short fasts with careful feeding rather than to attempt a long fast.

One school teaches its students that "Generally speaking, the use of several fasts of four to seven days each is just as effective as one fast for several weeks." While there are cases where we are compelled to employ a series of short fasts in this way, it has not been my experience that a series of short fasts is as effective as one long fast. I do not know of any one who has had long experience with fasting who claims that such has been his or her experience. Dr. Hazzard does not favor this view. Neither does Carrington. The works of Macfadden are full of contrary expressions, as are the works of Tilden.

Those who cater to popular fears and prejudices and those without experience, favor short fasts, often a series of them. This plan is also preferred by those who desire to drag a case out as long as possible in order to get more money out of the patient. It is not always easiest and best for the patient to take a series of fasts. In his experiments with salamanders, Morgulis found that a single protracted fast was less injurious than intermittent fasting—a series of short fasts. With exceptions to be noted elsewhere, this is also our experience in fasting men, women and children. It should be known, also, that weak and underweight patients often stand fasting much better than strong and overweight patients.

The alternate fasting and feeding program is not as satisfactory as the one long fast and tends to be more difficult for the patient to carry out. He tends to reach a stage where he rebels against undergoing another fast. He hesitates, he draws back, he even dreads it. In many of these fasts, they last just long enough for his body to become adjusted to the fasting process and then they are broken. Each time he fasts he is forced to go through the same experience. Thus, he never experiences the comfortable stages of the fast. It has been my experience that in all cases, where the long fast is possible, one long fast is far more effective and more satisfactory than a series of short ones. No plan of feeding between the fasts will accomplish what the fast will do, if continued. The length of the fast must be governed by the patient's condition and by the results obtained.

There are those who object to a long fast on the ground that it constitutes such a shock to the nervous system and such a drain on the vital resources that lasting injury results. I have not personally observed any of the evils attributed to the long fast and do not find such results described by those whose experience with fasting entitles them to speak on the subject. On the other hand, I find that when some of the examples cited, as showing that a long fast injures the body, are checked upon, they are found not to prove any such thing, but the opposite.

—293—

In 1886 the painter, Merlatti, fasted fifty days in Paris. It is asserted that he was in bad condition at the end of the fast. I have been unable to check up on this assertion and do not know how true it is. His heart action and body temperature remained normal throughout the fast. Pashutin records that he was watched after the fast. The statement is sometimes made that after his forty-two days fast in 1877, Dr. Tanner was in such bad condition he had to be placed under medical care. This statement is very misleading. Dr. Tanner had been in very bad health for years preceding his fast and undertook the fast to recover health. He was under the observation of a physician through the whole of the fast and thereafter for some time. He actually regained his health by and through the fast. Dr. Tanner occupied a room in the home of Dr. Moyer, in Minneapolis, Minn., during his fast and was attended daily by Dr. Moyer. According to his own testimony he "had given up hopes of ever regaining what might be called normal health" and undertook the fast only after he had "virtually collapsed" and "was at such a low ebb physically and mentally that" he "did not care whether" he "lived or died" and "determined," as he says, "that, since my drugs gave me no relief, I would starve myself to death ere I again would suffer the physical misery that had been mine for months preceding."

At the end of ten days of fasting all symptoms of his disorder disappeared and Dr. Moyer attempted to induce him to discontinue the fast. Tanner persisted to the end of the forty-second day. His health was distinctly improved. His medical colleagues refused to believe that a man can go so long without food, so, "in order to relieve myself," he writes, "of the odium heaped upon me by the medical enemies" of his claims to have gone without food, in 1880, he underwent another fast of forty days beginning June 28, and ending at noon August 6. This fast was public and observed by many medical men and the whole story flashed to the world daily by the newspapers and telegraphs. Tanner's health was not impaired by this fast.

In general, it may be safely advised that if a fast is undertaken it should be done with satisfactory results as the end in view and stay with it until results are forthcoming. Thousands of sufferers attempt to do with a fast of two to four days what can only be accomplished by a fast of two to four weeks or more. "I tried fasting and it did not help me," they say. Playing around with short fasts and semi-fasts will seldom give satisfactory results. Fast for results or forget it—this is my advice. The body cannot undo, in three to four days of fasting, the results of years of surfeiting and of un-*Hygienic* living. The most rapid recoveries are seen in *acute* "diseases" and three to four days of fasting are seldom enough in these. Longer fasts are required in chronic forms.

If the pathological condition of the patient does not demand or permit of a complete fast, it should not be insisted upon. The patient must be carefully watched and if any danger signals arise, the fast should be broken despite the fact that hunger has not returned and the tongue is still foul. These are cases in which it is better to be safe than sorry. Long fasts are seldom or never advisable in advanced tuberculosis. Short fasts can aid but little in cancer. Catarrhal troubles are seldom or never overcome during a short fast. A long fast is usually required in rheumatism, arthritis, and gout. Long standing digestive complaints usually require a long fast. Diabetes and Bright's "disease" call for a long fast, as do most forms of heart trouble. In inflammation of the digestive tract, such as gastritis, enteritis, peritonitis, dysentery, diarrhea, typhoid fever, typhus, cholera, typhilitis, appendicitis, etc., it is essential that fasting be continued for several days after fever and other symptoms have subsided. Even in mild acute disease, it is well always to continue the fast for at least twenty-four hours after the symptoms have subsided.

Hunger and Appetite

CHAPTER XXIV

Hunger is the great safeguard of all life. It impels the organism in need of food to search for and procure food. It may be safely inferred that if there is no hunger, there is no need for nourishment. Hunger is a normal expression of a physiological need and when it is absent, we may take it for granted that the physiological need that gives rise to it is also absent. In proportion to the need of the body for food will hunger be present, and precisely in proportion to its lack of need for food or to its inability to digest and assimilate food will there be an absence of hunger. When hunger is absent, therefore, no food should be taken. It seems vital, therefore, that we learn to distinguish between hunger and other common sensations— that we learn to properly interpret the language of our senses.

The sense of hunger is little understood, perhaps because it has never really been studied. What little attempt has been made by physiologists to study hunger has been made on sick and ailing men and women, with the result that all kinds of morbid sensations have been and continue to be mistaken for hunger, not merely by the layman, but by the expert, who is presumed to know. Science, at present, teaches that hunger is expressed in the stomach, registered especially in the upper part of the stomach, and is manifested by various discomforts. That this is a fallacy will become readily apparent when, and if they make their investigations upon really healthy subjects.

Physiologists have accepted the theory advanced by Cannon that the contractions of the stomach that are concomitant with what they call hunger pangs are the immediate cause of the sensation of hunger. They say that these contractions of the stomach are definitely associated with the sensation of hunger and are more marked, the more intense the sensation. Cannon records the results of his studies of hunger and his conclusions from these studies in his book, *Bodily Changes in Pain, Hunger, Fear and Rage.* In this excellent book he says:

"The sensation of hunger is difficult to describe, but almost everyone from childhood has felt at times that dull ache or gnawing pain referred to the lower mid-chest and the epigastrium, which may take imperious control of human action. As Sternberg has pointed out, hunger may be sufficiently insistent to force the taking of food which is so distasteful that it not only fails to arouse appetite, but may even produce nausea.

"The hungry being gulps his food with a rush. The pleasures of appetite are not for him—he wants quantity rather than quality, and he wants it at once.

"Hunger may be described as having a central core and certain more or less variable accessories. The peculiar dull ache of hungriness, referred to the epigastrium, is usually the organism's first strong demand for food; and when the initial order is not obeyed, the sensation is likely to grow into a highly uncomfortable pang or gnawing, less definitely localized as it becomes more intense. This may be regarded as the essential feature of hunger. Besides the dull ache, however, lassitude and drowsiness may appear, or faintness, or violent headache, or irritability and restlessness such that continuous effort in ordinary affairs becomes increasingly difficult. That these states differ much with individuals—headache in one and faintness in another, for example—indicates that they do not constitute the central fact of hunger, but are more or less inconstant accompaniments. The 'feeling of emptiness' which has been mentioned as an important element of the experience, is an inference rather than a distinct datum of consciousness, and can likewise be eliminated from further consideration. The dull pressing sensation is left, therefore, as the constant characteristic, the central fact, to be examined in detail."

It will be well, before going deeper into our study of hunger, to view briefly what the physiologists have to say about the sensation of hunger and its cause. I quote: "it is well known that during hunger certain general subjective symptoms are likely to be experienced, such as a feeling of weakness and a sense of emptiness, with a tendency to headache and sometimes even nausea in persons who are prone to headache as a result of toxemic conditions. Headache is likely to be more pronounced or perhaps only present in the morning before there is any food in the stomach." He speaks of "hunger pangs" and of their "greatest intensity."—Macleod's *Physiology in Modern Medicine*.

In this same standard text, the author discusses what he calls "hunger during starvation," by which he means hunger during a period of four days of abstinence from food undergone by Carlson and Luckhardt, "who voluntarily subjected themselves to complete starvation, except for the taking of water, for four days." He says "during enforced starvation for long periods of time, it is known that healthy individuals at first experience intense sensations of hunger and appetite, which last, however, only for a few days, then become less pronounced and finally almost disappear."

Of Carlson's and Luckhardt's four days of self-imposed "starvation" he says "sensations of hunger were present more or less throughout the period*** on the last day of starvation a burning sensation referred to the epigastrium was added to that of hunger." They found that their sensations of hunger and appetite both became perceptibly diminished on the last day of "starvation" (their fourth day without food) the diminution being most marked in the sensation of appetite. They found that instead of an eagerness for food developing, there developed on the last day a distinct repugnance, or indifference to food. They also describe a distinct depression and a feeling of weakness which accompanied appetite during the latter part of their "starvation" period.

They also found that after partaking of food, after their prolonged period of four days of "starvation," their "hunger" and appetite sensations rapidly disappeared. Also, practically all of their mental depression and a great part of their weakness disappeared. Complete recovery of strength did not occur until the second or third day after resumption of eating. From that time on, both men felt unusually well; indeed, they state that their sense of well-being and clearness of mind and their sense of good health and vigor were as greatly improved as they would have been by a month's vacation in the mountains.

These investigators point out that since others who have "starved" for longer periods of time (than four days) unanimously attest the fact that, after the first few days, the sensations of hunger become less pronounced and finally almost disappear, they must have experienced the most distressing period during their four days of "starvation." Although the hunger sensation was strong enough to cause some discomfort, it could by no means be called marked pain or suffering, and was at no time of sufficient intensity to interfere seriously with work. Mere "starvation" cannot therefore be designated as acute suffering.

Howell's *Textbook of Physiology* tells us that the sensations of hunger and thirst are of such a vague character that it is difficult to analyze them by methods of introspection. He adds that the sensation that we commonly designate as appetite or hunger "is referred or projected more or less definitely to the region of the stomach." "When the sensation is not satisfied by the ingestion of food, it increases in intensity and the individual experiences the pangs of hunger." He also refers to "hunger pain." The sensation of hunger is described as "more or less disagreeable."

Best and Taylor point out (*Physiological Basis of Medical Practice*, page 495), that in an investigation of hunger and hunger contractions in a human fasting subject, extending over a period of five days, the hunger contractions showed no diminutions. In fact they actually increased in amplitude, yet the "hunger pangs" and the general sensation of "hunger" lessened after the third day.

Whatever may be the true relationship of these gastric contractions to the sense of hunger, the physiologists from Cannon to Carlson, have blundered in that they have accepted certain pathological symptoms as the sense of hunger. The primary error in all of their reasoning is that of accepting morbid sensations for hunger. No genuinely healthy subjects have been used as subjects of experiment. Any man of experience, reading the foregoing, will recognize at once that not one of these men has ever seen a hungry man and has mistaken the morbid sensations of a food-drunkard for the normal expressions of life. Real hunger, rather than producing "lassitude and drowsiness," or "faintness," produces alertness and activity in the search for food.

Mr. Hoelzel tells us that Dr. Carlson changed his views considerably about hunger before his death. Unfortunately he does not seem to have published his changed views. It may be that his changed views were more in line with what those of us who have had greatest experience with fasting regard as a true indication of the need for food.

In attempting to arrive at an understanding of what the sensation of hunger is and is not, I think it wise to give attention to the observations of those who have had greatest experience with fasting, especially with long fasts, rather than to the experiments of those who have conducted a few rather short fasts in their study of hunger. A man who has carefully observed a hundred or more fasts of forty or more days duration would seem to be in a better position to evalute the various "feelings" that are thought to represent hunger, than is the man who has observed one or two fasts of four to seven days duration.

I also doubt the validity of studies of "hunger" that are made on subjects who swallow balloons which are subsequently inflated with air and left in the stomach. No physiologist would admit that the behavior of a stomach, stretched by the presence of an inflated baloon, would be the same as the behavior of an empty stomach. The balloons were part of a contrivance designed to register and measure the frequency and vigor of the contractions of the stomach, but they could tell nothing of the sensation of hunger. Another element associated with these experiments that vitiates the conclusions was the constant preoccupation with food and thoughts of hunger, even the constant direction of attention to the stomach. This preoccupation with thoughts of food and of the stomach conjured into existence sensations that would not otherwise have developed. The very psychological factor involved also kept alive the fictional desire for food that is so common.

Let us try to arrive at an understanding of hunger by seeing what it is not. Headache is not hunger. Pain in the abdomen is not hunger. Gnawing in the stomach is not hunger. Lassitude is not hunger. Drowsiness is not hunger. Weakness is not hunger. Faintness is not hunger. A "dull pressing sensation" is not hunger. Restlessness is not hunger. In forty-four years of conducting fasts, during which time I have conducted thousands of fasts that have extended over periods that have ranged from twenty days to ninety days, I have yet to see a single individual in whom pain, headache, drowsiness, a "feeling of emptiness," etc., accompanied the development of genuine hunger. These observations should be worth something. They are certainly more dependable than those that are made on individuals abstaining from food for three to five days.

Dull ache in the epigastrium, violent headache, irritability, restlessness, lassitude, drowsiness, faintness and a decreasing capacity for continuous effort—how like the effects that follow the missing of the accustomed cigar, pipe, cup of coffee or tea, glass of whiskey, or dose of morphine are these symptoms! How did Prof. Cannon miss their true significance? The "feeling of emptiness," and the gnawing that he describes, are not accompaniments of hunger. Neither is the "dull pressing sensation" which he has left as the "central fact" of hunger, any part of the physiological demand for food, which we call hunger. These are both morbid sensations. "No person," says Page, "feels faint upon passing a meal, or has a gnawing stomach, except it be occasioned by an irritated or unduly congested state of that organ. It is a sure proof of dyspepsia (using this term in its popular sense, as implying the condition of that organ). Strictly speaking the term is a synonym of indigestion."—*Horses, Their Feed and Their Feet*, p. 28.

A pang is a short, sharp pain. Carlson says that "it has been definitely established that 'hunger pangs' are caused by contractions of the empty stomach." This was "established" by having subjects swallow balloons which registered the frequency and intensity of the gastric contractions. We cannot doubt the contractions: we doubt the validity of the interpretations that have been placed upon them. "Hunger pangs" would seem to be cramps and these are certainly abnormal. Normal muscular contractions, even if vigorous, are not painful. On the contrary, if they are registered in consciousness at all, and gastric contractions are normally not so registered, they tend to be pleasurable.

Think of thirst. Is it pain? Is it a headache? Is it irritability? Is it faintness? Is it drowsiness? Is it any of the sensations described by Prof. Cannon as belonging to hunger? It is none of these things. Thirst is felt in the mouth and throat and there is a distinct and conscious desire for water. One does not mistake headache for thirst. The sensation of thirst is too well-known.

The irritation caused by the passage of the tube through the pharynx and œsophagus and the presence of the inflated balloon in the stomach are such as to occasion abnormal behavior. To think of such behavior as physiological is absurd; to expect to study the normal activities of life in this manner is foolish. The behavior of a stomach filled with a distended balloon and its behavior under normal conditions are not exactly identical. It contracts under both conditions, but its contractions are not likely to follow the same patterns under the two conditions. Certainly its contractions upon a foreign object cannot be regarded as manifestations of hunger.

It has been demonstrated by more than one experimenter that, after a few days of fasting the stomach contractions tend to increase rather than to diminish, although the sensations that are commonly mistaken for hunger lessen and cease altogether. This should reveal that the "hunger contractions" are not that at all, but merely the regular peristaltic movements of the stomach.

Carlson also says that there is a "generalized weakness and restlessness, referred to no special part of the body" in hunger. In genuine hunger, instead of the weakness commonly associated with it, there is alertness and often, if not always, a distinct feeling of wellbeing. Dr. Claunch said "a healthy person will get hungry before he gets weak while a sick person will get weak before he gets hungry." This rule was based on close observation of hundreds of fasting people. As many of these fasts were of considerable duration and were not confined to three or four days of abstinence, his conclusion is to be trusted above that of the scientists who arbitrarily restrict themselves to inadequate experiments.

Those who feel a gnawing in the stomach, as they describe it, should know that this is not hunger but a morbid symptom. Instead of eating to palliate the symptom, they should fast until they are comfortable. Irritation of the stomach, due to indigestion, is frequently mistaken for a desire to eat. That eating affords relief from these symptoms proves that they were hunger in the same way that a shot of morphine proves that the pains of the addict are genuine demands for morphine.

Dr. Susannah W. Dodds had quite an extensive experience with fasting and her observations are worthy of consideration. She says that "the sense of all-goneness in these cases is not from lack of nutrient material, but owing to the absence of the habitual stimulus."—*The Diet Question*, p. 87. If an orthodox writer were considering these same symptoms in dealing with drug addiction, he would call them "withdrawal symptoms." In the case of the supposedly hungry person, they are commonly due to the withdrawal of salt, pepper and other condiments, and *irritants* or *stimulants* usually taken with food. Why have physiologists consistently refused to consider the observations of those who have had greatest opportunity to observe the sensation and evidences of hunger? Why should headache be considered hunger? Why is it ever associated with hunger? It is true that eating will sometimes "relieve" a headache, just as the accustomed cup of coffee will do the same. In these cases, is it the food or the drug that is taken with the food that "relieves" the ache? So long as we refuse to separate our foods from our drugs, how can we know whether we are suffering the *symptoms* of the disease called *hunger* or the *withdrawal symptoms* of a poison disease—addiction? Why shall we continue to define a normal sensation of the living organism in terms of symptoms of pathology?

Carrington referred to these symptoms as "habit hunger," Dewey as "hunger of disease," Oswald as "poison hunger." As they do not represent hunger at all, I see no reason to describe such sensations as hunger of any kind. As they are always abnormal, just as much so as are the alleged *cravings* of the morphine addict for his customary *narcotic,* and are most marked in those individuals whose stomach has been habitually subjected to the *excitement* and *irritation* occasioned by condiments, spices, etc., they should be recognized for what they are—symptoms of disease. The stomach, suddenly deprived of its regular occasions for excitement, by the fast, manifests the same signs of distress as do the nerves of the tobacco addict when these are deprived of their accustomed *narcotic.*

It is true that eating will allay these sensations, just as a shot of morphine will "relieve" the morphine addict, and there is just as much sense in taking food in the first instance as there is in taking the morphine in the last. Page says: "The fact that the meal affords immediate relief argues nothing against this position; it is the seventy-five or eighty per cent of water taken with the meal that relieves the digestion. It forms a *poultice,* so to say, for the congested mucous membrane of the stomach; but, unfortunately, it cannot, as when applied externally upon a throbbing sore thumb, for example, be removed when it becomes dry."—*The Natural Cure,* p. 202.

Why should morbid appetites be indulged? Is there any more reason for indulging a morbid appetite for food than there is for indulging a morbid appetite for clay or filth? If we refuse to indulge the morbid "craving" for glass, stones, bullets, pins, earth, etc., why shall we not restrain the morbid appetite for bread, beef, candy, fruits, etc.? In many of these cases several large meals a day are eaten and still the possessors of such appetites are not satisfied.

"False hunger," "habit hunger," "poison hunger" and similar phrases are misnomers. The term hunger should be reserved for the normal demand for food and other and more appropriate terms should be employed to designate those abnormal sensations that are commonly mistaken for hunger and for those sensations of discomfort and unease that are mistaken for a call for some poison that one is accustomed to taking. It should be known that there is no such thing as a poison hunger or a craving for poison.

Dr. Cannon is wrong again in asserting that the hungry person gulps his food, or that he seeks for quantity rather than quality. Evidently he carried out his researches on a group of neurotics, dyspeptics and food drunkards. He never permitted any of them to go without food long enough for full adjustment to follow. The hungry person, at the completion of a long fast, commonly finds that half a glass of fruit juice is all that he wants. If he is given this quantity of juice every hour during the day, he may find that by about four o'clock in the afternoon, he has had all the food he desires. He is content to wait until the next day to take more. Dr. Oswald wrote: "Only natural (normal) appetites have natural (normal) limits," and nowhere is this more true than in the truly hungry person.

Hunger has been said to be selective rather than indiscriminate, frequently demanding a specific food or a specific type of food. This, it seems to me, better describes the characteristic of hunger, than Cannon's description. On the other hand, unlike *appetite*, hunger is not finicky, but is satisfied with plain fare and readily accepts another food if the one desired is not available.

A vast experience with fasting has taught us that the morbid sensations that are mistaken for hunger are likely to be most severe in the diseased, especially in those with disease of the stomach. We know, also, that these sensations soon subside and cease altogether when one fasts. After a few days perfect comfort is experienced. This should not be so if they were indications of a genuine need for food. When it is said that hunger ceases after a few days of fasting, it is not hunger that is meant at all; but the symptoms of disease that are mistaken for hunger. I doubt that genuine hunger would cease upon a fast.

Being ravenous is no indication that the eater can digest what he eats. Hearty eating is frequently seen to be accompanied by a gradual decline in weight. Many of these cases put on weight when they reduce the amount of food they eat. How often do we see patients who are always eating and who complain that they are "always hungry." They eat several times a day and three or more times at night, but they never seem to get enough to eat. Of course, these people are never hungry; they are food drunkards who employ food as palliation. Eating temporarily "relieves" their gastric and nervous distress. They are merely extreme cases of what physiologists mistake for hunger. There are wasting "diseases" in which there is an insatiable appetite, the craving being constant, no matter how much food the patient eats. These people eat despite the fact that they have no ability to digest and assimilate the food eaten. Indeed, their constant eating helps to perpetuate their functional and structural impairment and aids in keeping them emaciated.

Neither the all-gone, faint feeling, nor the sensation of gnawing in the stomach, nor a feeling of emptiness, nor of weakness, nor a headache, nor any other morbid symptom is hunger. These are morbid sensations representing gastric irritation, a neurosis, gastric ulcer, indigestion, gastric inflammation, reaction from withdrawal of stimulation, etc., rather than hunger. That faint sinking feeling at the pit of the stomach, with a morbid "craving" for something to eat, is due to chronic inflammation of the lining membrane of the stomach. Such symptoms of gnawing and faintness and all-goneness are seen in their height in cases of acute gastritis as well as in gastric ulcer. Indeed,, a bowel movement may induce them in cases of colitis. There is no end to these morbid sensations that are mistaken for hunger, although the surest and speediest means of getting rid of them is to fast. It is significant in this connection that these abnormal sensations are strongest in those of gross habits, in those who have been accustomed to highly "stimulating" viands, in those of intemperate habits and in the obese. In the neurotic, also, they are likely to be severe. The healthy person, the person of more moderate habits, the vegetarian, etc., is not troubled with such sensations and discomforts. If left alone these morbid sensations sooner or later pass away, but if palliated by eating or by taking more condiments or by drink, they are but temporarily smothered. As soon as the stomach is again empty of food, they are back again, perhaps with renewed intensity.

Graham says: "This peculiar condition of the stomach (the feeling of abnormal hunger) will pass away much sooner and with less uncomfortableness of feeling in the pure vegetable eater of regular habits, when the ordinary meal is omitted, than in the flesh eater; and he who makes a free use of stimulating condiments with his food, experiences still more inconvenience and distress at the loss of a meal, than he who eats flesh simply and plainly prepared. Hence, the pure vegetable-eater loses a meal with great indifference, fasts twenty-four hours with little inconvenience or diminution of strength, and goes without food several days in succession without suffering anything like intolerable distress from hunger. The flesh-eater always suffers much more from fasting, and experiences a more rapid decline of muscular power; and he who seasons his food with highly stimulating condiments, feels the loss of a single day severely; a fast of twenty-four hours almost unmans him; and three or four days abstinence from food completely prostrates him, if he is cut off from all stimulants as well as aliment."—*Science of Human Life,* p. 559.

There is another theory that hunger is due to the accumulation of gastric juice in the stomach. In fasts that I have undergone, I have experienced a number of instances in which considerable quantities of highly acid gastric juice have been regurgitated from the stomach, but no feeling of hunger was present. In a few cases in patients there has been stomach discomfort until the eructations of the acid gastric contents have brought relief, but no desire for food was complained of. Indeed, pain is incompatible with hunger.

Whatever may be the ultimate interpretations placed upon the experimental findings of Cannon, Carlson and others, they will not, I am sure, be mistaken for true indexes to the body's need for food. Neither gastric acidity nor gastric contractions, but blood and cellular depletion, give rise to the sensation of hunger.

As most men and women, including scientists, declare that hunger is always felt in the stomach, therefore, the "stomach hunger" must be normal, it has been argued that to take the view that normal hunger is manifested in the mouth and throat, we must be prepared to take the position that most men and women have never experienced normal hunger since infancy. This is precisely what we contend. Mr. Carrington says: "most persons have never experienced normal hunger in all their lives! Their appetite and taste are perverted by overfeeding in infancy, and have never had a chance to become normal during the whole course of their lives—owing to the overfeeding being continued ever since." Dewey pointed out that with many people the "evil work" of inducing disease began with the very first meal which was forced upon them by the mother or nurse before they were ready for it. As the forcing process was continued, he says "in due time trouble began," and, thereafter, every outcry of nature was interpreted as a signal of hunger." He says that the meals of the infant "all through the first year of life are regulated by the tunes of crying." Happily, the so-frequent feeding of infants is not as common today as when Dr. Dewey wrote these lines, but it is still all too true that gastric impairment and gastric distress are built in infancy by wrong feeding.

People do not know the sensation of hunger because they have never experienced it. At least genuine hunger is a rare experience among present-day Americans. Even the poor commonly over eat and do so day after day, although they are likely to eat foods that do not adequately meet their needs. The practices of feeding by the clock, started at birth, of stuffing babies at all hours of the day and night, of feeding children between meals, a practice that tends to be kept up throughout life, guarantees that these young people shall never experience genuine hunger. Appetite? Yes. They have all kinds of appetites, but hunger is foreign to them.

The average person, never having experienced true hunger and having suffered many discomforts in the region of the stomach, will object that hunger is always felt in the stomach. But if, from infancy, these people have never experienced genuine hunger, how can they know that what they mistake for hunger has any relation to hunger at all?

Hunger is the language of the body calling for materials—food. This call is made necessary by the depletion of the blood of materials. The blood, in circulating through the capillaries, gives up its materials to the tissues, thus depleting it of supplies. Why should this call for food be painful or uncomfortable? Why should we attempt to define or describe hunger in terms of pathology? Even physiologists have accepted the popular notion that hunger is a disagreeable sensation, one verging on actual suffering.

In many quarters there is fear of hunger. There is the belief that hunger is an evil. Not hunger, but the lack of means of gratifying its demands, is the evil. Hunger is as normal and as serviceable as thirst, tiredness, sleepiness and all other sensations by which the body makes known its needs. It is one of the great protectors of the welfare of the body, not one of life's enemies. A lack of food may prove to be an evil, the way in which the body makes its need for food known is certainly not evil.

Contrary to the prevailing view, I must insist that real hunger is a genuinely pleasant, even an exquisite sensation, one that is worth experiencing for its own sake. How do we describe sensations? We know that hunger is felt in the mouth, throat, nose and to some extent in the whole body, and that there is no pain or suffering associated with it. We know, on the contrary, that suffering tends to repress the desire for food and to make digestion impossible. In real hunger there is a distinct and conscious desire for food. The condition is one of comfort, not of discomfort and suffering. There is a "watering" of the mouth (flow of saliva) and often a distinct desire for a particular food. Hunger is a localized sensation and is not in the stomach. The healthy person is not conscious of any sensations in or about the stomach when hungry.

As everyone who has had an extensive experience with fasting knows, true hunger is felt in the mouth and throat and nose and is related to the senses of taste and smell. It is indicated by a watering of the mouth for plain food—even for a crust of dry bread. Also, almost everybody knows from personal experience the gnawing sensation or other sensation that is commonly thought of as hunger usually comes on at meal time, or when the stomach is empty, and subsides after an hour or two, if no food is taken. As we see in thousands of cases of fasting, these morbid sensations subside and completely cease after two or three days of fasting, not to recur after the fast is broken.

For over a hundred years Shew, Graham, Trall, Page, Dewey, Oswald, Haskell, Macfadden, Carrington, Eales, Tilden, Weger, Claunch, Shelton and hundreds of others, who have had extensive experience with fasting, have been calling attention to the fact that hunger is a mouth and throat sensaton rather than a stomach sensaton, but the professional physiologists have persisted in ignoring their work and their testimony and have accepted popular superstitions about the sensation of hunger and have "confirmed" these by limited experiments on sick men and women. Cannon, Pavlov, Carlson, etc., have all based their conclusions on inadequate data and on experiments that are too short to be conclusive.

Certainly if one is ever hungry, he is so at the conclusion of a long fast. Fasting experts insist that hunger is invariably manifested at the conclusion of a long fast, like thirst, in the mouth and throat. We employ this fact as a complete and satisfactory test of the sensations observed during a fast—it reveals whether it is true hunger or morbid sensations. Never under any circumstances following a fast, is hunger felt in the stomach. Always it is manifested in the mouth and throat and always there is an entire absence of distress or of morbid sensations associated with the stomach.

APPETITE

One of the most frequent dietetic errors is that of mistaking appetite for hunger. Appetite is no more hunger than sexual passion is love. Graham made a sharp distinction between an "appetite" which is merely the expression of habit (the habit of eating at certain times) and "that natural and healthy hunger which is a physiological manifestation of the real alimentary wants of the body" and asserted that it "is of the utmost importance that this distinction should ever be kept in view," when considering man's dietary habits. Appetite, which is so much a matter of habit, has sometimes been referred to as "habit-hunger," but I do not think the inclusion of the word hunger in this compound term is correct. As has been previously pointed out, habit may be morbid, true hunger never is. Bulimia, or an ox-like appetite, is seen in a number of states of disease, but it has no more relation to true hunger than a headache has to the appreciation of music.

Horace Fletcher says that the "mark of distinction" that differentiates real hunger from appetite is the "watering of the mouth for some particular thing." Appetite is indiscriminate and often finicky. "Natural hunger is never in a hurry," declares Carrington. Appetite is often in a big hurry. Pavlov showed that appetite for food, which cannot be hunger, may be induced by swallowing a mouthful of wine. He says that at the moment the wine reached the stomach, he "perceived the onset of a very strong appetite." What he mistook for a demand for food was irritation of the stomach. He made the same mistake here that Cannon made in mistaking similar irritation for hunger.

Contra-Indications of Fasting

CHAPTER XXV

The dangers of fasting are so slight as to be almost negligible or insignificant. When Purinton declared that "an extreme fast, say from twenty to forty days, is just as apt to wreck a man as it is to rescue him, unless, as I have mentioned before, it is properly conducted and completed," he plainly had in mind the many mistakes that the ignorant and inexperienced can and often do make, both during the fast and in breaking the fast. Books on fasting list a number of contra-indications to fasting. These need clarification. They follow:

(1) *Fear of the fast on the part of the patient*: Fear may kill where the fast would be of distinct benefit. If fear of the fast can be overcome there is no reason why it should not be instituted.

(2) *Extreme emaciation*: In such cases a long fast is impossible. A short fast of one to three days may be found beneficial, or a series of such short fasts with longer periods of proper feeding intervening may be found advisable.

In extremely emaciated patients I do not favor pushing the fast to the return of hunger, but favor a process of careful nursing with one or more short fasts. Whereas, Carrington points out that such patients may die before the return of hunger, I am convinced from experience, that with a careful nursing program and but limited fasting, these patients may be restored to health in many cases that would otherwise die. I have repeatedly fasted such cases, even for as much as twenty-two days at a time; always with distinct benefit. Indeed, the fast is often the only thing that will enable these cases to overcome their emaciation.

(3) *In cases of extreme weakness or of extreme degeneration*: Even in many such cases a series of short fasts, as mentioned before, may often be beneficial. In the latter stages of consumption and cancer, the fast can be of no value except to relieve the patient's suffering. It may prolong life a few days. Fasting is of distinct benefit in the earlier stages of both of these conditions, however.

Great weakness is not always a danger signal; rather it may often prove to be a "false alarm." More often than otherwise, weakness signifies poisoning or a crisis. It is essential that the weakness be considered in union with all other symptoms present. Indeed, this is true of all the danger signals. No one of them, considered by itself, constitutes an evidence of real danger. Carrington regards periods of great weakness that are often seen in fasting patients as crises, or periods of great physiological change going on in the body. He says that "the fact that hitherto weak hearts are actually strengthened and cured by fasting proves conclusively that any such unusual symptoms, observed during this period, denote a beneficial reparative process, and not any harmful or dangerous decrease or acceleration, due to lack of perfect control by the cardiac nerve." In this connection I may add that I have never seen a death from "heart failure" during a fast, although I have seen many crippled hearts make complete recovery during a fast. Prostration and weakness are part of the process we call disease, and are not due to the lack of two or three meals. Hence it is that, as the patient returns to normal, strength returns even when no food has been eaten or digested. It has been pointed out in the preceding pages that great weakness is not necessarily a bar to fasting; that it is in such cases that we often see the greatest gains in strength.

(4) *In cases of inactive kidneys accompanied by obesity*: In such cases it is said that the tissues may be broken down faster than the kidneys are able to eliminate them. This I doubt. I know of no reason why the tissues of the body should be used up faster at this time than at other times. It is true that there is increased elimination during the fast but this is not so great as to constitute a great burden upon the kidneys. I have repeatedly fasted cases of Bright's "disease" and cases of kidney stone, kidney abscess and pyelitis with distinct benefit in all such cases.

(5) *In marked "deficiency diseases"*: Some advocates of fasting do not advise fasting in these conditions; but hold that, since they are due to food deficiencies, these patients need a changed diet rather than a fast. It was shown in previous pages that fasting is distinctly beneficial in rickets, anemia and other deficiencies, and that a failing appetite in these conditions plainly indicates the need for a brief fast. It should also not be overlooked that in all deficiencies there are toxic states that must be overcome before the best of diets

can do its perfect work. Deficiency is not always due to faulty diet. It may be due to impaired nutritive machinery and function from a variety of causes. Physiological rest is frequently the first essential of recovery in such cases.

(6) *Difficult Breathing:* This symptom is sometimes seen in two types of cases; namely, nervous cases and cases of heart impairment. In nervous cases it constitutes no warning of danger. In heart cases, it should cause a careful watching of heart action. Should this show signs of weakening, the fast should be terminated at once.

I have fasted many cases, with nothing but benefit, which would not have been placed on a fast by others who employ this measure. I have continued fasts in cases where others would have discontinued the process, with no development in any case of any of the troubles or evils against which we are so frequently warned. I have fasted cases for more than twenty days who were advised by Dr. Hazzard not to fast more than five days. I have fasted cases that Dr. Hazzard had previously placed on lemon juice and honey rather than on a fast. Fear of legal consequences, should something go wrong, prevents many advocates of fasting from using it to its greatest advantage.

There are cases in which it is well to proceed cautiously and in which the inexperienced person should not attempt to conduct a fast; but in general there is seldom any such thing as a contra-indication to fasting, just as there is seldom or never a contra-indication to any other form of rest.

Fasting in Special Periods and Conditions of Life

CHAPTER XXVI

Special periods of life and certain conditions of the body are often regarded as bars to fasting, even by those who profess a belief in the beneficial efficacy of the practice. Let us consider a few of them. But first let us consider:

WHY FAST

A temporary expedient of this nature must be recognized as a fundamental and radical process that is older than any other mode of caring for the sick organism, for it is employed on the plane of instinct and has been so employed since life was first introduced upon the earth. It is hardly conceivable that both animal and human instinct would lead to the continued adoption of the process throughout the ages if it failed to meet some urgent need in the organism of the sick. It may be said, with Dr. Robert Walter, that fasting "liberates vitality (energy) to be used in the process of purification" and that this energy, in health, would "otherwise be used in the process of appropriating food materials." He said of the fast that it "is exceedingly beneficial in the great majority of diseases. Indeed, in many of them the capacity to appropriate food is entirely destroyed, the very thought of it becoming repugnant to the individual."

WHEN TO FAST

I take the position that the time to fast is *when it is needed.* I am of the decided opinion that delay pays no dividends; that, due to the fact that the progressive development of pathological changes in the structures of the body with the consequent impairment of its functions does not cease until its cause has been completely and thoroughly removed, putting off the time for a fast only invites added troubles and makes a longer fast necessary, if indeed, it does not make the fast futile. I do not believe that any condition of impaired health should be tolerated and permitted to become greater.

Now is the time to begin the work of restoring good health; not next week, next summer, or next year.

There has been much discussion of what time of year is best in which to fast. Mr. Purinton advises all prospective fasters to "choose summer or spring for the conquest fast," but while I agree with him that warm weather is, on the whole, the best time for a fast, I advise that no sufferer delay a needed fast until spring or summer, but to take it when needed. As Oswald says: "Winter is not the worst time for a fast, it may even be the best, to judge from the phenomena of hibernation."—*Fasting, Hydrotherapy and Exercise,* p. 65. Louis Kuhne called attention to the fact that many animals eat far less in winter than in summer. Theoretically, at least, less food is required to maintain body heat in summer than in winter; but the winter faster who is kept warm may fast with the greatest of ease.

I agree with Carrington that it is easier to fast in summer than in winter. The sense of chilliness that the faster experiences is greater in winter than it is in the warm months. Although this sense of chilliness does not correspond with the real *cold* of the outside or room temperature and, curiously enough, a thermometer will often show that the temperature of the faster is one or more degrees higher than before he undertook the fast, in spite of the fact that he has the feeling of being *cold.* This, in my opinion, should not deter the man or woman who needs a fast from taking one at any season of the year. A fast should not be delayed because of some slight discomfort. If the faster is kept in bed, as he should be, with a hot jug to his feet, the feeling of *coldness* is easily controlled.

FASTING BY VEGETARIANS

Certain advocates of flesh eating, particularly one who lectures on the radio and gives away hams as a means of securing an audience, cautions vegetarians against fasting. They tell vegetarians that they are the last who should fast. Why? Because fasting is "more likely to cause serious acidosis in vegetarians and others with low protein reserves. Diets high in protein of poor quality may be more harmful than low protein diets which provide the essential amino acids in good proportions."

This objection to fasting by vegetarians is not based on experience and observation, but is purely theoretical. This is one of those instances where "the facts of experience silence the voice of theory." It is not only true that vegetarians stand fasting better than heavy flesh eaters, it is equally true that light meat eaters stand fasting better than heavy consumers of flesh. Every advocate of fasting from Jennings, Graham and Trall to the present is in agreement on this.

Trall said of his observations in conducting his establishment, "containing more than a hundred inmates on the average, about half of whom were either vegetarian in principle, or were restricted to an exclusively vegetable diet by special prescription, that such patients can bear fasting for a time much better than the flesh eaters; and they usually suffer but little, in comparison with those who enjoyed a mixed diet, from the craving sensation of the stomach, on the approach of the dinner or supper hour. To this rule I have never known one exception."

FASTING IN INFANCY AND CHILDHOOD

Replying to the question: may babies be safely treated by fasting, Carrington says: babies not only can be "treated safely by this method, but it is unsafe not to treat them by this means, when they become unwell." Fortunately, few infants require more than two to three days of fasting. I have had but few cases that required an extended fast. When nature cuts off the appetite of the infant, it should be permitted to fast until there is again a demand for food. If there is pain, fever or inflammation, no food should be given. Infants may fast for days without harm. They lose weight rapidly and regain it equally so. They seldom have to fast as long as an adult. I have never hesitated to permit a sick infant to fast, and I have yet to see one harmed by it. The sick child that is not fed rests peacefully and sleeps most of the time. Parents do not realize how much unnecessary suffering they cause their feverish children and how much avoidable anxiety they cause themselves by feeding them when sick.

Complications result almost wholly from feeding and drugging. They almost never develop in cases that are not fed and not drugged. If fasting is instituted at the very outset of whooping cough the child may never whoop. Vomiting does not occur in whooping cough when no food is given. Scarlet fever ends in four to five days and no complications develop. Measles, pneumonia, diphtheria, smallpox, etc., soon end if no food is given. I have fasted numerous children and babies, in both acute and chronic diseases (no infants in chronic disease) and it is my observation that they bear fasting well, often making much less fuss about it than adults. It has been noted by all fasting advocates that children rarely require as long a fast as an adult suffering with the same disease. Being young, they have greater recuperative power, they are less toxic, and their organs are commonly less damaged.

Babies and children are habitually over-fed. Indeed, over-feeding is perhaps, the greatest curse of infant and child life. As over-feeding builds disease in babies, it helps to account for a great amount of sickness among them and for many otherwise avoidable deaths. Certainly our children should be as healthy and vigorous as the young of other species, but such is not true. Our children are fed more, on the assumption that, as they are growing, they need much food to supply the materials of growth. How absurd are our feeding practices, based on this assumption, may be demonstrated by a little mathematics. A child growing twelve pounds a year grows but half an ounce a day, or less, and he certainly needs but little extra food with which to provide this increase in growth.

When the overfed child has become sick nature indicates in every possible manner that food is not desired. The pain, fever, dry mouth and tongue, coated tongue, foul breath, lack of desire for food, nausea, vomiting, and other evidences that digestion is impossible, indicate in the strongest possible manner that no food should be urged upon the baby or child. Infants and children recover more rapidly while fasting than do adults and do not require to fast so long. There should be no hesitancy in withholding food until they are again ready to take it. To feed them under conditions of acute disease is not to nourish them.

"In childhood," says Dr. Oswald, "chronic dyspepsia is in nearly all cases the effect of chronic medication. Indigestion is not an hereditary complaint. A dietetic sin *per excessum*, a quantitative surfeit with sweet meats and pastry, may derange the digestive process for a few hours or so but the trouble passes by with the holiday. Lock up the short-cakes, administer a glass of cold water, and, my life for yours, that on Monday morning the little glutton will be ready to climb the steepest hill in the country. But stuff him with liver-pills, drench him with cough-syrup, and paregoric, and in a month or two he will not be able to satisfy the cravings of the inner boy without 'assisting nature,' with a patent stimulant." — *Nature's Household Remedies*, p. 60.

Where their troubles are light and there is still some demand for food they will not fast without considerable fuss. In such cases fruit juices or vegetable juices (raw or broths) may be permitted them. At one period I attempted to use diluted milk (50-50) instead of these juices, but it was never satisfactory. A short fast when baby is irritable, "out-of-sorts," or feverish, instead of the usual feeding and drugging, will save much suffering and prevent small discomforts from developing into more formidable bonfires.

It has been fully demonstrated that repeated short fasts, of one to three days, in growing animals, when *recovery* is complete between fasts, produce better growth and greater strength. Children are not harmed by fasting, but only by starvation.

FASTING IN OLD AGE

We often meet with the objection that a patient is too old to fast. I have conducted a number of fasts in patients from seventy years to over eighty-five years of age and I have found no reason to consider aged persons to be in a class by themselves. Adult animals of any species, including *Homo Sapiens,* can fast much longer than the young of the same species. Old people actually stand fasting best. Growing children stand it least, although they stand it well. Patients do not get too old to fast. The regenerating effects of fasting are especially apparent in the old.

I have conducted numerous fasts in both men and women whose ages ranged from sixty-five to eighty-five. Many of these patients have had long fasts of from thirty to over forty days. Dewey reported several cases of elderly people who fasted under his care with positive benefit. Carrington says that he has observed several such cases. I agree with Carrington when he says: "Notwithstanding, I should recommend fasting with great caution in persons over sixty years of age," but not for the same reasons he adduces. I do not hesitate to place old people upon a fast, but I watch them more closely than I do younger people, not because they do not stand fasting well, but because they are often possessed of hidden weaknesses that render it inadvisable to carry the fast to great length.

FASTING DURING PREGNANCY

In another volume we have called attention to the fact that *chronic "disease,"* even that form called tuberculosis, frequently abates during pregnancy. Great changes, developmental changes akin to those of puberty and adolescence, take place in a woman's body during pregnancy. Weak hearts, weak lungs, weak kidneys, weak nervous systems are strengthened. Glands long dormant awaken to activity. Her whole body undergoes a strengthening, renovating process.

This is the meaning of the nausea, vomiting, ("morning sickness"), lack of appetite and other symptoms that so many women experience during the early weeks of pregnancy. No woman in good health, who is living sensibly, ever has the slightest trace of these symptoms. No woman who has undergone a thorough renovation just prior to becoming pregnant, and who lives sensibly during this time, ever experiences these "symptoms of pregnancy."

They are not symptoms of pregnancy. They are symptoms of renovation. They indicate that nature is undertaking a house cleaning, that the body is to be put into its best shape preparatory to pregnancy and parturition. If they are heeded all will be well. If they are not heeded, nature will usually succeed in her work in spite of opposition and interference. Sometimes she fails. Always her success is more complete and more satisfactory if we cooperate with her.

The development of these symptoms is a sure sign that a house-cleaning is necessary. When anorexia, nausea and vomiting develop, absolutely no food but water should be taken until these have disappeared and there is a distinct call for food. There should be no fears about fasting. You may be sure that these symptoms will end and nature will call for food as soon as her renovating work is completed and long before there has been any damage to mother or fetus. A fast is just what she is calling for in the plainest possible manner, and a fast she usually gets even if she has to keep throwing the food back into the woman's face as often as she eats it for days. Rest is called for as loudly as the fast and should be taken.

If this renovating work is permitted full sway and the woman will eat and live sensibly afterward, there will be no necessity for another fast during pregnancy. She will continue in good health. But if she "eats for two" (six), and lives the conventional, unhygienic life, she will suffer from a sour stomach, gas, dizziness, headaches, constipation and frequently more serious difficulties. She may develop an acute "disease." In such a case the hygiene of the *dis-*

ease is the same as it would be were it to develop in any other period of life. The pregnant woman should not hesitate to fast for as long as nature indicates, if she is suffering with an acute eliminating crisis. Let her be assured that to do so will shorten her period of illness, and that it will harm neither her nor her child. On the other hand, to eat will not help either her or the child.

The ridiculous advice to pregnant mothers to "eat for two," is beginning to lose its assumed validity. Suppose a baby weighs nine pounds at birth (three pounds too much); this is an average gain of a pound a month during the period of pregnancy. To meet the requirements of the baby growing at such a relatively slow rate, the mother is urged to eat two, three or more extra pounds of food a day. Instead of this being helpful to her and the evolving baby, it helps to make her sick, provides for a fat, hence oversized baby, reduces the health and elasticity of her tissues, and provides for great pain in childbirth. During pregnancy she has nausea, vomiting, sour stomach, swollen ankles, varicose veins, etc., as a consequence of such unintelligent eating.

In vomiting during pregnancy, physicians are afraid of both starvation and dehydration, hence they keep the woman plied with fluids and foods. All manners of clean and unclean things are introduced into the woman's stomach, in addition to the inordinate drugging that usually accompanies such cases when cared for by regular physicians. There should be no wonder that the vomiting continues.

There is no danger of starvation and we may be sure that the vomiting will cease before any marked or dangerous dehydration can occur, providing the woman is not fed. Indeed, in the absence of food, she will usually be able to take water. Nothing succeeds like fasting in morning sickness.

Chronic "disease" should not be handled differently during pregnancy from the manner in which it is handled at other times. The author would object to a long fast in chronic "disease" during this period. There can, however, be no objection to a short fast, but a long fast involves elements that one should seek to avoid.

Dr. Hazzard says: "When a pregnant woman fasts, her tissues, even including such essential ones as the heart and brain, will be utilized as may be necessary to properly nourish the child." This can be true only after the exhaustion of her internal reserves; for, true to the principle that the tissues are sacrificed in inverse order to their importance, the essential organs are not damaged until it becomes necessary to sacrifice them for the child. But a woman does not want to lose her hair or nails or teeth, nor should she be asked to where this can be avoided. Under the modern plan of feeding, most women lose a tooth and develop a few cavities during pregnancy, anyway.

A short fast, where one is necessary, or will be of benefit, should be entered upon without hesitancy by the pregnant woman suffering with a *chronic "disease,"* but a long one should be avoided unless *acute "disease"* makes it necessary. Feeding in *acute "disease"* does not feed, anyway.

FASTING DURING LACTATION
If fasting is necessary during lactation, it should be done, but if not necessary it should be avoided, for the reason that it stops the secretion of milk and even the diminution of this secretion resulting from a fast of three or four days is seldom overcome by a return to eating. If only one of the essential elements of nutrition is withdrawn from the diet of hens, they immediately cease laying. By these means the great amount of food lost to the body through the production of eggs is conserved and life prolonged. A similar thing is seen in fasting mammals in which milk production ceases. In all animals, scarcity of food limits reproduction.

FASTING BY THE STRONG AND THE WEAK
It is usually readily granted that the strong may fast for a certain length of time, perhaps with impunity, but it is usually objected that the weak should not fast. Here, again, we are met with the contention that these weak individuals need to be nourished. They require to be "built up." The fact that these people have grown weak while overeating on "plenty of good, nourishing food" is completely overlooked. If food builds and maintains strength, how do the well-fed become weak?

Mr. Sinclair says that people would write him and say that they would like to try a fast but that they were "too weak and too far gone to stand it." Everyone who employs fasting meets this objection quite frequently. Mr. Sinclair's answer to this objection, with which I fully concur, will therefore, be interesting. He says: "There is no greater delusion than that a person needs strength to fast. The weaker you are from the disease, the more certain it is that you need to fast, the more certain it is that your body has not strength enough to digest the food you are taking into it. If you fast under these circumstances, you will grow not weaker, but stronger. In fact, my experience seems to indicate that the people who have the least trouble on the fast are the people who are the most in need of it. The system which has been exhausted by the efforts to digest the foods that are piled into it, simply lies down with a sigh of relief and goes to sleep."

There is the foolish notion, fostered by the medical profession and shared all too faithfully by nurses and fond relatives of the sick, that the weak patient must be fed, and that if he cannot eat, he must have some medicine, some digestant or some tonic to "give him an appetite," or else he must be coaxed and cajoled, even forced, to eat. It is argued that if the patient does not eat, his strength can not be sustained; that he must, therefore, inevitably sink from weakness; he must be fed, even if he cannot digest what he eats.

The patient is so weak in many cases that he is unable to turn over in bed, he can hardly move hand or foot, there is little muscular action, yet it is insisted that he be fed three times a day. His digestive system, though equally prostrated, is expected to go on with its regular work as though there is the regular need for food. Will such a patient die of starvation? Never. Will he recover if fed? Not so surely as if he is permitted to fast. He may die of intestinal intoxication if he is fed; he may die if not fed, but he cannot be nourished by feeding, no matter what foods are given. He may be so weak that he will die if he gets much weaker, still he should fast. The surest way to make him weaker is to feed him.

It is a fact that has been demonstrated hundreds of times, that many invalids, instead of losing strength while fasting, gain it. Invalids that are growing weaker on the many and varied "nourishing diets" prescribed by physicians will frequently grow stronger as soon as fasting is resorted to. Paradoxical as it may seem, the weakest persons often derive the greatest benefit from a fast. The weakness of the average person is not due to lack of food but to toxin poisoning. The elimination of these during abstinence often registers a great increase in strength while the fast is in progress. This is to say, the patient grows stronger while he is still fasting and completes the fast stronger than when he began it. No matter how strong the man, if he becomes ill, he is weak. A Hercules may be prostrated in pneumonia or typhoid fever. Muscular strength is suspended during such periods.

The notion that the more food we can get a sick person to swallow the better for him is wholly wrong and is the source of much mischief. The very reverse represents the truth. When digestion ceases, nothing but misery and danger can come out of pouring food into the stomach. The fact is that it is in those cases that are the weakest that we often see the most surprising gains in strength.

Eating appears to give an amazing amount of strength to certain chronic invalids. These may feel weak and exhausted. They eat a meal and immediately they are energetic and strong. This is more likely to be the case if they are suffering from disease of the stomach than if the stomach is in near normal condition. This "gain of strength" is undoubtedly mere stimulation. Experimental fasts have shown that after a fast less food is required to maintain physical energies, physiological activities, weight and nitrogen balance. Fasting produces a more efficient "machine."

FASTING BY THE EMACIATED

Shall emaciated persons fast? By all means. Emaciation is rarely due to a lack of food, but almost always is a result of sickness. Dewey, Carrington, Macfadden, Rabagliati, Sinclair and many others have pointed out that in numerous instances, the first gains in weight some of these emaciated individuals make, despite much effort and many different kinds of weight-gaining diets, comes after a fast. I have seen many such cases in my own experience. It is easily possible to exaggerate the importance of weight in any consideration of fasting. Some extremely emaciated patients surprise us by the length of fasting they can safely and profitably undergo.

Great emaciation is not a bar to fasting. I have fasted numerous very thin people. One man, an asthmatic, who was veritably "skin and bones" when reaching my institution, fasted seventeen days and became practically free of asthma of nine years' standing. A subsequent fast completed his restoration. This man actually grew stronger during the fast. Indeed, in some cases of wasting "disease," no amount and kind of feeding produces any improvement until a fast, or a greatly reduced diet (a starvation diet), has first been employed. Page, Rabagliati, Kieth, Nichols and others record many such cases. Many deaths in tuberculosis are the result of starvation from overfeeding.

Sinclair records the case of an Episcopal clergyman who, "was so emaciated that he could hardly creep around" and was contemplating suicide. "He fasted eleven days and then gained thirty pounds." Dr. Eales says: "If you are thin and below normal weight, a fast will help you. Do not think that fasting is beneficial only for fleshy people. Thin people, as well as fleshy people are in an abnormal condition, and will derive great benefit from a fast. Numerous instances are on record of thin people fasting and gaining rapidly in health and weight after a fast."

I had one case to gain thirty pounds in four weeks, after a fast of nine days. This gain was made on a diet that few people would consider sufficient to meet their needs. This patient had suffered with gastric hyperacidity, gastro-enteritis, colitis, gas, constipation, poor circulation, emaciation and mental depression for seven years before consulting me. The fast, particularly a complete fast, remedies both emaciation and obesity. After a complete fast the body tends to attain and then maintain its ideal weight. Formerly fat patients do not regain their excess weight; whereas, those who were thin often gain a pound or more a day for a month or longer.

Prof. Agostino Levanzin, B.A., Ph. C. says: "It is contended in many quarters that thin people do not need fasting; that what they need is 'building up' and 'nourishing' food. I am convinced, on the contrary, that many thin persons need fasting more than corpulent persons—for their condition shows that they have been undernourished as a direct result of over-feeding for years. This must be checked at once, and this is best done by a fast, which will allow the nutritive organs to return to a condition in which they are capable of appropriating the food."

If food builds flesh, how do the well-fed become emaciated? How many greatly emaciated people do we meet every day who are eating like harvest hands? Many of them are weak and unable to work. If food gives strength, why are they so weak and skinny? Often these people make their only gains in weight and strength after a fast. Carrington points out that in hundreds of cases of emaciation (cases that are slowly starving while overeating) fasting will enable them to gain weight; thus actually preventing starvation. In this connection it is worthy of note that nature cuts off the desire for food in deficiency diseases—a plain indication that no more food should be taken. The great improvement seen in anemia when fasting is resorted to, while overfeeding causes these patients to grow worse, should convince even the most skeptical of the superiority of the fast.

Great emaciation is due to impairment of health and the degree of emaciation is commonly proprotionate to the degree of impairment. Such cases frequently make no gains in weight until after a fast. "Starvation from overfeeding" is a common, but rarely recognized phenomenon. Large numbers of habitually over-fed individuals have long since lost their power of digesting food at all, or they do it in a very imperfect manner. Oswald said of this: "The overfed organism is under-nourished to a degree that reveals itself in the rapid emaciation of the patient."–*Household Remedies*, p. 57.

The objection is frequently made in the case of emaciated patients that they are already weak and under-nourished and need "building up," rather than a fast. "Plenty of good, nourishing food" is thought to be the great need in these cases. But "plenty of good, nourishing food" is precisely what these emaciated individuals have been taking in the majority of instances. Instead of fasting being suicidal and criminal, as the average physician contends in such instances, the results of taking "plenty of good, nourishing food" has proved to be suicidal.

The fact is that, we rarely see a man or woman who is emaciated from taking too little food. Most of them are heavy eaters, even eating excessively in an effort to gain weight. Their emaciation is due, not to a lack of food ingested, but to failure to digest, absorb and assimilate the food eaten. In order for these individuals to gain weight, they must be given, not more food, but added capacity to utilize food. This can be acquired only by remedying the functional and structural impairments that have crippled their nutritive powers. Too often this cannot be done while the patient is taking "plenty of good nourishing food." It is a curious fact that in great numbers of cases of emaciation, we must supply them with less food in order to nourish them *more*.

Emaciation may be so extreme that only a short fast is possible; but we are often surprised at how well the emaciated person holds up under a fast that goes much beyond the time we think is possible. Dr. Oswald once remarked: "Energy and emaciation seem to go hand in hand."

FASTING IN DEFICIENCIES

As knowledge of the causes of *"disease"* increases, it becomes increasingly evident that there are certain forms of *"disease"* which are in part due to food deficiencies—beri-beri, scurvy, rickets, etc. What these cases need is better nutrition, better food. Yet one can not always arbitrarily rule out the fast in "deficiency diseases." For, sometimes they are due to a lack of assimilating power on the part of the body and this is remedied by the fast. Dr. Weger, who has had much experience with fasting says: "If the body, because of its crowded nutrition, cannot assimilate vitamin-bearing food, it can be brought into the condition to do this by a purifying fast."

The value of the fast in rickets and certain *"diseases"* of childhood is well established. Its value in anemia has been discussed elsewhere. There is no reason why fasting cannot be employed in dietary deficiencies with great benefit. Indeed the loss of appetite seen in men and animals fed on greatly deficient diets indicates strongly that a fast is called for. The experienced practitioner need not hesitate to place his patients upon a fast although some of them will require careful watching. If he lacks experience, some of his patients may be handled without the fast.

Symptomatology of the Fast

CHAPTER XXVII

The symptomatology of fasting forms a most interesting study, which can be fully appreciated only by the man or woman who studies it at first hand, by carefully observing fasting individuals, and by personally fasting. The following studies of the fasting patient will, however, give the reader a good working knowledge of this vital part of the subject.

SUBJECTIVE SYMPTOMS

Under his discussion of "Subjective Impressions" arising during the fast, Benedict says, "It is commonly believed that the withdrawal of food for one or two meals results in dizziness, a feeling of faintness, and at times, in pains in and about the epigastrium." This is not only the common belief, it is also the professional belief. Physicians, even physiologists who should know better, attribute any discomfort that may follow the missing of food, to the lack of food. Benedict shows that, while in some cases some discomfort was noticed, in the majority of cases, no such symptoms were observed. On the contrary, unusual vigor and strength were observed. He says: "The fast of Merlatti, which was said to have continued 50 days, was characterized by extreme discomfort, pain, and sensations of coldness. During the 30-day fast of Jacques, the only marked discomfort noticed was a slight attack of gout which appeared on the sixteenth day. In the numerous fasts of Succi, no marked discomfort was observed. In fact, during his fast at Florence his cheerfulness and apparent good health were the subject of much comment. It should be stated, however, that both Jacques and Succi took small amounts of narcotics from time to time throughout their fasts, though, as Prausnitz has pointed out, this may have been as much to stimulate a popular interest in the concoctions as to dull the sense of any possible pain, except possibly during the early days of the fast. Celli experienced considerable discomfort during the first one and one-half days of his fast, but this suddenly ceased after a movement of the bowels. *** The records of the subjective impressions of J. A. in the experiments in the Stockholm Laboratory, show that on the first day of the fast he noticed no dizziness. On the second day, while his general condition was good, he observed unusual weakness following a slight muscular exertion. On the third day he was not in a little discomfort when climbing on a short ladder inside the respiration chamber. On the fourth day, the pain in the stomach disappeared and no dizziness was noticed in the experiment on the ladder. On the fifth day the general condition was excellent, and there was no pain or discomfort in the stomach. His strength, too, was greater although he noticed that if he arose suddenly from bed there appeared to be black spots before his eyes. *** In Prausnitz's opinion, the feeling of discomfort attending hunger is, in many instances, a purely physical condition. *** It seems, therefore, that from the experiments made in this laboratory, the conclusion can properly be drawn that fasting, *per se,* produces no marked symptoms of pain or weakness, at least during the first days of inanition."

Two factors must be taken into account in our consideration of this conclusion that fasting produces no marked symptoms of pain or weakness during the first few days of abstinence. One of these is that Benedict's tests were made upon comparatively well individuals and these do not develop pains when fasting; the other is that he says "fasting *per se,*" does not produce symptoms of pain or weakness in the first few days of fasting. Pain or weakness or both may, and often do, arise in the beginning of a fast due to a variety of causes, but not to the fast. That they are not produced by the fast is obvious from the fact that they cease while the fast is still in progress. These will be accounted for as we proceed.

FEELING OF CHILLINESS

Among the most common subjective symptoms is that of a feeling of chilliness. Despite the fact that the individual maintains normal temperature on a fast, or even has a slight rise in temperature, there is commonly a feeling of chilliness in a moderate temperature in which he ordinarily feels comfortable. This feeling of chilliness may be experienced, even when the body temperature is above normal, that is, when there is slight fever. We attribute this feeling of chilliness in individuals of normal or above normal temperature to decreased cutaneous circulation. Let a man strip nude in a cold room and remain there until he feels warm. Then let him walk nude into a warm room. Immediately, shivering results and he will feel cold.

It is well-known that heavy eaters are always complaining of the heat. They may be said to be constantly "feverish." Carrington suggests that the feeling of chilliness may be, in part, due to the absence of this feverishness. He suggests, also, that what is now regarded as normal temperature is a degree too high. The faster, the person on a fruit diet, the moderate eater, comfortable in summer, is likely to feel cold to the touch of the heavy eater.

Carrington records the case of a man whose temperature, by thermometric reading, was regularly, while eating, 2° F. below normal, yet he never felt chilly; but who on the twenty-third day of his fast, his temperature having risen to 97.8° F. (only .8° below normal), felt cold. He gives it as his opinion that the feeling of chilliness in this instance was due, in part at least, to decreased peripheral circulation—an anemia of the skin. But he also thinks that sharpened senses which, as we have seen, are rendered more acute in every instance of fasting, possess a keener perception to changes in body temperature.

We experience a sense of chilliness only when blood has been withdrawn from the skin; when, in other words, there is anemia of the skin, and we may actually be so chilly as to *shiver* on the hottest summer day. We may feel chilly while the thermometer shows our body temperature to be normal or slightly above normal. Geo. S. Keith, M.D., LL.D., records a case of a patient in which, he says: "The great peculiarity in the case was a chilliness coming on when he took anything like a meal."—*Fads of An Old Physician*, p. 168. This is somewhat a reversal of the chilliness seen in fasting, but it shows that the sensation of chilliness is not due to fasting, *per se*.

As pointed out before, whatever the explanation of the feeling of chilliness, it has nothing to do with the actual temperature of the body, which may really be above normal. Susana W. Dodds says of it: "In this cold paroxysm there is a rise in temperature (which the fever thermometer will detect) sometime before the chilling stage begins."—*The Liver and Kidneys*, p. 44.

THE PULSE

The pulse varies greatly during a fast. It may run up to 120 or even higher, or it may drop to as low as 40, per minute. Indeed, Mr. Macfadden recorded a case in his practice in which the pulse went down as low as 20 and was so feeble it could scarcely be felt. It is the usual thing to have the pulse rate increase at the beginning of the fast and then, after a day or two, to drop. In chronic cases that are confined to bed during the fast, the pulse usually, after its temporary rise, drops to 48, or 40, where it may remain for a day or two days and then mounts up again to 60. After a few days it will settle at 60 and remain there until eating and activity are resumed. It is, of course, understood that the pulse is subject to all the variations, while fasting, as at other times of life, and that where there is "disease" of the heart, or nervous troubles, it will often vary greatly from the above standard. Where stimulants are employed during a fast, these occasion more heart activity than if taken when one is eating.

Discussing what, to the uninitiated, are alarming heart symptoms which may arise during a fast, Mr. Carrington says: "I may here remark, however, that such extreme variations invariably denote some profound physiological change taking place at the time—a crisis, in fact. The fact that hitherto weak hearts are actually strengthened and cured by fasting proves conclusively that any such unusual symptoms, observed during this period, denote a beneficial reparative process, and not any harmful or dangerous decrease or acceleration, due to lack of perfect control by the cardiac nerve."—*Vitality, Fasting and Nutrition*, p. 464.

Mr. Macfadden recorded the case of a man whose heart beat fell to twenty and was so faint it could scarcely be felt, after three weeks of fasting. It quickly rose after the patient took some nourishment. (*Natural Cure for Rupture*—p.p. 36-37). Abnormally slow pulse is seen in rare cases of extreme debility, especially in those who have for weeks, months or years prior to the fast, been in the habit of taking stimulants. A complete withdrawal of the stimulants results in a great slowing up of the habitually excited activities of the body. Mr. Carrington says that some of these cases die, although I have not seen it. He says: "The long-deferred crisis is at hand. Either the patient will recover the expended powers, and live; or, if wasted to such an extent that recovery is impossible, will die, during the fast. This is the most frequent, if not the *only* cause of death that occurs during cases of protracted fasting, when death occurs before the return of natural hunger. Such cases never die from starvation; it is a physiological impossibility for them to die during a fast before the return of natural hunger—unless the vital powers have previously been so wasted as to render their recuperation impossible—death being due to this failure; and it will thus be seen that the real cause of death is, again, previous mal-treatment—death occurring in spite of, and not on account of, the fast. Had the fast been instigated, in such cases, at an earlier period, the vital powers might have been sufficiently strong to have withstood the shock—recuperation instead of failure would have resulted; *i.e.,* instead of death."—*Vitality, Fasting and Nutrition.*

A very rapid pulse is seen in exercise, excitement, nervous shock, and gas pressure, etc. Exertion may increase the pulse rate more in the faster than in the regular eater. As there is nothing essentially abnormal about this and the pulse rate soon settles back to its regular fasting level, there need be no concern over it.

Let us not forget, in considering the unusual cases, that the vast majority of patients will not experience any of these inconveniences during a fast. Abnormally high or low pulse rates during a fast are exceptions and not the rule and do not denote any danger from the fast in itself. They should cause no alarm, so far as fasting, *per se,* is concerned. As a rule, the heart beat is steady, forceful and in keeping with the activities of the body.

While in acute disease it is usual to have temperature and pulse rate rise and fall together, in fasting and chronic disease this is not always so. For example, in many cases of heart disease or in goitre, the heart may be beating at an enormous rate and temperature remain normal or fall below normal. In fasting, on the other hand, the pulse rate may fall very low and temperature remain normal. Or, if the fasting patient becomes active, his pulse rate may rise to 110 or 120 a minute and his temperature remain normal.

APPETITE

It is doubtful if the sick man or woman is ever truly hungry, although appetite may be present, even irresistible, as in *bulimia.* There is a myth abroad that hunger ceases on the third day of the fast. This implies that hunger has existed during the preceding days. This is commonly not true. Indeed, a common complaint of chronic sufferers is that they have "lost appetite." Dr. Eales says: "Hunger left me on the third day, and from that time on to the time of breaking my fast I never knew what hunger was." This is the universal testimony of all who fast, but there seems to be no reason to doubt that they have mistaken appetite for hunger.

The faster soon loses all desire for food, if there is any desire at the outset, and often develops an actual repugnance to it. But there is no uniformity about the time that is required for the loss of appetite. It may be lost on the first day, the second day, the third day or the fourth day. On the other hand, some fasters complain of hunger after having fasted several days. When asked to describe their hunger, they describe symptoms that are not related to hunger. Like the physiologists, they mistake morbid symptoms for hunger.

More than a hundred and thirty years of conducting fasts have convinced most *Hygienists* that the "appetite" which sick persons frequently allege they have, and often those who are not sick say they have, is purely in the mind—a spurious hunger, which in great numbers of people, is the only hunger they have ever known, since overfeeding and frequent feeding by the clock and between-meals eating, was started in infancy and continued throughout their lives. But they are deceived by it and are honest in believing they are hungry.

From the cessation of appetite onward, for many days the body ceases to call for food, until a time arrives when food must be taken. During this period, we often observe the development of a positive repugnance to food, even the sight, odor or thought of food resulting in nausea and sometimes vomiting. If food is eaten under these circumstances it may be vomited. After these preliminary remarks it may be well to consider the experiences of others.

Sinclair says, "I was very hungry the first day—the unwholesome, ravening sort of hunger that all dyspectics know." Such "hunger" soon ceases and fasting becomes easy. There is no desire for food. He also tells us:

"I recollect reading a diverting account of the fast cure" "in which the victim was portrayed as haunted by the ghosts of beefsteaks and turkeys. But the person who is taking the fast knows nothing of these troubles, nor would there be much profit in fasting if he did. The fast is not an ordeal; it is a rest; and I have known people to lose interest in food as completely as if they had never tasted any in their lives."

Large numbers of individuals go on a fast and never experience any desire for food from the start. Indeed, many of them have no desire for food before going on the fast. Levanzin, who fasted several times in his life, says he never felt hungry on the first day of his fasts. The demand for food during the first two days of fasting has been over-emphasized by many writers on the subject. Much of the supposed demand for food experienced during this time is not that at all, but the "craving" for the accustomed stimulants. John Smith says: "The more stimulating the food, the sooner does the demand for it return."—*Fruits and Farinacea*, p. 175.

Fasting patients sometimes complain of being hungry, when the experienced practitioner knows that they are not. Occasionally one complains of hunger through the whole length of the fast. These sensations are due to irritative conditions or to the mind.

Dr. Guelpa in his book, *Auto-intoxication and Dis-intoxication*, says that food taken into the stomach serves to absorb and neutralize the toxic material in the stomach and intestine and thus relieves the sinking, empty, gnawing, etc., sensations which are caused by active auto-intoxication, but mistaken for hunger. Major Austin points out that drinking a large glass of saline purge "causes the disappearance of hunger instead of increasing it" and thinks this is due to the cleansing of the alimentary tract of toxins. Of course, the disappearance of hunger after taking a purge may be accounted for in another way, but I would remind my readers that these toxic symptoms are not hunger sensations.

These "hunger sensations" may be relieved in such a variety of ways—lavage, water drinking, heat applied to the upper part of the abdomen, abdominal massage, etc.—or will pass away in a short time without anything being done to relieve them—that only the inexperienced and uninformed can think of them as representing a physiological demand for food. A patient informs me that he was very hungry during the night and could not sleep. Upon being questioned he says the hunger has passed away—a sure indication that it was not real hunger.

Pashutin says: "Some of the experiments which we will have an opportunity to speak about below led to the conclusion that this desire for food and water is great only at the earliest stage of inanition. Manassein, however, mentioned that the animals also at the last period of starvation manifested great thirst." Again, quoting from Albitzky, he says, "At the later days of starvation *** only violent force by means of a cage or chain holds the animal undertaking to hunt for something edible."

In fasting steers, as in man, the so-called "hunger feeling" ceases after the second day. This feeling is believed to be caused by the physical contraction of the alimentary tract in adjusting itself to the diminished bulk of its contents. We do not accept this explanation of hunger. These animal experiences coincide exactly with human experiences in fasting. The so-called "hunger contractions" of the stomach increase in vigor in both man and animals during a fast, but do not give rise to hunger. Dr. Trall observed that vegetarians can "bear fasting for a time much better than the flesh eater; and they usually suffer but little in comparison with those who enjoy a mixed diet, from craving sensations of the stomach, on the approach of the dinner or supper hour. To this rule I have never known an exception."

Dr. Oswald says: "In my experiments on the operation of the fasting-cure, I have noticed the curious fact that for the first day or two the clamors of the stomach are restricted to certain hours, and can be induced to waive a disregarded claim."

Appetite is often accompanied with various feelings of discomfort, even actual pain. There may be a general feeling of weakness or there may be mental depression. Frequent complaints of gnawing in the stomach, an "all gone" sensation in the stomach, rumblings in the abdomen, actual abdominal pain, nausea, headache, weakness and other morbid sensations accompanying appetite are made by Mr. Average Citizen. Indeed, I meet many who refer to distress in the stomach as hunger. These symptoms are identical with those experienced by the drug addict who is deprived of his accustomed drug. The symptoms of drug addiction are usually more intense. Food drunkenness (gluttony) produces its symptoms and these symptoms are mistaken for hunger. The symptoms are temporarily relieved by eating, just as a cup of coffee temporarily relieves the coffee-induced headache, and this leads to the idea that food was needed. Such symptoms pass away if their owner will refrain from eating for a few days. Indeed, in many cases, they will pass away within an hour after the accustomed meal time has passed if no food is eaten.

True hunger is accompanied by no symptoms. In true hunger one is not aware that he has a stomach. There is no headache, or other discomfort. There is merely a consciousness of a need for food, which, like thirst, registers itself in the mouth and throat. Dr. Claunch thus differentiates between appetite and hunger: "The difference between true hunger and false craving may be determined as follows: When hungry and comfortable it is true hunger. When 'hungry' and uncomfortable it is false craving. When a sick person misses a customary meal, he gets weak before he gets hungry. When a healthy person misses a customary meal he gets hungry before he gets weak."

THE TONGUE AND BREATH

These are interesting studies during a fast. The tongue becomes heavily coated in almost every instance (I have seen five or six exceptions) and remains so throughout the fast, gradually clearing up, beginning at the edges and the point, until, when hunger returns, it is clean.

The breath becomes very foul and remains so during most of the fast, gradually becoming less so as the work of purification proceeds, until, with the return of hunger, it is sweet and clean. The more foul is a man's body, the more foul will be his breath and the more heavily coated his tongue. "The breath smells faintest when the stomach is emptiest" was a maxim that could have been legitimately employed only among a truly healthy people.

TEMPERATURE

When we observe body temperature during a fast, we are presented with a paradoxical series of phenomena which prove both interesting and highly instructive. For example, temperature tends to remain normal in most cases of fasters suffering with chronic disease, to fall in acute disease and to rise in those patients who have sub-normal temperature. Benedict points out that during the fast, for a period of seven days at least, there is an occasional tendency for it to increase as the fast progresses.

Temperature does not rise as high in fever patients who are not fed as it does in the same patients when fed. Invariably, the temperature falls to normal as the fast progresses. Indeed, in acute "disease" where there is high temperature, the fever subsides somewhat as soon as eating is discontinued and seldom rises high thereafter.

In rare cases of chronic disease there is sub-normal temperature. This is most likely to be observed in the morning before the patient has become active. It is striking evidence of the value of the fast that in these patients, as the fast nears its natural termination, the temperature rises to normal and remains there. In those chronic sufferers whose temperature is habitually below normal, it will surely but slowly rise until it reaches normal by the time the fast naturally ends. "Thus," says Carrington, "supposing the patient's temperature to be 93.8° at the commencement of the fast, it will gradually rise until about 98.4° is reached—though the fast may have extended over forty or more days . . . Time after time, in case after case, I have watched this gradual rise in the bodily temperature of the patient, and in every case the temperature has not failed to rise as the fast progressed. At first, it is true, the temperature sometimes tends to fall, but let the fast be persisted in, and a return or rise to normal will occur in every case."

Carrington records several cases where temperature was sub-normal while eating, but gradually returned to normal while fasting. In some of these, premature eating resulted in an immediate drop in temperature. One case he records had a temperature below 94° F. before the fast. At the end of a thirty-four days fast the temperature had nearly reached the normal standard. A. Rabagliati, M.A., M.D., F.R.C.S., Edinburgh, made this same discovery, and says of it: "In point of fact, I raised the temperature of a man who was, besides thin, emaciated, and attenuated by constant vomiting, lasting for seven years, from 96° F. to 98.4° F. by advising him to fast for thirty-five days. On the 28th day his temperature had risen to normal, and remained so."—*Air, Food and Exercise*, p. 261.

Low temperature is often the result of too much food, or lowered vitality due to habitual over-eating. The case just quoted from Dr. Rabagliati was, as he remarks, "dying on the plan of frequent feeding." He lost 13 pounds during the fast and gained health although he had been sick and taking a "highly nourishing diet" for seven years. Carrington noted a few instances of long fasts where the temperature dropped a degree or two immediately upon resuming eating.

Dr. Hazzard records a case in which body temperature was constantly at ninety-four degrees at the beginning of the fast. No change in temperature was noted until the twentieth day, when it increased nearly a degree, it reached ninety-seven degrees ten days later and remained at this standard thereafter. She also says that in a few subjects the temperature was so low that it could not be determined on a clinical thermometer, but "invariably normal individual average was reached before the end of the treatment."

Experiments upon fasting animals show that the temperature remains normal through the fasting period and then begins to fall rapidly for from 2 to 6 days before death supervenes. It is the rule, in chronic troubles, for the temperature to remain normal. Dr. Eales' temperature remained normal throughout his fast. Dr. Tanner's temperature dropped at the end of his fast, although he survived. This drop in temperature, both in man and in animals, undoubtedly marks the exhaustion of the body's reserve resources and the beginning of actual starvation.

I have had but one such case in my own experience, the sudden drop occurring on the 36th day of the fast. I broke the fast immediately and kept the patient warm with heat applied externally. He made a quick recovery and suffered no ill effects. Carrington thinks that the fact that temperature falls to normal when above it and rises to normal when below it and that it reaches the normal point, in either case, just as the fast is completed and ready to be broken, is further proof that "fasting is a natural process, counselled by nature, with landmarks clearly defined, and but waiting to be recognized by man." This, it seems to me, is the only logical conclusion that can be drawn from the facts.

"FAMINE FEVER"

In famine "fevers," often typhus develop. As fasting is not identical with famine, we do not see the development of typhus or other serious fever in fasters. In many cases, particularly of overfed individuals, we do have what is falsely called "famine fever" when a fast in entered upon. It is a slight elevation of temperature which may last from one to several days. I agree with Carrington that "it is, as in the case of all other diseases, a curative crisis, and should be regarded as a favorable sign, in consequence." Dr. Rabagliati also regarded it as remedial and added: "If we cannot fast without fever, it is because we have been previously improperly fed."

SLEEP

It is the usual thing for the fasting person to sleep no more than three to four hours out of each twenty-four hours, and this frequently causes worry. Three general causes for this sleeplessness are recognized: (1) It may be due to general nervous tension. The faster cannot sufficiently relax. (2) Sleeplessness is often due to a deficient circulation. The feet become cold and the faster finds it difficult to maintain warmth. A hot water bottle or jug placed at the feet will usually remedy this. (3) The fasting person does not require the usual amount of sleep In a general sense, the amount of sleep one requires is proportioned to the quality and quantity of one's food. If you are comfortable and relaxed, you may be quite certain that you will sleep as much as you require.

In his narrative, from which I have previously quoted, Mark Twain records the case of one man who went without sleep for twenty-one days at a stretch, noticing during this period of fasting, no desire for sleep and no ill effects from not sleeping. Horace Fletcher frequently pointed out that when he ate less food he required less sleep. The sleepiness and sluggishness that follow a heavy meal are well-known to everyone. If we are to be mentally alert, we must eat lightly or not at all. Such facts would seem to indicate that the digestion of large quantities of food is an exhausting process.

The faster who does not sleep is likely to fret and fuss about how long the nights are, but he does not feel the loss of sleep. It is true, of course, that all fasters who complain of not sleeping, like all other patients who declare that they never closed their eyes all night, sleep much more than they think they do. I have visited the rooms of fasters who complained of not sleeping and found them fast asleep, only to have them tell me the following day that they "never slept a wink all night."

A few patients sleep more while fasting than when eating. Insomnia victims are especially likely to do this. Fasting is perhaps the quickest and most satisfactory means of remedying insomnia, although there are cases in which it requires six to ten days to secure the sleep. Sinclair says, of his first fast: "I slept well throughout the fast."

I cared for one young man who slept sixteen hours out of twenty-four almost every day of a thirty days fast. Another man, an asthmatic, slept almost day and night for days during and following the fast. But asthma cases, like insomnia cases, having lost much sleep, usually sleep much as soon as fasting brings relief from the dyspnea so that they can sleep.

Progress of the Fast

CHAPTER XXVIII

Fasting is not the severe and trying ordeal that the uninitiated may think. It may be a very trying period or it may be a very pleasant experience; in the majority of cases it is not at all unpleasant, while in many instances the fasting individual is more comfortable than he was while eating. The man who suffers after every meal is likely to find the fast to be a period of welcome comfort. Popular fancy pictures the faster suffering the tortures of "starvation," whereas, it is often true that the faster is much more comfortable than the individual who imagines that the faster is undergoing severe suffering.

One author puts it this way: "Fasting is not always a pleasant experience, but, then, neither is it a pleasant experience to be sick." While fasting may be a period of comfort and pleasure (as one young woman expressed it after her fast was over: "It was the most thrilling experience of my life. I would not take anything for the experience and am looking forward to another"); but it is certainly no pleasure to go through a period of drugging. All of this is contrary to what may be thought by the individual who has never undergone a fast and has never had opportunity to observe a fast. He is likely to labor under the belief that the fast may be a very severe and harrowing ordeal. He may picture the faster as suffering the most intense agonies of starvation, his agonies increasing in intensity until, finally, the victim expires in the most excruciating pain. If this picture had any truth at all in it, it would certainly be impossible to induce any person to enter voluntarily upon a second, much less a third or fourth fast.

In his "Diary of a Faster" (*Physical Culture*, Feb. 1914), Fred Busch describes his fast of 17 days, day by day. He tells us that he was unable to eat even the simplest of foods without distress. He adds: "sound sleep is unheard of—work is a punishment—life in general a drudge." He records on the morning of the second day of his fast that he slept a full eight hours the night before and that he was feeling rather good. He slept well every night through his fast. Seventeen days of comfort, during which he carried on his regular work in his office, and did more work than while eating, reveals that fasting may be a very pleasant experience in many conditions of life.

I do not think that it can be too strongly emphasized that the bodily sensations of fasting are, in many cases, more pleasant than the bodily sensations of feasting. The patient who has suffered so much previously from being forced to eat when there was no desire for food, the patient who has suffered so much pain after all food, is likely to feel a great sense of relief and satisfaction from the time the fast begins. When a man goes on a fast, every abnormal sensation, every "craving," every ache and pain that he may develop immediately thereafter, is credited to lack of food. They are, in reality, due to the absence of his accustomed stimulants—coffee, tobacco, condiments, alcohol, etc. That they all disappear as the fast progresses, proves that they are not due to lack of food.

THE EARLY DAYS OF THE FAST

The first two days of the fast may be the hardest, due (1) to the persistence of the demand for food, and (2) to the sudden withdrawal of the accustomed stimulation. Headache, dizziness upon arising, spots before the eyes, nausea, vomiting and gnawing or an "all-gone" sensation in the stomach, are the chief elements of discomfort during the first few days of the fast. These symptoms are largely the result of the withdrawal of coffee, tea, tobacco, condiments and stimulating foods. Fat people and "good livers," suffer most in these respects. As a general rule, it may be set down that the more marked these symptoms are during the early days of the fast, the sooner the fast will accomplish the desired results.

If we compare the discomforts of the faster with those suffered by the alcoholic when he gives up his alcohol, I think we can arrive at a rational explanation of them. It must first be understood that, just as the non-drinker does not suffer any discomforts as a result of abstaining from alcohol, so the healthy man does not suffer discomforts when he abstains from food. But the alcoholic who fasts from alcohol, is greatly distressed, not by his abstinence, but as a consequence of his prior drinking. His suffering is not due to his abstinence from alcohol but to the fact that for a long time prior thereto he had been in the habit of drinking alcoholic liquors. If, because of his distress, which he may wrongly attribute to his abstinence, he may cast aside his good resolutions and return to drinking, his distress will vanish as if by magic, but we know that in so doing, he only lays the foundation for more and greater future suffering and renders it more difficult to abstain at some future time when he may again decide to give up his alcohol.

If, now we think of the patient who goes on a fast and suffers minor discomforts, especially in the first few days of the fast, are we not witnessing phenomena similar to if not identical with those suffered by the alcoholic who attempts to discontinue his drinking? The person who has previously habitually over eaten, who has eaten rich fare and taken a lot of spices and condiments with his food, who has indulged freely in coffee, tea, soda fountain drinks, tobacco, etc., and is deprived of all of these sources of injury at the same time he is deprived of food, is almost certain to suffer some discomfort. Nervousness, headaches, gastric distress, insomnia, weakness, etc., that may develop are similar to the nervousness, gastric distress, insomnia, weakness, etc., that the alcoholic experiences when he discontinues drinking.

In this way and for this reason a faster may find the early part of a fast as trying as the effort of the alcoholic to totally abstain. But, it would be as unwise to break the fast because of such discomforts as it would be for the alcoholic to return to his drinking. If he does not sleep for a few nights, if he experiences a disagreeable aching void, if he has a headache, he is very unwise if he throws the whole thing up and returns to his overeating, his coffee and tobacco.

Crises that may and sometimes do develop in a fast, most often after the fast has been in progress for two to three weeks or more, but rarely in the early days of the fast, are of a somewhat different character to these early discomforts that are experienced by a certain percentage of fasters. Nausea, vomiting, diarrhea, skin eruptions would seem to result from a more or less sudden release into the blood stream, from the broken down fat and other broken down tissues, of stored toxins, so that the body is forced to resort to some means of compensatory elimination to free the blood of them.

Dr. Shew says of the first few days of fasting: "A feverish excitement of the system, together with a feeling of debility, faintness and depression is generally experienced. The patient becomes discouraged and melancholic, and is very excitable and sensitive to surrounding influences. He also experiences pains and soreness in the loins, feet, and sometimes in the joints. He becomes very tired of the sitting posture and leans to one side or the other for support. But all of these disagreeable symptoms, which are necessary in the process, grow by degrees less and less, as the morbid matter is eliminated from the vital economy. And when the body has at last grown pure, these unpleasant consequences disappear entirely, and the convalescent gains strength with inconceivable swiftness through the period of the after-care"—*The Hydropathic Family Physician*, p. 790.

As we almost never meet with fasters who present the picture here drawn by Dr. Shew, I am of the opinion that his description is a good index of the grossness of living habits of the people of his time. When we consider that the symptoms presented by the faster are in keeping with the unphysiological character of his mode of living, this seems to me to be a fair conclusion. Great changes for the better have taken place in our living habits during the hundred years that have elapsed since Shew wrote the foregoing lines. Any of the symptoms he enumerates may be met with, but we almost never see all of them in a single patient. Many patients never develop any of them.

Fasting does not cause fever. The so-called "famine fever" described in the earlier works on fasting, but which we seldom see today, is confined to those whose eating habits are gross. Older writers used to speak of the period between meals as fasting and of an increase of an hour or more between one meal and the next as the "*languor* of inanition and the fever of repletion," but they wholly mistook the nature of the sensations that arise when food is abstained from beyond the accustomed meal time. The healthy man does not have fever upon missing a meal or several meals. The habitually overfed and wrongly fed person may have a rise of temperature upon missing a meal or two. Fever and feverishness flow from the previous state of plethora and toxemia. If a person cannot fast without developing fever his mode of living has been very imprudent.

Although there are rare exceptions in which the tongue does not coat, it is the rule that the tongue becomes heavily coated almost immediately. The teeth become pasty, the breath is foul, and the taste in the mouth is very bad. These are somewhat similar to the condition of the mouth in acute disease and are indications of elimination. They are somewhat annoying, but should be welcomed as evidences of the efficiency of the organism in freeing itself of toxic materials.

DISAPPEARANCE OF SYMPTOMS

As the fast progresses, the symptoms grow less and less marked until they cease entirely. Many things that the sick customarily do are more disagreeable than the most disagreeable symptoms that ever develop during a fast. These things are disagreeable always; whereas the fast is so only in a minority of cases and not so throughout its length. The original symptoms, for which the fast was instituted, also gradually cease. Sinclair says in describing his first fast, "Previous to the fast I had a headache every day for two or three weeks. It lasted through the first day and then disappeared—never to return."

Thirty years ago a patient came to me from New York. All save one physician who had cared for him had insisted upon an operation for tumor of the brain. For months he had suffered day and night a severe headache that the drugs of physicians had failed to relieve, even temporarily. Twenty-four hours without food brought complete relief from the pain. The patient described the result as a miracle and wanted to start immediately for home.

Another remarkable example of the gradual disappearance of symptoms during a fast is presented by the usually rapid clearing up of skin eruptions. One example will suffice. A young man who had suffered with acne for ten years and tried medical and drugless methods to no avail, was placed upon a fast. In nine days his skin was as clear of eruptions as that of a baby. The remarkable changes that occur in the skin and the increased brightness of the eyes add greatly to the youthful appearance of those who fast.

INCREASE OF SYMPTOMS

I have emphasized the gradual disappearance of symptoms. I must also emphasize the fact that there is sometimes a temporary increase in symptoms during the early days of a fast. Headache may sometimes increase at first and then diminish. The gastric pains in hyperacidity and gastric ulcer are almost sure to increase during the first three days of the fast. Nervous symptoms are sometimes aggravated at first. It also occasionally happens that skin eruptions grow worse. Catarrh is most likely to increase at the outset. Streams of mucus may pour from the nose, sinuses, throat, vagina and colon.

An amazing quantity of mucus is often excreted through the uterine and vaginal walls. This is especially true in those women patients who had leucorrhea before the fast was instituted. In all cases, however, these increased symptoms are only temporary and the reverse process soon sets in, resulting in ultimate recovery.

In some forms of gastric abnormality, especially hyperacidity and certain nervous states, ulcer, etc., pain accompanies an empty stomach and is relieved by food. It is known to everyone of experience that the relief from pain afforded by eating is only temporary and is soon followed by the same pain and gnawing. Eating does not remedy the condition, which may persist for years of eating.

When such a patient is placed upon a fast, there are two to three days of suffering, often increased suffering, followed by relief. If the fast is persisted in, permanent relief or actual recovery follows. With the coming of relief the patient experiences greater happiness and peace of mind.

A very unusual case was cared for at the Health School while this revision was underway. A man with a large gastric ulcer, very nervous and irritable, depressed, emaciated and weak, whose ulcer was of several years' standing and who had marked hyperacidity of the stomach, experienced no relief from stomach distress for more than ten years and then only intermittently. For some reason which I do not know, gastric secretion continued in this man long after it customarily ceases and, after it had practically ceased, it would start up at times and cause considerable discomfort with eructation of gastric juice. It need hardly be added that this man's fast was far from comfortable. Fortunately, it was successful.

Increase of symptoms in the early days of a fast or the development of new ones should not cause the fast to be broken. The really healthy person experiences no reactions from the fast. Major Austin says: "A very good test indeed of a so-called perfectly healthy person's real state of health is the effect produced on him or her by missing one or two meals. If the tongue begins to get coated and the breath foul and the individual feels seedy and out of sorts, it is proof positive that the state of health is not as good as it was supposed to be." The more severe the reactions produced the greater is the real need for the fast. "In exact proportion to the severity of her fasting symptoms," says Dr. Dewey (*A New Era for Women*), "so is her need to persevere and for the reason that they all mean disease in course of development."

CRISES DURING THE FAST

Crises developing during the fast are not different from those developing at other times and are not to be cared for any differently. They are all orthopathic in character and, although often disagreeable, should be welcomed.

The increase in symptoms previously noted should be considered as critical action. Fever, dizziness, headache, vomiting, nausea, backache, skin eruptions of various kinds, but particularly urticaria (nettle rash), jaundice, diarrhea, etc., may develop.

Many of the symptoms experienced by the faster are due to nervous re-adjustment. Take the case of a woman patient who "suffered" from sensory paralysis in an area of skin about the size of the hand at the base of the spine, and who, after a few days of fasting, experienced severe pain in this part for about two hours, this followed immediately by restoration of normal sensibility in the part—the pain in this case was patently a part of the process of nervous readjustment.

The headache that follows the giving up of coffee and the headache that often follows immediately upon the cessation of eating are both processes of nervous readjustment. Depression and irritability that sometimes accompany the early part of the fast are processes of readjustment similar to the irritability and depression that follow the discontinuance of tobacco.

Since they are always followed by improved health, it seems certain that these symptoms are necessary parts of an essentially beneficial process that the fast has enabled the body to institute and consumate.

Not all fasting cases develop any appreciable crises and in the great majority of cases where these do develop, they are mild and of short duration and result in improvement in the patient's condition. For the guidance of the reader I will describe some of the more severe crises and crises that are of relatively rare development. Doubtless imperceptible crises occur in every fast in chronic "disease." Crises that make themselves felt by marked outward symptoms do not always occur. Whether evident or not, these crises always lead to better and ever better health.

Most of the symptoms here considered are of no special significance. Others are of such rare development that the person contemplating a fast need not expect them to develop. In no case do all of these symptoms develop. Indeed, many fasters go through a long fast without the development of any symptoms at all. The purpose of discussing these developments is not to lead the reader to believe that they indicate that fasting is dangerous, for they do not, but to acquaint him with possibilities (they are hardly probabilities in most cases) and to tell him how to deal with such crises if they do develop. They are not serious and they do not develop in more than a small percentage of cases. They need not be feared.

The varied symptoms that are seen in fasting do not represent any "turn for the worse," in the patient. On the contrary, they are symptomatic of certain internal vital or functional and organic changes, which are always for the better. Unfortunately, most people, including most doctors of all schools, are still laboring under the old delusion that symptoms are or represent destructive processes, hence there is no understanding of the actual beneficial character of these crises.

Spitting: What may be denominated a "spitting crisis" develops in a few cases. An almost incessant stream of mucus is poured into the mouth and throat necessitating constant spitting. Often this lasts for several days and it may be so persistent during this time as to prevent sleep. It is so obviosuly an eliminating process that we need not dwell on this part of the phenomenon. Like most crises it is uncomfortable and annoying while it lasts, and, like all crises, it is succeeded by marked improvement in the general condition.

Although there are occasional cases in which the saliva flows as freely during the fast as when eating, it is the rule that it is greatly reduced in amount and the other secretions of the mouth are so reduced that there is dryness of the mouth, lips and throat. In occasional cases the secretion in the mouth, chiefly mucus, may be so unpleasant, as to induce vomiting. This unpleasant taste will gradually lessen and will disappear altogether before the fast is to be broken. For immediate relief, the tongue may be thoroughly scrubbed with a brush and the mouth cleansed with water.

Nervous Crises: One case in my practice presented a nervous crisis which I believe to be unique. Fasting literature does not contain a description of another such case. Slight pain and severe burning would begin at the base of the skull and travel down the spine, the part above ceasing to suffer as the pain passed below it. When the pain and burning reached the base of the spine, it "jumped" to the knees, the back side of these, and from here it would "jump" to the base of the skull. This would last an hour or more, and then there would be a period of intermission during which the patient would secure rest and sleep before it would set in again. The patient was very weak during the three or four days the crisis persisted. As soon as it was over she was as strong as ever.

Catarrh: A cold may sometimes develop near the beginning of the fast. Soreness in the throat may also occur, though rarely. The elimination of mucus is almost always increased in the early part of the fast in *chronic "disease."*

Skin Crises: Skin eruptions may cover the whole body (I have had but one such case in my own practice) or they may be only local. The eruption usually itches. One case in may practice was that of a woman who developed a solid mass of urticarial eruptions on both forearms from hand to elbow. One arm itched intensely, the other itched not at all. Such eruptions may last but a few hours but usually they persist for from three to four days. They are processes of elimination.

In June 1956 I cared for a man with an enlarged prostate who broke out, after a week of fasting, with a generalized rash on trunk, arms and legs which, except for the absence of all acute symptoms, might have led to a diagnosis of measles. Much itching prevented the patient from sleeping for three nights. Then the rash subsided. This particular development was unique in my experience. I have never seen anything else just exactly like it in all my years of practice. My opinion is that such developments grow out of sepsis in the body somewhere.

Headache: Severe headache and backache are usually accompanied with considerable prostration. Sometimes the patient and family become frightened. The pains are severe but there is no danger. No attempt should be made to break the fast during this stage. The headache and backache may last for from one to three or four days. They represent nervous readjustment and are met with largely in nervous patients. Headaches are usually due to the withdrawal of tobacco, tea, coffee, drugs and stimulating foods. Head-

-347-

ache commonly develops from the first to the third day. By no means all patients present this symptom.

Aching Limbs: Besides pains in the back, usually in the lower spine, there frequently develop in the early days of the fast, pains in the hips, pains at the base of the skull and aching in the limbs, particularly in the joints. These pains and aches are often very annoying, but seldom last more than one or two days. They develop chiefly at night and cease during the day.

Nausea: This seems to be an expression of a sudden decrease of the normal tension of the stomach. It may be induced by a foul odor, a bad taste, a disgusting sight or an emotional shock. Severe pain, illness, fatigue, rapid descent in an elevator, etc., may produce nausea by lowering the tension of the stomach. These things bring about a loss of tension through a complicated "reflex" mechanism.

Continual emotional disturbances, such as prolonged worries, anguish, grief and repeated shocks, may result in a persistent loss of tone in the stomach and produce the "all gone" sensations or vague nausea often complained of. In many cases there is no doubt that the sudden withdrawing of all food, as in fasting, results in a temporary lowering of tone or tension in the stomach and this produces nausea. On the other hand, tall, thin, undernourished people are likely to suffer with a chronic lack of tension in the stomach and this becomes more noticeable when they fast. The presence of bile in the stomach also causes nausea. Its presence is very likely to lead to vomiting.

Vomiting: This develops in roughly about fifteen per cent of cases. The patient may vomit but once or he may vomit a few times in a day and this end the crisis, or he may vomit for two, three or several days. The vomiting may occur on the first, second or third day of the fast or at any time thereafter. There seems to be no rule about the time of its occurrence. It may come in the middle of the fast or near its termination. I had one case to vomit almost continuously for six days and nights and two others to vomit frequently during a period of two weeks. Much mucus and bile make up the contents of the vomitus. The case that vomited persistently for six days and nights developed persistent hiccoughing following the vomiting and this lasted for seven days before it ended.

One elderly lady vomited for four days and nights and made an excellent recovery. Mr. B., who underwent a thirty-one days fast in my institution in 1932, began vomiting on the twenty-third day of his fast and vomited day and night for seven days. He excreted large quantities of mucus and bile. Like all other cases, he was very weak while vomiting, but became strong again as soon as the vomiting ceased. It is the almost invariable rule that increased strength follows the cessation of the vomiting. Indeed, the patient is obviously so much improved in every way and feels it, that the conclusion is inescapable that the vomiting has served some very important office in freeing the body of accumulated waste.

Bile is an excretory product. The liver seems to increase its work of excretion and to throw bile into the intestine in great quantities at short intervals. Some of this is regurgitated into the stomach, where it occasions nausea and vomiting. I do not regard vomiting as a danger signal but as a cleansing process. Carrington says that vomiting spells occurring at the end of a prolonged fast have been known to terminate fatally. I have seen no such fatalities and am inclined to think that death in such cases must have been due either to heroic measures to stop the vomiting or to other causes. The unusual excretory activity of the liver can hardly be classed as a cause of death.

But there is a danger associated with prolonged and persistent vomiting. When a patient vomits frequently, day and night, for a number of days, and, as is usually true under these circumstances, takes little or no water, dehydration occurs and this may reach a dangerous stage. The patient refuses water for the reason that the taste in the mouth is so foul he finds water distasteful. He also finds that if he drinks water it is immediately vomited. In those rare instances in which the patient both vomits and has a diarrhea, the loss of water is even more rapid. Either of these crises may greatly weaken the patient. When they occur together, they leave him very weak and he recovers slowly.

I had one patient who refused water during his fast. He was an adherent of a religious sect that enjoined fasting and he refused water also. Urged to take water, he would do so, only to run his finger down his throat and induce vomiting as soon as my back or that of the nurse was turned. He refused to break his fast when I wanted it broken, but wanted to await instructions from God. He was induced to take some juice, but induced vomiting as soon as the nurse was out of the room. This man died. He did not die because his food reserves were exhausted, for he was still overweight at death, but, I am sure, from dehydration. After this death I resolved to accept no more patients for fasting who would not agree to carry out my instructions. These fanatically motivated individuals may hereafter kill themselves at home, not in the *Health School.*

Although it is often difficult to break a fast while a patient is vomiting and, in the great majority of instances, there is no reason why it should be broken; rather, it should be continued, I have made it a practice, for the past several years, to break fasts in these cases before the dehydration reaches a dangerous state. In a letter to Mr. Carrington, dated March 26, 1903, Dr. Dewey wrote: "Only God could break a fast where there is a sick stomach and there is no time to let nature perform the task. Taking food in such a stomach would be death-dealing. There is nothing to do but make the body and mind as comfortable as possible, and Nature will cure, if the seal of death is not set." Mr. Macfadden says of vomiting during a fast: "It is certainly inadvisable to break a fast at such a time. If food be administered at such a time, it most certainly will be ejected, and it may aggravate the vomiting all the more." Dewey records the case of a man who developed vomiting after fasting fifty days. Food was tried, but promptly ejected. He waited for the return of hunger, which came after a last spell of vomiting on the sixtieth day.

In general I agree that it is unwise to break a fast while vomiting is going on. But I do make exceptions and I have found that it does not take God to break it. If the patient can retain water, when taken in small, perhaps frequent sips, it is better that the fast be continued in all cases. But dehydration must be avoided. In such cases it may take two or three days to break the fast. I often have to try different juices before I find one that will be retained. I am of the opinion that Dr. Dewey failed in his efforts to break fasts while the patient was vomiting because he did not persist in his efforts long enough or else he did not find the right food or juice with which to break it.

Much mucus is often (usually) expelled in the vomiting process. I have seen no pus so ejected but Carrington tells of such. I have seen vomiting last for as long as two weeks after forty or more days of fasting and, while it leaves the patient very weak, there has in no case been any danger of death. Sometimes vomiting, headache and eruption will all come together. With a little experience in handling cases, one can judge fairly accurately in advance who is and who is not going to develop a severe crisis. Long standing cases of digestive troubles, particularly those accompanied with nervous disorders, are most prone to develop these.

Cramps: These may occur in the bowels of both sexes, or in the womb of females. In the bowels they may be due to gas, to bowel action, or to "pyschic" interference with sympathetic control of peristalsis. Uterine cramps are rare, occurring chiefly in those patients who bleed from the uterus. More rarely the cramps result from efforts to disgorge the womb of an accumulation of mucus.

Gas: Many patients have considerable intestinal gas while fasting. Those who suffer with digestive troubles, visceroptosis, colitis, enteritis, etc., and "nervous" patients are most likely to be troubled with gas. In not a few cases there is sufficient gas to cause distress, even sleeplessness. Most of these cases experience difficulty in expelling the gas.

In most cases, distress is probably not due to the presence of a large amount of gas, for this is seldom present in large amounts. It seems rather to be due to increased internal tension. A constant internal tension or pressure is maintained in the digestive tube. This is regulated by the sympathetic nervous system. Increased tension is felt, reflexly, as pain or discomfort in the muscles of the abdomen.

"Nervousness," shock, strong emotions, etc., may cause increased tension in the tube and the faster will experience some kind of discomfort. Subconscious fears also may cause the so-called gas pains. Those who have long suffered with digestive derangements are especially prone to changes in the internal tension of the tube.

Functional irregularities in the stomach and intestine may cause pain because of increased peristaltic contractions that often exist in these. Marked visceroptosis, with sharp angulations, may increase the internal tension and cause discomfort or pain.

Increased peristaltic activity of the stomach walls, due to "nervousness," may also result in discomfort that is mistaken for "gas pains". Increased tension may occur in any section of the tube and thus pain or discomfort may be either general over the abdomen or may be more or less localized.

Fasters who so suffer generally complain that the "gas" makes them nervous and keeps them awake at night. It seems that the opposite of this is the truth—the nervousness causes the increased tension and resulting discomfort. Where these patients are able to completely relax, their "gas pains" cease. Although I no longer employ any of these: suggestion, abdominal massage, hot water applications to the abdomen, a drink of warm water and other measures, will usually relieve this distress, at least temporarily without actually lessening the amount of gas.

Gas rumblings in the intestine mean unstable nerve control of this organ. Cathartic drugs will almost always produce these rumblings. This is due to excitement produced by the irritating drugs.

The gurgling and rumbling often heard in the abdomen is due to the movements of gas from one section of the intestine to another. It may often be due to emotional interferences with the normal sympathetic control of the gut. A nervous patient may exhibit such rumbling on the slightest provocation. Enemas, due to the excitement they occasion, often produce these symptoms.

Diarrhea: This is a rare development, although it is more common in fasting than some advocates of fasting know about. This is due to the fact that their use of the enema hides the actual development. It comes, when it does, only as a house-cleaning process, and only because there is an imperative need for it.

Enlargement of the parotid gland: (the salivary gland that lies at about the angle of the jaws, one on each side of the mouth), rarely seen in a fast, but sometimes developing immediately after the fast is broken, has been variously interpreted. It is a common development in famine victims and is said to be due to "semi-starvation" and to deficient protein. Undernutrition and malnutrition frequently result in this enlargement, fasting rarely. Studies so far made of the development leave much to be desired. It is an evanescent development, lasting from two or three days to as many weeks, but rarely more than a few days. I have seen no mention of it in fasting literature, other than that of Mr. Hoelzel and his experimental work often lacked many elements of proper care of the body. This was permissible in experimenting, but would not be so in the care of the sick.

Dizziness: This is a very frequent symptom and manifests chiefly in the early part of the fast, or when one arises suddenly.

It lasts but a few seconds and may be prevented by rising slowly. It is a common development during the fast and arises out of the sudden withdrawal of blood from the brain. If the faster will "take it easy," he will rarely experience any dizziness.

Fainting: This may occur in the early days of a fast. It should occasion no alarm or apprehension, and the patient should be cared for merely by stretching him, or her out and loosening all tight clothing and admitting plenty of fresh air to the patient.

Although relatively few fasters faint, many of them do at some time or other during a fast. Often this may occur on the first or second day and not again thereafter. Carrington mentions a case in which "a practical suspension of all consciousness resulted from the ingestion of the first meal, after the breaking of the fast, and lasted some hours." He emphasizes the fact that such occurrences are merely rare curiosities rather than "pathological phenomena likely to occur." He says that "it is doubtful if precisely the same effects will ever again be observed in fasting patients—being due, in every case, to a peculiar combination of causes, all but impossible to duplicate again."

When a fasting patient faints he should be cared for precisely as if he fainted while eating three square meals a day. All he needs is fresh air and time. He should not be set up, but should be left in a prone position. No stimulants or smelling salts need be given. Let him alone and he will soon open his eyes and look around, then get up and go about his business. Dashing cold water in his face is equally unnecessary. Rest, not shock, is the need of the person who has fainted.

Sore throat: Although sore throat is most often seen following immediately upon breaking the fast, it occasionally develops during the fast. The soreness is never great, lasts but a day or two, at most, and need occasion no concern.

Palpitation: "Pain in the heart" and palpitation of this organ are due to gases in the digestive organs. These symptoms are of rare development and are not dangerous, although they are usually the source of much needless apprehension on the part of the patient. Palpitation may be the result of "nervousness," fear or exertion.

Pain felt in the heart is rarely actual pain in the heart. It is usually pain in the chest. It may be due to gas, it may be of "psychic" origin, it may be of toxic origin. Unless it is accompanied with other symptoms that indicate heart trouble, it should be ignored. It is not serious and soon passes.

Insomnia: This is most often due to a lack of need of sleep. Little sleep is required by the average fasting individual. In a few instances sleeplessness is due to nervous tension or to discomfort. Sleeplessness should cause no worry.

While few fasters sleep as much as when eating, all of them sleep much more than they realize. This is also true of all patients who suffer with insomnia. Ten hours of sleep seem like fifteen minutes because we are not conscious of the passage of time while we are unconscious; an hour of wakefulness seems like a whole night, because time drags so slowly when we are waiting to go to sleep.

Visual defects: While it is no uncommon thing to see great and lasting improvements in vision develop during a fast, particularly during a long fast, there are somewhat rare instances in which there develops temporary weakness of vision. Carrington mentions what he regards as a "curious development" which he says may never be seen again. A patient saw double for a time just prior to breaking the fast. Two visual images were perceived instead of one. I have seen one or two such developments myself at the end of a very long fast. What is seen more often, but still only rarely, is weakness of vision, so that the faster can see but little. He is forced to discontinue reading, or his vision may become weaker, even, than this would indicate. Much of this seems to be due to a temporary loss of coordination between the two eyes, as they do not focus upon the object viewed. That no real injury to the nerves or mechanism of vision occurs is shown by the fact that the weakness and defect soon disappear after the fast is broken and vision is soon better than it was before the fast. I had one case in which this development occurred, in a man who had worn heavy lenses for years prior to the fast. After the fast was broken he was able to discard his glasses and got along without them. Another case is that of a woman who wore glasses but who saw double (without her glasses) before the fast, and regained normal vision while fasting. She was able to discard her glasses on the sixteenth day of her fast and could see to read, sew, thread needles, etc., without her glasses. She did not return to the use of glasses until about seven years later.

DANGEROUS COMPLICATIONS

Under the head of danger signals or complications, works on fasting usually list uncontrollable vomiting, persistent hiccoughs, a persistent, very erratic pulse, extreme weakness, fear of starvation, or an unreasonable and persistent determination to break the fast. The last three of these, I think, may be properly considered as signs of possible danger.

Great Weakness: This is not always a danger signal; but may be in some cases. Although it usually causes the practitioner to terminate the fast, this is due more to fear on his part than to any actual danger to the patient. Persistent extreme weakness is more likely to prove a danger signal, although this is so rare that I have seen but one such case.

Erratic Pulse: This may sometimes be a danger signal, but is not so in most cases. The heart will bear careful watching in such cases, and the fast may be terminated if the practitioner deems this advisable. An erratic pulse is usually of short duration, and should be taken seriously only when it is lasting.

A very rapid pulse or a very low, feeble pulse is usually considered a danger sign. This is certainly not always so. I have frequently continued fasts with a very rapid pulse, and I have continued others when the pulse was so low that one could hardy count it. All such symtpoms must be considered in relation to the general condition of the patient and not in isolation.

Difficult Breathing: Dr. Kritzer lists the following symptoms that should be carefully watched because "they are nature's warnings to discontinue the fasting:" "palpitation of the heart; dyspnea (difficult breathing); vomiting; hiccoughs, night sweats, a rapid, thin, wiry pulse, extreme nausea." The experienced practitioner knows that these are not indications for breaking the fast, and that they are not danger signals. I have witnessed the development of difficult breathing during a fast in but few cases and I have not seen it mentioned in any of the literature on fasting. It must be an exceedingly rare occurrence and, if and when it does occur, must be considered in relation to the general condition of the patient.

Retention of Urine: This is a very rare occurrence. I have never seen it develop. Authors attribute it to insufficient water drinking; but this cannot be the cause. Hot sitz baths and hot enemas are advised to secure relaxation. I do not favor their use.

A catheter may be employed if necessary. Dr. Christopher Gian-Cursio reports a few cases of suppression of urine. In one case he secured a flow of urine by resort to a vaginal douche. No catheter was used. He says he much prefers fasters to have other reactions as this creates a great amount of fear in the patient and their panic-stricken "friends." Carrington mentions one case in which there was "prolonged retention of urine toward the end of a prolonged fast."

Delirium: This condition is of very rare occurrence; but may develop in those who have taken large quantities of nerve paralyzing drugs, or who are very toxic. The delirium is of short duration, and by itself should cause no apprehension. Should it develop in connection with suppressed urine, extreme weakness, rapid, feeble pulse and other signs of prostration, it should be considered a sign of danger. Such dangers do not arise from the fast, but from other causes.

Petechiæ: These are small purplish hemorrhagic spots in the skin which are chiefly associated with severe fevers, such as typhus, and are supposed to be indicative of great prostration. I have seen them develop in about a dozen fasters during more than forty years of conducting fasts. Only two of these fasting patients have been young; the remainder have been well past middle life. They appear in patients who are in very low states of nutrition. This development has not been observed in any of the longest fasts I have conducted, while three or four of them have been in comparatively short fasts. The patients have at no time been prostrated. They probably mean great weakness of the capillary walls so that these break easily, permitting the blood to flow into the skin. It has been my practice to break the fast immediately upon their appearance. Only in one instance was the fast carried several days beyond their appearance. In this patient no harm resulted from extending the fast.

There are really few danger signals that develop during a fast and these are extremely rare. Perhaps in all cases these are due to something other than the fast. Due to popular prejudices against fasting and to the violent opposition of the medical profession to the procedure, practitioners who employed fasting hesitated to continue a fast in the face of developments they considered danger signals. Should the patient die they are likely to be accused of starving him to death and sentenced for manslaughter.

Ten thousand patients may die after swallowing poisonous drugs or after having one or more of their organs removed and no one is held responsible; but let one patient die while fasting and an autopsy is at once ordered to fix responsibility for death. This hindered, for a long time, progress in knowledge of fasting and prevented the discovery that what were thought to be danger signals often were not.

STRENGTH AND WEAKNESS

Benedict devotes consideration to strength tests during the fast. He says: "The tests made by Luciani on Succi in which a dynamometer was used to measure the strength of the right and left hands, showed results seemingly at variance with popular impressions. Thus, on the 21st day of the fast Succi was able to register on the dynamometer a stronger grip than when the fast began. From the 20th to the 30th days of the fast, however, his strength decreased, being less at the end than at the beginning of the fast. In discussing these results, Luciani points out the fact that Succi believed that he gained in strength as the fast progressed, and hence probably did not exert the greatest power at the beginning of the experiment. Considering the question of the influence of inanition on the onset of fatigue, Luciani states that the fatigue curve obtained by Succi on the 29th fast day was similar to those obtained with an individual under normal conditions . . ."

Levinson says: "Many people think that during a long fast you have to sit down on a Morris chair reading newspapers or dozing because you have not sufficient strength for doing any work at all. If you weigh two hundred pounds and your normal weight should be one hundred and thirty-two you can fast for sixty days and for each day you increase your strength, because you are coming back to your normal point. I started this fast from my normal weight; I have gone through thirty-two days of continuous scientific hardships and tortures, but I never felt that I was losing any strength and there are the dynamometer tests to show it.

"On the last day I could press up to one hundred and twenty pounds without any difficulty with my left hand and I never do any regular exercise except walking. I could go up and down a steep flight of steps to my balcony without support or shaking in the knees. I never lay down except during experiments.

"I used to pass the few spare hours that were at my disposal writing long letters and busying myself actively; on the evening of the last day I was dancing in the laboratory and laughing. In the afternoon the elite of the medical and scientific men of Harvard University and the medical colleges came to see me. I stood up for nearly two hours and for the whole time."

Telling of his discussion with the reporters at the end of his experimental fast he says: "I explained to them the impressions of my fast, compared them with those of my precedent fasts and answered many questions with my spirits up and without feeling the least exhaustion. Those that feel any lack of strength during a fast are to be classed in the same category with those who feel hungry. They are nervous, and very impressionable people, and their sufferings are only the baneful effect of their too vivid imagination.

"If you suggest to yourself that you are strong and that you can walk two miles on the thirtieth day of your fast, believe me, you can do it without great difficulty, but if you fix in your weak mind that you are going to faint and worry and persist to worry about it, be sure that not a very long time will elapse before you faint really, a victim of your wrong auto-suggestion."

What may, at first, seem paradoxical is the fact that when a patient becomes very weak in fasting, if he persists in the fast, the weakness ceases and he grows stronger. Indeed I have seen patients who were one day so weak they could hardly raise their heads from the pillow and, next day, still fasting, were so strong they wanted to get out and do things. Great weakness, bordering on prostration may be seen in certain crises, especially in vomiting, so long as the crisis lasts. As soon as the crisis has ended, strength returns with a rush.

Hygiene of the Fast

CHAPTER XXIX

Fasting is not a toy to be played with by the ignorant nor should it be looked upon as a stunt. There have been stunt fasters, but we do not advise one to undertake stunt fasts. Nor do we advise indiscriminate fasting of any kind by anyone. Anyone undertaking an extended fast should either be fully acquainted with all the details of fasting, or he should be directly and immediately supervised by one who has had much experience in conducting fasts. As elsewhere, but "a little knowledge is a dangerous thing." The fast is such an unusual experience for the average person, and his feelings and sensations, while undergoing it, are so entirely different from his previous experiences, his mental condition is often so perturbed, due to unfounded anxiety, that the development of any insignificant symptom, such as palpitation of the heart, faintness, gastric discomfort, vomiting, etc., may cause alarm. It is here that the experienced man can offer the faster the support and reassurance that is so helpful under the circumstances.

Carrington has emphasized the fact that fasting is a great deal more complicated than is commonly supposed, or than is involved in the mere idea of "going without food." "There is a science of fasting," he says, "which we are just now (1909) beginning to realize." While expressing the view that the dangers of fasting are so slight as to be insignificant, and its benefits, when rightly applied, far-reaching and immeasurable, he says: "fasting should be applied by skilled hands; or rather, practiced only under the close supervision and observation of one skilled in" conducting the fast. He says: "the average physician is no more qualified to undertake the supervision of a protracted fast than is any other man who has a good working knowledge of physiology." He advises that the fast be undertaken under the supervision of a good reputable *Hygienist*.

When one undertakes to fast, one reasonably desires to obtain the greatest possible good in the shortest possible time. To accomplish this requires that the fast be conducted in strict accordance with a few simple and easily understood principles. These few principles must be known and observed in abstaining from food, by either the well or the sick. Tilden says: "Fasting as a remedy requires great knowledge and experience, and should not be assumed by laymen, nor by professional men who have given the subject no thought from a fundamental point of view." Fasting must be fully understood, rightly applied, it must be conducted with skilled hands, if full results are to be expected. There are many factors that must be considered while the patient is abstaining from food. If the sick person's condition represents years of abuse by bad habits and treatment, great skill is required to take him through a fast to perfect health. Many of the evils ascribed to fasting have resulted from the attempts of unskilled and inexperienced men to conduct fasts.

No greater truth was ever uttered than that contained in Oswald's statement that, "Fasting is a great system-renovator. Ten fast-days a year will purify the blood and eradicate the *poison-diathesis* more effectively than a hundred bottles of expurgative bitters." But to achieve ideal results the fast must be properly conducted. The *Hygiene* of the fast does not differ from the hygiene of "disease." Indeed, we must learn to regard fasting as a *Hygienic*, not as a therapeutic measure. I do not like the terms "fasting cure" and "therapeutic fasting," or "curative fasting."

WHERE TO FAST

A close student of fasting once remarked: "The trouble with fasting is, there's no place to do it in." He meant that the surroundings are so important, the possibilities and the liabilities are so great, that we need to have a proper place for the fast. One of the biggest obstacles in the way of the man who attempts to fast at home is the fact that his family, his relatives, his friends and neighbors will not let him alone. They constantly urge him to eat, tell him that he is going to starve to death, that he is looking bad, that he will be sure to injure himself, etc., etc. Members of the family may become very angry with him and quarrel with him, thus exemplifying the truth of the old adage that a man's enemies are of his own household. They call in a physician who tells him that he is injuring himself; sometimes the police are called and a threat is made to have him committed. Food is brought to him and offered him; tasty tidbits are made for the purpose of tempting him. They make a nightmare of his fast. Result: he throws in the sponge and resumes eating.

Home should be an ideal place to fast, but owing to the prevailing ignorance of and opposition to it, this is rarely the case. Home is also commonly located amid the noise and fumes of a city where the water is drugged until it is as unfit to drink as the air is unfit to breathe. The fast should be undergone amid quiet, peaceful surroundings, where the air is pure, pure water is available and the people are congenial. As it should be also properly supervised, the best place to fast is in an institution, preferably a *Hygienic* institution, located in the country. In Winter, this should be in the South. The new school, the *Hygienic*, requires supervision by men and women who are perfectly familiar with all of the symptoms, changes in flesh, and in mental changes which fasting makes possible. The *Health School* or *Hygieian Home* for the reconstruction of the patient. will not be in the hands of a group of sleek, fat, indulgent men and women who reveal, by their own condition and their own ways of life, that they do not know the laws of life, and who have never disciplined themselves, but in the hands of healthy, clear eyed, men and women who serve as inspirational examples of the health they are helping to build in their patients.

CONSERVATION

All of our care of the faster should be designed to conserve in every possible manner, his energies and reserves. Every method of care and every influence in the environment of the patient that occasions a dissipation of the patient's energies and reserves should be carefully avoided. Much harm results from the use of drugs and measures of treatment that are not conservative and there is everywhere, in the ranks of those who oppose fasting, a tendency to credit this harm to the fast, rather than to the enervating measures employed in mis-caring for the patient. Let conservation, rather than dissipation, be our watch-word. The instructions that follow, if carried out conscientiously, will prove conservative; hence, they will definitely shorten the period of time the patient will have to fast, and will leave him in better physical condition at the end of his fast.

REST

In the closing years of the last century and the early years of this, many fasters seem to have tried to ascertain how much work they could get out of their bodies while fasting. They were proud of winning foot races, of the amount of weight they could lift, of the greater amount of mental work they could do, of the longer hours they spent in work, of the late hours in which they engaged, and of similar feats of activity. Tanner's race with a reporter, Sinclair's greater mental output, the weight lifting of Macfadden and Low, all while fasting, are examples of this nature. All such examples of the ability of the faster to perform mental and physical work, all examples of mental acuteness and of physical endurance are valuable in revealing the strength of the faster and the resources and capacities at the command of the body abstaining from food, but they are not examples to be emulated by the sick person who fasts for the purpose of improving his health. Conservation of his resources will provide far better results. Let him rest—mentally, sensorially and physically, while he is resting physiologically.

The hibernating animal possesses sufficient reserves to maintain a minimum of physiological and little or no physical activity throughout a prolonged period of abstinence, but in the case of a fasting man, there is no hibernation and there is no reduction of phsiological activity to such low levels. Rarely, even, does he discontinue all physical activity, even for short periods, to the same extent as does the hibernating animal. Usually, also, there is considerable mental and sensorial activity. Prof. Morgulis describes the winter sleep of Russian peasants in trying years of famine, when entire families are "massed closely together," on top of a wide stove. "Deprived practically of every means of subsistence," "well-protected against loss of heat by close contact as well as by their fur coats." He says "members of the entire household and frequently of entire villages remained with occasional interruptions, in a state of winter sleep, *preserving their energy by limiting its dissipation.*"

Nature does the same thing when she prostrates the patient and suspends all digestive activities. She preserves energy by limiting its dissipation. The energy thus saved is available for use in the temporarily more important work of healing. If we are wise we will take our cue from nature and also conserve our energies, while fasting, by curbing their expenditures. I favor the plan of putting the fasting individual to bed. I am sure that better and quicker results are thus obtained. Nature puts her hibernating animal to bed and to sleep. Seals and salmon are, of course, very active during their months of fasting, but they are exhausted at the end. The salmon usually die and the seals sleep for weeks.

Observations made during the fasts of Succi and others show that the body wastes less rapidly when the patient is kept warm and at rest. Rest conserves the body's energies and substances and hastens the process of healing. I agree with Purinton, who says in his *Philosophy of Fasting*: "Not an ounce of energy shall be dissipated during the extreme fast. This means loafing, resting, lazying along and not caring." The best place for the faster is in bed. Talking, laughing, listening to the radio and viewing and listening to television prevent genuine rest. They are noisy, disturbing, and emotionally upsetting. A newspaper or a novel may be disturbing, exciting or depressing. I went into the room of one of my young women patients and found her crying. I asked why she was crying. "She died," she sobbed. "Who died?" I asked. "The woman in the picture," was her reply. She had been viewing a movie on television and the heroine had died at the end of the picture. The patient had become so emotionally involved with the heroine that her death seemed real. Emotional involvements with the characters in the soap operas and other picture can be very enervating. Wisdom admonishes that such things be avoided while fasting.

In hibernation, due to the extremely low degree of metabolic activity, the nutritive reserves are consumed very slowly, but fasting may be associated with vigorous physical activity—witness the fur seal bull and male salmon during their mating seasons. It is quite obvious that, given the same amount of nutritive reserve, the active individual will consume his internal food stores sooner than the resting individual. For this reason, if for no other, the fasting patient who rests while fasting will emerge from the fast in better condition than the faster who is active during this period. At the same time, if a prolonged fast is essential, rest will enable the patient to conserve his reserves to the utmost and thus lengthen the period over which he can safely fast. The nutritive materials stored in the tissues supply the minimum amount of sustenance indispensable to keep up the necessary activities of life until a more favorable condition of life is produced. The less physically active organism expends less of its reserves, not alone due to reduced physical work, but, also, due to decreased physiological activity.

The great value of rest in all pathological conditions is well established. Beyond a certain minimum of physical activity (and even this is profitably dispensed with in most acute and a few chronic conditions) the more rest the sick organism receives, the more rapidly is good health restored. This principle does not cease to be true when the sick organism is fasting. Rest (physical, mental and physiological) is equally important and beneficial during a fast. By physiological rest in this particular connection, I have reference to freedom from stimulation—excitation.

In insects the condition of perfect quiescence is accompanied by the most wonderful changes. The worm-like caterpillar becomes, within its cocoon, the butterfly with locomotive powers immensely greater and with a totally new and different organism. Growth and repair are most efficient in man when he rests and sleeps most. The nearer the faster can approach the quiescence of the *pupa*, the greater will be the conservation of his energies and the more rapid and efficient will be the repair of his damaged structures. Even reading, writing, talking, listening to the radio and similar forms of activity should be avoided as much as possible. The noisy radio with its jazz music, its emotionally exciting soap operas, exciting or depressing newscasts, etc., is especially bad.

MENTAL INFLUENCES

Somewhere in the Bible is the statement that "a man's foes shall be they of his own household." How true this is may be discovered by anyone who undertakes a fast at home. Even missing one meal is often enough to cause a family alarm that results in a near-panic. Every form of pressure will be brought to bear upon the faster to persuade or even to coerce him to return to eating. Well-meaning though these members of the faster's family may be, they are actually the enemies in his own household. It is wise, therefore, to get away from family and friends when undertaking a fast.

Fasting is an unusual experience for most patients. The first fast, in particular, is likely to be filled with unfounded anxiety, uncertainty, mental perturbation, and even fear. The faster will experience new and formerly unknown feelings and sensations and these will disturb him. Nausea, faintness, pain, vomiting, headache, and other symptoms that occasionally arise may give rise to panic and result in injurious treatment or in a premature and hurtful breaking of the fast. The faster needs to be under the care and constant supervision of one who understands these developments and who can give him encouragement and explanation. He is even helped by being with other fasters, as these support him by their own experiences.

Levanzin says that at the start of the fast, if the patient concentrates his thinking upon his privation from his accustomed pleasures, he suffers mentally. He advises that the patient try to find a diversion so that he may have his mind on something else. He advises drinking a glass of water when the accustomed meal time arrives, but I do not advise this unless there is actual thirst. If the patient will not worry about his "deprivation" he will be less likely to experience any discomfort at all. The Bible advises: "When thou fastest, anoint thine head and wash thy face that thou appear not unto men to fast."

Fear of the fast, broodiness and other phases of mental depression are especially to be combatted. While fasting, as at other times, one's thoughts and emotions profoundly affect the organs and functions of the body. A cheerful attitude is especially important at this time. Literally, millions of people have fasted and many thousands have fasted for long periods, and we know that there is no danger associated with prolonged abstinence from food. Disabuse the mind of all fear and apprehension. Do not imagine that you are going to grow weak or starve to death. Fear in particular is dangerous.

Prof. Morgulis says: "The practical value of inanition (emptiness) will never be fully utilized until both laymen and the medical profession lose their instinctive fear of fasting." I do not believe the fear of fasting is at all instinctive, but that it is due to misinformation and false training. An instinctive fear of fasting, it seems to me, would, of itself, be a strong reason for rejecting the measure altogether. Morgulis adds that "the experiences of recent years which through the medium of the press have reached a large audience will in course of time, alleviate the entirely unjustifiable fear of abstention from food for longer periods."

The hunger strikes and a few similar experiences which have been published are as nothing compared to the many thousands who have fasted for long periods under the care of those whom Morgulis refers to as "amateurs" and "enthusiasts." Nor has the daily press, in carrying such stories, done a hundredth part as much in breaking down this "entirely unjustifiable fear" of fasting as have the "enthusiasts," through their lectures, writings and successes in fasting the sick. For sectarian reasons, Morgulis, who belongs to the self-styled "regular" medical profession, would minimize the work of these men and refers to them as "crank reformers who see in inanition a panacea for all ills of the flesh."

FEAR

Sinclair says: "There are two dangers to be feared in fasting. The first is that of fear. I do not say this as a jest." "The faster should not have about him terrified aunts and cousins who will tell him that he looks like a corpse, that his pulse is below forty and that his heart may stop beating in the night. I took a fast of three days out in California, on the third day I walked fifteen miles, off and on, and except that I was restless, I never felt better; and then in the evening I came home and read about the Messina earthquake, and how the relief ships arrived, and the wretched survivors crowded down to the water's edge and tore each other like wild beasts in their rage of hunger. The paper set forth, in horrified language, that some of them had been seventy-two hours without food. I, as I read, had also been seventy-two hours without food, and the difference was simply that they thought they were starving. And if at some crisis during a long fast, when you feel nervous and weak and doubting, some people with stronger wills than your own are able to arouse in you the terrors of the earthquake survivors, they can cause their most direful anticipations to be realized."

The fast should not be continued if the patient is in dread of it—living in fear. Fear may kill. It certainly inhibits elimination. Scientific works on the mind and emotions are replete with well authenticated cases of death resulting from fear, anger, grief, shock, etc. Instantaneous death has resulted more than once from the reading of a telegram. In other cases, grief or fear has sent people to the grave in a few days. Only recently in this city, grief over the death of his father resulted in the death of a young boy in three month's time.

MAINTAIN POISE

Physical and emotional activities cause a rapid expenditure of the stored reserves. The fasting man is more or less active—physically, mentally, emotionally, sensorially—and this activity consumes his reserves at a much more rapid rate than the reserves of the hibernating bat, for example, are consumed. This results in a more rapid exhaustion of reserves. For, while man's metabolic rate is greatly reduced, it is not lowered to the same extent as that of the hibernating or estivating animal.

FRESH AIR

The effort to keep warm should not cause one to exclude fresh air from the room. Fresh air is even more imperative during the fast than at other times. See that the room is well ventilated both day and night.

WARMTH

Hibernating animals manage to live despite the low temperature of their bodies, but man and, perhaps, most other non-hibernating animals would freeze to death if subjected to such prolonged low temperatures without food. Resistance to cold is greatly reduced by the low metabolic rate of the faster, so that he feels cold at what may be, under ordinary circumstances, a comfortable temperature. This causes a more rapid using up of his reserves. Therefore, the faster should be kept warm in order that his reserves may be conserved to the greatest extent.

Chilling causes discomfort, prevents rest and sleep, and checks elimination. It may, in some cases, cause nausea, vomiting and pain. Warmth promotes comfort and elimination. The patient who is kept warm recovers more rapidly. A hot jug to the feet will usually be sufficient to insure comfort and prevent chilling. The faster should not be overburdened with bed clothing. Fasting patients should not be permitted to remain cold. They are inclined to chill easily and if nurse or doctor is careless, such patients can freeze to death even in July or August; and they certainly will freeze to death in the winter unless they are carefully attended to. It is the rule that those persons who suffer constantly with cold hands and feet lose this complaint as a result of fasting. During the fast, however, the feet particularly, are likely to feel cold much of the time.

Fasters must be kept warm. It requires nerve force to warm the body, and the patient should not be permitted to waste his nervous energy in keeping warm, but should be kept warm by artificial heat. The fasting patient who throws off the covers and kicks his feet and legs out, declaring he is too hot, yet who has cold extremities, as revealed by feeling his feet, must be carefully warmed and kept warm. Such patients are actually in danger. Tilden says of such: "unless that patient is carefully warmed and kept warm, death will ensue within twenty-four to forty-eight hours. And if the case has advanced very far before receiving this attention, death will certainly take place." Again: "After fasting has gone beyond a certain point—after the patient has reached a point where the rectal temperature goes one or two degrees below normal—there will be great difficulty in resuscitation." Where such a condition as he here describes has been permitted to develop, and it should be known that its development is due to ignorance or carelessness, artificial heat and much of it must be applied to the faster. Food will have to be given in very small quantities and at frequent intervals. Rest and quiet are very important in such a condition.

EXERCISE

For a number of years I continued exercise through the fast of most chronic sufferers. My rule was: "Chronic sufferers, unless otherwise contra-indicated, should have daily exercise while fasting." I insisted that the exercise should be mild and carefully adapted to the strength of the patient and preferred those forms of exercise that could be taken while lying in bed. I employed the corrective exercises that may have been needed in most cases during the fast. My rule was that fatigue should be avoided.

I became convinced that this was not good practice in most cases. It is now my practice to require all sick fasters to rest. Only those vigorous individuals who are undergoing a fast of ten days to two weeks as a Spring house-cleaning, and fat individuals who are fasting for reduction of weight are now given exercise while fasting. While the fast is in progress, the emphasis is placed on rest. After eating is resumed, exercise is given.

WORKING DURING THE FAST

On general principles working during a long fast is to be severely condemned. It has been done. It can often be done. But it should not be done. Perhaps the first fast of any length in which the faster worked was the twenty-eight days fast undergone by Mr. Milton Rathburn, a wealthy grain dealer, in 1899. Mr. Rathburn, who was a very fat man, took this fast to reduce, upon the advice of Dr. Dewey, and continued his daily work throughout the entire length thereof. According to the New York Press, of June 6, 1899, "he worked and worked hard. He came down earlier to his office and went away later than usual. He made no effort to save himself. On the contrary, he seemed determined to make his task as hard as possible."

Others have done this same thing and some of them were even more remarkable. In 1925, a weaver in Jersey City, N. J., fasted forty days and worked as a weaver throughout the time. On January

18, 1926, George Hassler Johnston, of New York City, a friend and co-worker of the author, began a fast which lasted thirty days, during which time he was unusually active. Mr. Johnson underwent this fast, under my supervision, purely as a publicity stunt and not because he was in need of a fast. He was an athlete of no mean ability and was in excellent physical condition at the beginning and at the end of the fast.

During the entire period of the fast, Mr. Johnson arose each morning at 5 o'clock and went to a radio broadcasting station, where he broadcasted three classes in exercises, each class lasting fifteen minutes. From here he usually walked a distance of twenty-five blocks to the office of the Macfadden Publications, where he entered upon his editorial duties. At 11:30 A.M. each day he visited one or the other of the three Physical Culture Restaurants in New York, where he remained until 2 P.M., meeting the people and answering their questions and giving advice upon fasting, diet and exercise. From the restaurant he would return to the office where, at 3 P.M., he conducted two classes, composed of Macfadden employees, in calesthenics. After this he resumed his editorial duties, remaining at his desk until 5 P.M. During most of the fast he would walk home in the evening, a distance of 72 blocks, and spent his evenings at Madison Square Garden, watching the boxing and wrestling bouts. It was not until the end of the first week of the fast that he gave up his training at a down-town gymnasium and his track work—running.

This fast ended on the evening of Tuesday, Feb. 16, just 30 days after it had begun. On June 2, just three and one-half months thereafter, Mr. Johnston started from Chicago, in an effort to walk from there to New York without food. This stunt, I warned him against, but he made a brave effort and ended it June 20th at Bedford, Pa., having covered a distance of 577.8 miles in the 20 days.

This walk carried him over hills and valleys, through wind, rain, and the summer's heat and through crowds that flocked along the way. Handshaking, interviews, posing for pictures and making short health talks consumed almost as much of his energy as the walking. These often delayed him so that his walking on several days began late in the forenoon, although it often extended far into the night. I warned Mr. Johnston before he left to conserve his energies and predicted that he would go 20 days and no longer. He would have covered more miles in the same time he walked had he done more walking and less of other things, but he would still have ended on the 20th day.

This thing can be done, but it is damaging, even dangerous, and should never be undertaken. Gandhi, the Hindu Nationalist leader, who has probably fasted more than any other man in modern times, learned the necessity of conserving his energies while fasting. A painful mistake, which almost left him an invalid for life, taught him this lesson. It was while in South Africa that he took his second long fast, lasting fourteen days, that he foolishly imagined he could do as much work as while eating. On the second day after breaking the fast he began strenuous walking. This caused excruciating pain in the lower limbs, but he did the same the next day and for several days thereafter. The pains increased. His health was gravely injured by this and he was years in fully recovering from it. Of this he said: "From this very costly experiment I learned that perfect physical rest during the fast and for a time proportionate to the length of the fast, after the breaking of it, is a necessity, and if this simple rule can be observed no evil effects of fasting need be feared. Indeed, it is my conviction that the body gains by a well-regulated fast, for during fasting the body gets rid of many of its impurities."

This warning against working throughout a long fast does not apply to a short fast. I have on several occasions worked both at hard physical labor and at prolonged and exacting mental work for three or four days without food, and I have had hundreds of patients to do the same up to as high as nine days. But I do not think this should be prolonged beyond the tenth day, and where it is possible to absent oneself from work, it is best that all the time be spent in rest.

The practice pursued by many, of spending the whole day in activity, retards recovery from "*disease.*" Conservation of energy should be the guiding principle. Dr. Eales worked throughout his fast devoting eleven to twelve hours a day to the labors of his profession. He was very energetic during the whole time. Regular and frequent strength tests were made. The tests on the eleventh, sixteenth, twenty-first, twenty-third, twenty-fifth, twenty-ninth and thirty-first days of his fast showed his strength to be as great as at the beginning of the fast. The doctor reports that he could have competed in athletic work on the thirtieth day.

BATHING
Bathing during the fast should follow the rules laid down for bathing in a preceding volume. The faster in particular should avoid extremes of temperature. Wash the body quickly and do not stay in the tub or under the shower for a prolonged period. A sponge bath should be used if the patient is too weak to take his or her own bath. Objections have been raised to tub and shower baths while fasting on the grounds that the bath washes away substances from the skin, that must be made good by drawing upon the body's food reserves and that the bath is enervating. The sponge bath is advocated instead, although this also washes aways substances from the skin. A too hot bath, a too cold bath, a too prolonged bath may prove enervating, but a bath near body temperature and that is not prolonged will not prove more expensive to the body's nerve energy than a sponge bath. If the patient is too weak to take a shower or a tub bath, the sponge bath should certainly be employed. In extremely weak cases, the frequency of the bath may profitably be reduced.

SUN BATHING
Sunbathing is beneficial during the fast, but must be indulged with greater caution. Certain precautions are essential. As the fast progresses the sunbath may be increased up to a point, after which it should be decreased. The faster should always avoid the heat of the day and the sunbath should be of short duration. Nervous patients, heart patients, asthmatics and sufferers with pulmonary tuberculosis should be more careful in sunbathing than other patients.

Objections have been raised to the sunbath during the fast. It is asserted that the anabolic processes are at a standstill during this period; that the sunbath causes corrugations in the finger nails; that sunbathing accelerates calcium metabolism and in some way, this is supposed to be undesirable; that the sunbath is enervating. None of these objections appear to be valid. I have previously shown that there is an intense anabolism during the fast. What harm can come from an acceleration of calcium metabolism is not apparent. The sunbath does not cause corrugations of the finger nails. It may prove very enervating if it is too prolonged or if it is taken in the hottest part of the day.

Patients should not be permitted to remain in the sun until they are depressed. If the patient is irritable or nervous after a sunbath, it has been too prolonged or has been taken when it is too hot. A little intelligent supervision of the sunbathing of the faster will prevent the enervating effect. Enervation is the result of excess, not of sunning within the capacity of the organism to make constructive use of the sun. My rule is to start the sunning with five minutes of exposure on the front surface of the body and five minutes exposure on the back surface for the first day and to increase the exposure time one minute on each side each day until the twentieth day, after which I decrease it. There are individuals in whom this rate of increase is not insisted upon and a few who are not given sunbaths while fasting. I do not think that such inflexible rules of care as are insisted on in some quarters can be made to fit all patient's needs.

FOR THE BAD TASTE

Through most of the fast, the fasting individual is annoyed by a very bad taste in the mouth. This may be alleviated somewhat by a daily scrubbing of the tongue with a toothbrush. This should not be done, however, until after the tongue has been examined by the doctor who is conducting the fast. Mouth washes, lemon juice, etc., are not to be recommended. Gargling the throat is certainly of no value. As the fast progresses and the tongue clears up, the taste becomes less and less offensive, until, when the fast should be broken, the taste in the mouth is very pleasant.

GUM CHEWING

It has been determined experimentally, that the chewing of gum occasions an inhibition of gastric secretion. This, instead of enhancing digestion, as gum chewing is popularly and professionally supposed to do, actually retards the digestion of protein foods. As there is no digestion going on during a fast, it may seem unimportant if the faster chews gum, but this is far from true. I have permitted fasters to chew gum and I have noted a tendency to chew it in large quantities, the faster chewing three or four packages of gum a day. I am inclined to think that he chews it until he extracts all the sugar from it, then takes fresh gum, doing the same with this.

Gum chewing serves no useful purpose. It is an evidence of weakness, the foundation for which is laid in infancy and early childhood. Mothers give their babies bottles, nipples, crackers or cookies to keep them quiet. Later in life these perpetual sucklings trade their nipples or their cookies for chewing gum or the cigarette. Gum chewing is a mental habit that is needless and foolish, as well as a wasteful practice under any and all circumstances. It is not the innocent practice it is commonly regarded. There can be no doubt that it exhausts the salivary glands. It does not seem probable that any useless habit can be regularly indulged by anybody with impunity. Gum chewing is certainly wasteful of the patient's energy and the energy wasted in this useless practice may be, at least in very low states of health, just enough to mean the difference between recovery and death. It is particularly essential in all serious states of disease, and in fasting, that all nerve-leaks and all sources of enervation be discontinued. Energy must be conserved in every possible way. The faster should certainly refrain from chewing gum.

WATER DRINKING DURING THE FAST

Most fasting advocates advise drinking much water while fasting. This is done on the theory that water aids in eliminating toxins from the body. Levanzin expresses this theory as follows: "as a rule, it is certainly advisable to do a good deal of water drinking during a fast—since this serves to flush out the whole system and wash through the accumulated impurities." He also states that water "carries along with it many impurities from the blood." Both Carrington and Macfadden advocate drinking more water than thirst calls for while fasting. Mr. Carrington advocates drinking water as a means of relieving morbid sensations in the stomach that may arise during the early part of a fast. Water-drinking for this purpose is the use of water as a palliative and not to serve any need of the body. Water taken in excess of need must be thrown out speedily lest the excess result in harm, and it does not occasion any increase in the elimination of toxins.

This is a mistake that the early *Hygienists*—Graham, Jennings, Trall, Alcott, etc.—did not make. They frowned upon much water drinking. The fact is that there is neither need for so much water, nor benefit from taking it. Drinking water as a mere matter of routine is not advisable. One may rely upon the instinct of thirst to tell him when he should drink and how much. Drink when thirsty. Do not drink when not thirsty.

Prof. Levanzin seems to have been a bit confused on this matter of water-drinking during a fast. He says that generally the faster desires "very limited quantities of water." He tells us that in 1911 he fasted five days without taking any water; that he suffered no discomfort, and that he busied himself with his usual occupations throughout this period. He also tells us that during his experimental fast undergone in Carnegie Institute he was compelled to take a quart of water a day, which was too much for him. In spite of all this he advocates much water drinking by fasters.

In this connection the following bit of information is both interesting and instructive. The *Popular Science Monthly*, 36:540, February 1890, carried the following, from Prof. M. Charles Richet, which appeared originally in the *Revue Scientifique* (edited by Richet) and quoted as part of a course on physiology at Faculty of Medicine, Paris: "Falck's dog went 61 days without drinking or eating. Starving dogs usually drink but little, as if warned by instinct not to drink more than they have to. Water, in fact, expedites the wasting of the tissues and accelerates the drain of the salts in the organism. Hence, by drinking, we excrete more chloride of sodium, phosphates, urea, etc., so that, although in general animals deprived of water do not live as long as those which can drink, there is some difference between those which can drink a little and those which drink a great deal. The last die sooner."

Any increased excretion of urea and sodium chloride that might result from the drinking of water should prove distinctly beneficial. If phosphorus and other minerals are lost in greater amounts when much water is taken, this should prove to be detrimental. If it is true, as he asserts, that fasting animals that drink large quantities of water die sooner than those that drink small amounts of water, this should be regarded as confirming our objection to drinking large quantities of water during this period. That dogs that are given no water while they fast die sooner than those who get moderate amounts of water, should come as no surprise. Although hibernating animals, æstivating animals, and the fasting fur seal bull do not drink while abstaining from food, most animals, fasting under ordinary conditions, do drink. In man thirst is present in and water is needed while fasting. If the faster does not take water, he tends to become seriously, even dangerously or fatally dehydrated.

Dewey, on the other hand, took a decided stand against water in the absence of thirst. Thirst, he said, should be the only guide to the amount of water to drink. He insisted on drinking only as much water as demanded by thirst and was convinced that much water drinking, except when indicated by thirst, is definitely harmful. During the first fourteen days of his second fast (taken in New York City) Tanner took no water and suffered no inconvenience. He became stronger when he took water and won a race with a young reporter who refused to believe that one could maintain one's strength while not eating. He tells us that after taking the water he "ran up-stairs like a boy."

Fasting animals take but little water and some of them none at all. For example, the Alaskan fur-seal bull takes no water throughout the whole of his three or four months fast. Hibernatnig and estivating animals do not drink water during their period of dormancy. It is the rule that sick animals (this is especially true of acutely sick and seriously wounded animals) will not drink much water. I have repeatedly seen sick animals take no water at all for days at a time, or take but a few sips once or twice a day. For the most part, they refuse to drink large amounts of water.

Thirst is seldom great during a fast. I have watched fasters go for two and three days at a time and take no water, simply because there was no demand for water, and they have not suffered as a consequence. Others take but little water; sometimes not more than half a glass a day. Then, there are those who drink much water. In some of these there may be thirst; in others it appears to be nothing more than a result of a desire to get something into the stomach. Others drink because they have been taught that they must. In occasional fasters, there will arise a great thirst that may last a day or two or three days, during which time they will drink so much water that their tissues become water-logged and they gain in weight as a result. The thirst subsides and they do not drink so much thereafter. Large quantities of water should be taken when thirst calls for much water, as it sometimes does; otherwise, there should be no effort made to take large amounts of water. Excesses of water are simply eliminated without increasing the elimination of waste—perhaps, on the contrary, with an actual decreased elimination of waste.

A frequent development while fasting is a dislike for water. This is particularly true if the water is "hard". "Hard water" that, while one is eating, tastes pleasant enough, is rejected by the sharpened sense of taste. In such cases we find the use of distilled water, to be satisfactory. The loss of weight when no water is taken is about three times as rapid as when water is taken—the loss averaging about three pounds a day instead of the usual pound a day. This is especially helpful in dropsical cases and greatly shortens the duration of the fast in fat individuals who are fasting merely for reduction of weight. Tanner found that he lost but one and a half pounds a day while abstaining from water. He took water after the fourteenth day and lost a little less than half a pound a day.

Writing in *This Week's Magazine,* which is a Sunday supplement of the *New York Tribune,* under the title *They Never Have to Drink,* Roy Chapman Andrews, Director of the American Museum of Natural History, tells us that "many desert animals, particularly rodents," never drink after they are weaned. He mentions the "desert-living mice, rats, hares, and ground squirrels," that "not only do not drink but few, if any, perspire." He tells of installing a group of live desert pocket mice in the museum that "live among the vast dunes of nearly white gypsum in New Mexico" and tells of these, that they were "fed a diet of thoroughly dried seeds. They thrived on this unappetizing food and would never touch water." Each time liquid was offered they filled the dishes with sand. He adds: "In the Gobi Desert we found that even the wild ass rarely, if ever, drinks. On one vast stretch of the Gobi where there was no water for hundreds of miles, except for a few deep Mongol wells, there were literally thousands of wild ass and gazelle."

He recounts some experiences of the Central Asiatic Expedition, while at Wolf Camp in the middle of the Gobi Desert. A Mongol brought in a young gazelle which they nursed on a bottle for a time, after which it was adopted by a she-goat. He tells us that "When old Nanny finally weaned Skippy (the gazelle), he lived on camel sage and the leaves of thorny bushes scattered in clumps over the desert. I was particularly interested to see whether Skippy would drink water. During the six months he was with us he never touched a drop. He would sniff at the pan from which the goat was drinking and then turn away without even moistening his lips." Then, as if he might have been thinking of the creed of the physicians and dairymen, that we are never to be weaned, he adds: "We never offered him milk after he was weaned but I feel sure that no liquid would have tempted him."

Mr. Andrews thinks that "this is one of the marvelous adaptations of nature." He adds: "The ability to exist without water appears to be peculiar to rodents and other herbivorous mammals. As far as I know, all flesh eaters must drink." It is, of course, true that all animals must have water. These desert animals obtain large quantities of carbohydrates from their vegetable fare and when these are broken down in the process of digestion, they yield enough water to supply their bodily needs, and, in the case of the nursing mammal, to supply enough extra water for milk production.

While man dissipates considerable water in sweating, he certainly does not have any need for the large quantities of water advised in many quarters for both fasters and those who are eating. Nor does the consumption of large quantities of water produce all the beneficial effects commonly claimed for the practice. Certainly nothing is to be gained from forced drinking or the practice of routine drinking. The taking of water for which there is no physiological demand, as expressed in thirst, is of no value. The practice may prove decidedly harmful.

Prof. Carlson says that "an adult man fasting can live fifteen to twenty days without water. If food is taken, death from water deprivation comes quicker. If there is body fever or great external heat leading to sweating, death from water deprivation is hastened. Foods require water for elimination of waste products." It is not definitely known how long a fasting man may live without water. A few criminals have died in a few days to seventeen days when they denied themselves both food and water. But there were emotional and nervous factors in all such cases that hastened death.

Our aim is not, of course, to determine how long a patient can go without water. The aim is to provide for the patient the best possible conditions under which to carry forward the healing processes and to complete these in as short time as possible. The death of a woman from dehydration in New York state in the early part of 1950 at the end of a thirty days fast, as a consequence of having gone for the whole period without water, is not only a lesson about the need for water, but also a warning to those who attempt a long fast without proper supervision. Had this woman been under experienced expert supervision, she would not have been permitted to make this grave mistake. When food is not taken the need for water is lessened and there is a corresponding lessening of thirst. Although it is asserted by many fasting advocates that drinking large quantities of water, despite lack of desire for it, increases elimination, I have seen no proof of this, while, my own experience fails to substantiate the assertion.

SEASONINGS FOR THE WATER

Due to the bad taste in the mouth while one is fasting, the water is likely to appear to taste badly. At other times patients complain of the water being too sweet. They frequently request permission to add salt or lemon juice or other substances to the water to flavor it. The evils of salt using were discussed in the chapter devoted to "Objections to the Fast." The use of lemon juice means that the patient is taking food, and although he takes but minute quantities of the juice, it is enough to interfere with the fasting process and is often enough to cause a return of hunger and thus makes the fast much more difficult, or compels its premature breaking. It is never wise to add anything to the water. For the bad taste in the mouth one needs only cleanliness. The teeth, tongue and mouth must be cleansed. The tongue should not be brushed before it has been examined each day.

COLD WATER

In the summer time patients are likely to demand ice-water to drink. Drinking very cold water is not a good practice under any circumstance; it is especially harmful during a fast. Indeed, giving very cold water to fasters seems to almost stop their progress. There can be no objection to giving them cool water to drink.

FEEDING INTERVALS

Tilden says: "A fast must not be continued when the patient is suffering greatly, it matters not in what way. °°°

"Some patients will start without food and within a week they are very sick—sick because of great enervation. They have been overstimulated so long that when the stimulating food is removed they soon evolve a severe prostration. Most intelligent people know how much the inebriate suffers when he is compelled to go through delirium tremens. Delirium tremens is the acme of prostration. People who are tremendously prostrated or enervated, from years of overstimulation from food, do not suffer just the same as the inebriate but they suffer, many of them, just as greatly. A good many will become very sick at the stomach and vomit almost unceasingly. This must be avoided. When such a patient starts on a fast, the physician must recognize the coming symptoms, and break the fast by giving a small amount of fruit. As soon as the symptoms of irritation have subsided, the fast will be resumed, until other symptoms indicate that the system is suffering too greatly from the effect of going without food, when a little fruit may be given for two or three days, and sometimes a week. The fast can then be resumed; but, as soon as the patient begins to show the appearance of suffering, and the haggard state begins to develop, feeding must be resumed."

He says that "little by little, such cases can be piloted into perfect health." I give Dr. Tilden's plan for what it is worth. It is my own plan not to break a fast while there is vomiting. I have broken fasts when there is great prostration and resumed the fast after strength has been recovered. The remedy for delirium tremens is not more whiskey. Just so the remedy for the great prostration caused by long-continued food drunkenness is not more food. If we would not give a dose of morphine to the morphine addict who suffers when deprived of his morphine, or the coffee addict a cup of coffee to "relieve" her headache, why should we give the food drunkard more food to relieve his suffering? With all due respect to Dr. Tilden, whose experience with fasting was very great, I do not find this plan essential or helpful, except in a very few cases.

Tilden also urges daily enemas and lavages. He says: "the bowels should be looked after from the day the fast is started until it is ended. A retention of excretions will poison and make the patient very sick, and there is a possibility of his becoming so prostrated from the effect of the poison absorbed that he will die. Nausea and vomiting following fasting are a very good indication that there is too much absorption taking place. Then the bowels must be moved by enemas, or whatever is proper to do, until they are thoroughly cleaned out." My experience does not bear this out. I have seen more vomiting and nausea in cases that received daily enemas than in those who have received no enemas at all. Nor have I seen prostration and death as a result of absorption of retained excretions. Indeed, it seems clear to me that absorption does not occur. Tilden also says: "But fasting must not be continued if the patient begins to present a haggard appearance or if nausea and efforts at vomiting develop. When a patient under a fast begins to show a depressed state and haggard look and the tissues begin to droop down, and a decided discomfort begins to manifest, feeding must be resumed and the patient must be brought back to a reasonable state of comfort. Then fasting can be resumed; or if it is not thought best to go without food entirely, then the patient may be put on a small amount of fruit for a week or more. It requires a great deal of skill to assist nature back to a normal state when the health has been outraged almost to the point of dissolution. Fasting is not a remedy that should be trusted in the hands of laymen, nor in the hands of ignorant professional men. Putting such a remedy as fasting into the hands of laymen, to be applied to sick people, is equivalent to putting an insane man to work in a barber shop, especially if the barber's hallucinations are on the order of homicidal mania." We are not convinced that laymen cannot make excellent use of fasting in minor troubles and the less advanced pathologies; but we are sure that Tilden's warning should be heeded by those who suffer with advanced stages of pathology.

THE ENEMA DURING THE FAST

Dr. Hazzard, Mr. Carrington, Mr. Sinclair and others, regard the enema as almost indispensable during the fast. This arises out of a distrust of the body's powers of self-adjustment. There is no more need for, nor benefit to be derived from the enema during the fast than at other times. What is more, if no enema is used, normal bowel action will be established much sooner after the fast than if the enema is employed. Levanzin, who often advocated the frequent use of the enema during the fast, says that he uses the enema only when he desires to get faster results. If the enema really gives faster results, there would seem to be no reason, at least in the great majority of cases, why it should not be used in every fast. But *Hygienists* dispute that it gives faster results. We are convinced, on the contrary, that it retards recovery and impairs bowel function. Mr. Carrington voices the same view in these words: "we can readily see that frequent flushing of the bowels—say once a day—will materially assist a return to health, and effectively shorten the fast. It is a most important hygienic auxiliary to the main treatment; and, though so essential, Dr. Dewey hardly mentions the enema in any of his books; but its omission seems to me a very great fault, since we can see that its use will both shorten and lighten the period of fasting." This is an *a priori* conclusion that is not borne out by actual test and experience. It is based on the mistaken assumption that bowel action is elimination, and the added assumption that poisons are absorbed from the colon. Dr. Hazzard, who should have known better, was so possessed with her fear of auto-intoxication from the re-absorption of waste from the colon that she conjured up such symptoms resulting therefrom as mild delirium, stupor, hiccoughs, etc. The fact is, as all may know who have given both plans a thorough test, that the enema neither shortens the fast nor makes it more comfortable.

While connected with the Macfadden Publications, I once had a controversy with a member of the staff of *Physical Culture* over a statement in an article of mine dealing with fasting, to the effect that no enema should be used after the fast, but that one may safely wait a week or more for a spontaneous movement. He said: "Surely steps must be taken to move the bowels at least once a day under any circumstances. If the movement is held up for several days or a week, or fourteen days, so much poison is produced in the organism that the advantage of the fast is counteracted and all its benefits lost. °°° It seems to me that the failure of the bowels to move for a week or more would be almost fatal. It certainly would lead to all sorts of complications dangerous to health." These words voice the prevailing view of the matter, yet this view is wholly false. The fact that patients have gone for over thirty days without a bowel movement and have developed no complications, but have grown steadily better during these periods, proves positively that "failure of the bowels to move for a week or more" is not "almost fatal." One does not lose the slightest bit of the benefits of fasting nor does one develop "all sorts of complications dangerous to health." This is equally true when we wait upon the bowels after the fast is broken. The enema should not be employed when eating is resumed.

Dr. Hazzard claimed the dubious credit of having introduced the enema practice into the procedure of fasting. Dewey rejected the enema up to the time of his death. Dr. Tanner also rejected it. So did Jennings and Page, Dr. Claunch did not employ it. I have not employed it for over thirty-seven years and find this more satisfactory than its use. Dr. Page observed: "Tanner had no movement during his fast; Griscomb's experience was similar, and Connolly, the consumptive, who fasted for forty-three days, had no movement for three weeks, and then the temporary looseness was occasioned by profuse water drinking, which in his case, proved curative"—*The Natural Cure*, p. 112.

It is rare that the colon ever fully empties itself of the water ingested. Carrington says of the retained water, that, since it is perfectly harmless, and will be absorbed and eliminated by the system in exactly the same manner as water that is drunk is eliminated, no alarm should be felt over its retention. But one case I observed that retained water for twenty-four hours did not absorb it and eliminate it through the skin and kidneys. On the other hand, if the fear of toxic absorption from the colon is based on fact, such absorption of water would certainly result in far greater absorption of toxins than could ever occur without the water. Carrington mentions cases in which there was considerable difficulty in expelling the water (enema) and says that "retention beyond even a few minutes is impossible." In this connection, he is mistaken. Retention for considerable periods, even twenty-four hours, is possible, and we see it often.

Prof. Levanzin says that when enemas are not used during the fast, a "plug of hard feces is formed in the rectum, and another one at the duodenum (upper part of the bowels) is formed by the newly ingested food. The intestines are empty and full of air." To avoid the rectal plug, he advises the enema. The rectal plug is a myth. Were there an upper-bowel plug, the enema would never reach it.

Although a strong advocate of the use of the enema in the fast, Mr. Macfadden says: "enemas are somewhat enervating, and when the patient is already weak, he may find it a drain upon his vitality to take these"—*Encyclopedia of Physical Culture*, Vol. III, p. 1374. It does not seem to me necessary to resort to enervating practices in our conduct of the fast and for more than thirty-seven years I have refrained from the use of the enema. The enema is at all times a drain upon the patient's powers and its use during the fast not only weakens the patient and thus prolongs his illness, but it impairs his colon and he is often weeks and months getting over the effects. The employment of laxatives, as advocated and practiced by some, has the same weakening and debilitating effects upon the colon and they exert their irritating influence upon the stomach and small intestine, also.

Major Austin conducted an experiment upon himself to determine the relative values of the enema and purgation during the fast. He fasted for sixteen days taking nothing but water and half-an-ounce to an ounce of epsom salts every morning. He was energetic and carried out his ordinary duties, even engaging in and winning a walking match of two miles, most of the distance uphill, on the sixteenth day. He felt a little faint and giddy in the mornings upon arising and had the same sensations at times during the day upon arising after he had been sitting for some time. Some months after this fast he underwent a second fast of ten days, taking nothing but water and employing a three-pint enema of water each morning instead of the saline purge. He again carried out his regular duties, as before, but had less energy, his tongue was more heavily coated and he did not sleep as well as during the previous fast.

Some weeks later he took a third fast, this one also ten days long. He again used the saline purge each morning instead of the enema. His experience during the third fast was the same as that during the first. He says: "Thus I proved to my own satisfaction, that the use of saline purgatives during a fast makes the ordeal a very much less trying one than is the case when only the enema is used." He advocates as do others (Dr. Wm. H. Hay, for example, in this country), the use of both the enema and the purge and also advocates drinking large quantities of water.

I realize that the foregoing experiment is not sufficient to establish Major Austin's contention; that the experiment would have to be repeated many times on many patients with uniform results, to prove what he claims to have proven. I have repeatedly seen the same excellent results, that he records for his fast during which the purge was employed, in patients who received neither purge nor enema. Patients who have previously fasted under the care of others and who were purged during the fast, have described to me their experiences during this time and often they have had more discomfort and weakness than Major Austin had during his second fast when he employed the enema. Individual actions vary so much during the fast and in the same individual at different times, that the apparent "effects" of purging and the use of the enema in one case cannot prove anything. Let those who perform these experiments now conduct an extensive series of experiments without the use of either enema or purge. I know the evils of the enema as well as those of the purge. I know that the enema does not reach the small intestine, as the purge does. If we grant the need for either, the purge may be preferable, but I do not grant their need.

Major Austin says: "I may here explain that during a fast waste products and toxins are being continually deposited in the stomach and intestines, and unless these are washed away by large drinks of water and enemas or a saline purge, some of the morbid material is re-absorbed; this causes auto-intoxication and its attendant discomforts, weakness, headaches, etc." It has never been explained how the re-absorption of a small amount of the large amounts of toxins thrown out will cause symptoms that the whole amount of the toxins failed to produce before they were eliminated. Re-absorption is assumed and symptoms are arbitrarily referred to this. I agree that if re-absorption occurs, it would occur in the intestine and not in the colon and the waste matter could easily be reached by a purge and not by the enema. But does re-absorption actually occur? If so, why does it occur?

I suggest that the practice of drinking large quantities of water, to "wash away" toxins to "flush the system," may cause re-absorption of toxins. The water is absorbed. It does not pass out through the colon; but through the lungs, skin and kidneys. It will "pick up" and hold in solution, the waste and toxic matter in the stomach and intestine (it does not reach the colon) and it doubtless carries some of this into the body with it when it is absorbed. Drinking only when nature demands water and only so much as she demands will reduce this absorption to a minimum. Until my plan is thoroughly tested all argument to the contrary is wasted words.

Major Austin advises cold abdominal packs and cold sitz-baths to "tone up and improve the condition of the colon, which is left in a more or less flabby state after the warm-water wash-outs."

Reverse peristalsis, starting in the middle portion of the transverse colon and passing backward to the cecum, first noted by Prof. Cannon and now known to be constant in both man and animals, is normally confined to the colon; but in constipation, particularly in colitis, with spastic contraction of the descending colon, these reverse peristaltic movements are greatly exaggerated and when the ileocecal valve is incompetent, these reverse movements push the contents of the cecum into the small intestine. Water, feces, toxins, waste matter—the whole foul collection—may be forced into the intestine and from here be absorbed and poison the body.

The daily enemas and the purges and laxatives employed by many during the fast, undoubtedly contribute to the nervous depletion against which they often warn us. The fast certainly does not. The claim is made that fasting patients recover more quickly from their ailments if they are given enemas than if their bowels are left to their own resources. This claim is not made by those who have thoroughly tested both methods. For five years I employed the enema in all fasting cases, giving from one to two and occasionally three enemas a day. For thirty-seven years I have left the colon alone. If anything, patients who do not have the enema make the quickest recoveries and it is certain that their bowel function is a hundred per cent more efficient after the fast, if the colon has been permitted to attend to its own function in its own way.

Mr. Pearson, who thinks "enemas comprise 60 per cent of the treatment in fasting" and who, himself, took as many as three to four enemas a day during his own fasts, says: "The large quantity of water introduced into the bowels will cause a rapid infusion of the toxic poisons from the bowels to the surrounding tissues, thus inducing headaches" and that "it is advisable to use an antiseptic in the water to reduce these poisonous substances as far as possible." He says he "probably took two to four teaspoonfuls a day" of baking soda, "for about five years in enemas." With Pearson, as with Hazzard and Sinclair, the enema is a fetish. Dr. Hazzard, Mr. Pearson and others advise the use of two, or three and more enemas a day. Fasting animals do not employ enemas nor anything that may be regarded as serving the same purpose. Fasting seals and salmon, hibernating bears and snakes, fasting sick and wounded animals, regardless of the lengths of their fasts, employ no measures to force bowel action. Since this thing has been tried out on the plane of instinct for unnumbered thousands of years, and has been approved by nature, we need have no fear of fasting without the employment of enemas.

THE GASTRIC LAVAGE DURING THE FAST

Certain advocates of fasting employ the lavage as a routine practice. Dr. Tilden formerly employed it as a daily measure. This proved to be too great a tax upon his patients so he reduced its use to three times a week. From my own experience with the measure, I consider even this too great a tax upon the energies of the patient. Others employ the lavage only when there is actual nausea and gastric distress. They wash out the stomach to relieve the faster of discomfort. This measure often brings considerable relief, but at a big price. The insertion of the stomach tube is a severe enough tax on most patients. Pouring a gallon or more of water, with or without soda or other drug, into the stomach, also taxes them. The retching and vomiting occasioned by this procedure leaves the patient weak and nervous for hours. The relief afforded by the lavage is short-lived and the cost in nerve force is too great to justify it.

Many who employ the fast have the patient drink large quantities of water and then induce vomiting, where vomiting does not occur from the use of water alone. I do not employ and do not approve of forcing measures. Vomiting can and does occur when a real need for it exists without resorting to forcing measures. Nausea and gastric distress are most often due to lowered gastric tone and there is, in such cases, nothing to be expelled.

FALSE TEETH

Fasters who have false teeth should keep their teeth in during the fast and should bite on them sufficiently often to keep the gums tough. The gums will shrink somewhat in the general loss of weight so that the plates will not fit after the fast, until the gums have filled out again. This makes chewing, especially of uncooked foods, rather difficult, unless the gums have been kept tough.

FORCING MEASURES

The lingering faith in forcing measures is a hold-over from the time we still had faith in the drugs of the physician. When we lost our faith in his poisons, we adopted a heterogeneous array of drugless measures that are intended to force the body to do what we, in our almost infallible wisdom, think it should do under the circumstances. Hence, we find many advocates of fasting employing in conjunction with it, many measures that are intended to force the body to disgorge.

The one great "need" that is so frequently stressed is that of increased elimination. For example, Prof. Levanzin says that "it is important to remember that all avenues of elimination should be constantly open during a long fast—that the system may have a chance to cleanse and invigorate itself by throwing out a mass of impurities. Enemas, deep breathing exercises, frequent baths, proper water-drinking, etc.—all these are essential and greatly assist in the cleansing of the organism and the shortening of the fast." He advocated the use of the Turkish bath while fasting because of the mistaken assumption that sweating, thus induced, constitutes an eliminating process.

Dr. Hazzard had the thought that in "organic disease of more than ordinary degree," it is "virtually certain that the avenues of elimination will prove inadequate to exacted demands" in a long fast. The thought is inherent in this statement that fasting over-burdens the eliminating organs, if they are weak. Yet she says that "autointoxication takes place more often when feeding than when fasting." The chief fault I find with Mr. Carrington's monumental work on fasting is the fact that he strongly urges forcing measures—enemas, sweatings, excessive water-drinking, exercise, hydrotherapy, etc. He thinks that by the use of these forcing measures the fast may be shortened and recovery may be effected in cases in which it may otherwise be impossible. His insistence upon exercise while fasting is based on the thought that exercise stimulates the excretory organs. He thinks that those who take more exercise while fasting will be able to totally eliminate bodily impurities more rapidly. This was also Macfadden's view. Carrington said that those who exercise most will terminate their fast soonest. I would say that they will be forced to terminate their fast soonest, and often pre-maturely, because of the more rapid exhaustion of their reserves.

All of these forcing measures are not only unnecessary and futile, but they constitute a heavy drain upon the energies and substances of the fasting organism. All forms of stimulation are enervating and the more they are used the more enervation they produce. The activities of the organs of elimination are in keeping with the amount of functional energy with which they are supplied and all efforts to keep them "constantly active" in spite of a lack of energy, only renders them less able to act. For, everything that we appear to gain in the increased activity occasioned by the forcing measures, we lose in the inevitable reaction. Every new source of enervation becomes an actual check to elimination. Our efforts should all be directed to the end of conserving the energies and reserves of the patient in every possible way, and not to dissipating them as rapidly as possible. Rest, quiet, poise, warmth—these are far more important than any method of treatment ever devised.

Mr. Carrington, himself, in dealing with drug stimulants, urged the necessity of refraining from them and pointed out that the weaker the organism, the greater the necessity of doing nothing. It is strange that he should abandon this principle in dealing with the drugless stimulants. These various drugless stimulants may be as wasteful of the body's energies as drugs. The sweat bath, the hot bath, the cold bath, the alternate hot and cold bath, the salt rub, massage, etc., are all very wasteful of the patient's precious energies. The same is true of the enema and the gastric lavage. The reader is well aware that I do not approve of the chaotic mass of nonsense that is called drugless medicine. The methods of treatment employed by drugless practitioners are especially to be avoided during the fast. I could hardly do better at this place than to quote the following from Purinton: "The Conquest Fast doesn't harmonize with the Kneipp Water Cure, or the Macfadden School of Physical Culture, or any other regime that demands large expenditure of energy and vitality. These methods may be ever so good—they are not timely.

"I knew a man that had chronic rheumatism. He consulted a fasting specialist, and stopped eating, began to feel better, wondered if he couldn't be improving faster—consulted a Turkish bath specialist; and began bathing. Presently he died. Then each specialist declared the other had killed the patient." The fasting individual should conserve his or her energies and not permit them to be dissipated by depleting—stimulating and depressing—treatments. Too often fasting has been held responsible for the results of the blitzguss, frequent massage, spinal manipulation and other forms of drugless hocus pocus. The actions of the body in relation to drugs are more prompt and vigorous when fasting than when eating. Due to this fact, fasting usually compels one to abandon his accustomed drug habits. The nervous system of the faster becomes more acute and also relatively larger than when eating. For these reasons the resistance to drugs is more prompt and vigorous. It is always more dangerous to use drugs when fasting than at other times. Drugs are bad at all times; the faster especially should avoid them.

Breaking the Fast

CHAPTER XXX

An important fact that needs emphasis is that fasting is a very much more complicated process than is commonly supposed, even by its advocates. There is much more involved in the process than merely going without food. There is an art of fasting, but, if this art is to be properly executed, it must be based on the science of fasting. Its uses seem, at times, to be almost unlimited, its inconveniences are not great, its dangers are few and rarely seen, but for the most satisfactory results, it must be conducted by one skilled in its application. It is too vital and too important to be carried out indifferently. It is not a process that should be left to the guidance of those who have but limited knowledge of its proper conduct and who have had no experience in conducting fasts. Breaking the fast is one of the most important elements of the fast.

It is possible to break a fast on any food that is available—bread, flesh, eggs, nuts, etc.—providing a few simple precautions are observed. Animals follow none of our routines in breaking their fasts. They eat whatever is at hand and do not regularly stint themselves at their first meal. From this, it may be thought that we are unduly cautious, but I do not think so. Not only are there differences between what the animal does and what the average patient tends to do, if turned loose, but there seems to be great differences in digestive power, in favor of the animal. There is also the possibility that the animal would preserve more of the benefits of the fast if it broke the fast more carefully.

We do not employ the foods previously mentioned in breaking a fast for the reason that better means of breaking the fast are available to us. At the end of a long fast digestive secretions are not abundant and small meals or small amounts of food are advisable. The amount of food fed to the patient is increased as secretion becomes more abundant. When this rule is observed, there is little difficulty in breaking a fast and no danger in doing so.

The proper conduct of the fast is vitally important. There are really very few practitioners of any school who know how to con-

duct a fast or how to properly break one. A naturopath in New York
City broke the fasts of a mother and a daughter, who had been fasting
sixteen and thirteen days respectively, on chocolate candy. The
gastric and intestinal acidity resulting from this caused great distress
throughout the body. I was called in on these cases, and it required
four to five days of fasting to get them back into a comfortable condition. This method of breaking a fast is nothing short of criminal.

A friend of my wife describes to me how she fasted seventeen
days under the direction of a chiropractor in California and worked
hard during the fast. She worked for the chiropractor and he would
not permit her leave from work while fasting. He broke her fast
with toast and acid fruit. This woman immediately developed a
case of malnutritional edema. This is one of the few cases of this
kind I have ever known to follow a fast.

This case should thoroughly emphasize the necessity of placing
one's self under the care of a competent and experienced man, if one
is to take a long fast. A chiropractor who knows nothing of either
fasting or dietetics, and few of them know anything of either of
these, and who experiments with patients in this manner, cannot be
too strongly condemned. If chiropractors want to practice *Hygienic*
methods let them qualify themselves for this by proper training. This
goes also for osteopaths and medical men. I would not attempt a
surgical operation without first qualifying myself for the work, and I
am certain that no chiropractor, osteopath or medical man should attempt a long fast, or attempt to employ any other *Hygienic* method,
without first equipping himself for the work. Chiropractors who go
to school and learn to punch spines and then, finding spine punching
to be inefficacious, attempt to prescribe diet, etc., after reading a
book or two on these methods, are in the same position as would be
the medical man who attempted to "adjust" spines after reading a
book on chiropractic. He is really dishonest and untrustworthy.

Dr. Wm. F. Harvard records the following cases: "A young man
twenty-four years of age who had suffered from chronic constipation
and indigestion, fasted twenty-seven days after reading an article in
a popular health publication. On the twenty-eighth day he ate a
meal of beefsteak, potatoes, bread and butter and coffee. He was
seized with violent vomiting spells and could not tolerate even a
teaspoonful of water on the stomach. When called on the case I
discovered an intense soreness of the entire abdomen and every

indication of acute gastritis." "A young man about thirty who had fasted on his own initiative for forty-two days attempted to break the fast on coarse bread with the result that vomiting occurred and the stomach became so irritable that nothing could be retained. There was marked emaciation and extreme weakness and every indication for immediate nourishment."

An Associated Press dispatch dated Aug. 28, (1929) recounts the death of Chris. Solberg, 40 year old art model, following a 31 days fast, which he broke by "consuming several sandwiches." The sandwiches, a later report said, contained beef. Ignorance and lack of self-control killed this man. The dispatch tells us that "his fast (of 31 days) had reduced him from 160 to 85 pounds," or an average loss of more than two pounds a day. This loss I believe to be impossible. The average losses for a fast of such length vary between twenty-five pounds and thirty-six pounds.

"Prof." Arnold Ehret tells of seeing two cases killed by injudicious breaking of the fast. He says: "A one-sided, meat-eater, suffering from diabetes broke his fast which lasted about a week by eating dates and died from the effects. A man of over sixty years of age fasted twenty-eight days (too long); his first meal of vegetarian foods consisting mainly of boiled potatoes."

Ignoring the absurd explanation for these deaths, given by the "professor," we would say that the diabetic patient threw too much sugar (from the dates) into his body and died as a result of hyperglycemia. He probably passed out in a diabetic coma. He explains that the second patient fasted too long for a man of his age, and that an "operation showed that the potatoes were kept in contracted intestines by thick, sticky mucus so strong that a piece had to be cut off and the patient died shortly after the operation." "Professor" Ehret was so fond of mucus he could never see anything else. This fast was badly broken but the patient, in all likelihood, would have lived had he not been operated on. The fast was not too long for a man of that age. "Prof." Ehret really knew but little of either fasting or dietetics.

These cases help to influence many against fasting and yet they are the results of the worst type of ignorance and inexperience. Who but an ignoramus would feed a diabetic case a meal of dates after a week of fasting? Surely fasting cannot be blamed for this result. Before we talk of the evils and dangers of fasting let us be sure that these really belong to fasting and not to something else.

Sinclair says: "I know another man who broke his fast on a hamburger steak, and this is also not to be recommended." I had one patient to break a fast of over twenty days by eating a pound and a half of nuts the first day. Although no harm, not even slight discomfort, came from it in this particular case, this method of breaking a fast is certainly not to be recommended generally.

In some cases of fasting where efforts are made to feed the patient towards the latter end of a prolonged fast, but before hunger has returned, there has been noted a failure of the stomach to function. Dr. Dewey mentions such cases, who were induced by friends or physicians to eat, and who were absolutely unable to digest food, but vomited everything eaten. Fasting was resumed and continued until the return of natural hunger, with the result that digestion proceeded nicely.

WHEN TO BREAK THE FAST

Early *Hygienists* said: When your tongue is clean, your rest peaceful, your skin clear, your eyes bright, there is no more pain, and you are very sharply hungry you may select from the store of wholesome articles of food described in works of *Hygiene,* that which pleases you, and eat with moderation. That is sound advice, but hardly detailed enough. The usual indications for breaking the fast (these help to determine the dividing line between fasting and starving), are as follow:

Hunger invariably returns.

The *Breath,* which during all or most of the fast has been offensive, becomes sweet and clean.

The *Tongue* becomes clean. The thick coating which remained on it throughout most of the fast vanishes.

The *Temperature,* which may have been sub-normal or above normal, returns to exactly normal, where it remains.

The *Pulse* becomes normal in time and rhythm.

The *Skin* reactions and other reactions become normal.

The *Bad Taste* in the mouth ceases.

Salivary Secretion becomes normal.

The *Eyes* become bright and *eye sight improves.*

The *Excreta* loses its odor. The *Urine* becomes light.

Besides the usual signs that it is time to break the fast, Prof. Levanzin lists a feeling of cheer and elation as a manifestation that the time has arrived for the termination of the fast. I cannot do better than quote Carrington's description of the feelings of the patient at this stage. He says, *Vitality, Fasting and Nutrition,* p. 544: "A sudden and complete rejuvenation; a feeling of lightness, and good health steals over the patient in an irresistable wave; bringing contentment and a general feeling of well-being, and of the possession of a superabundance of animal spirits." Circulation improves, as is seen by the resumption of the normal pinkness under the fingernails. The increased rapidity with which the blood flows back into the skin, when this has been forced out by pressure, is another indication of the rejuvenating effect of the finish fast.

The primary indication that the fast is to be broken is the return of hunger; all the other indications which I have enumerated are secondary. Often one or more of these secondary signs are absent when hunger returns, but one should not refrain from breaking the fast when there is an unmistakable demand for food, merely because the tongue, for example, is not clean. Inasmuch as all the signs do not invariably appear in each case, do not hesitate to break the fast when hunger returns. In general I agree with Carrington that "natural hunger, and that alone should indicate the terminus of the fast; when the fast is ready to be broken. °°° The artificial breaking of the fast; the taking of food in the absence of real hunger, for the reason that the ignorant attendant thinks the patient has 'fasted long enough,' is an abomination, and an outrage upon the system which cannot be too strongly deprecated." Most fasts are broken too soon; that is, before the work of renovation is completed.

HOW TO BREAK A FAST

The care that must be exercised in breaking a fast is in proportion to the length of the fast and to the general condition of the fasting individual. The approved plan is to break the fast on liquid food, using for this purpose fruit juice or tomato juice or watermelon juice or vegetable broths. Fruit juice—usually orange juice—is used most often.

Orange juice, grapefruit juice or fresh tomato juice are excellent with which to break a fast. Watermelon juice or the juice of the fresh pineapple or of fresh grapes may also be used. A half a glass may be given at the start. After an hour, another half glass may be given. Juice may be given every hour the first day. The second day a whole glass of juice every two hours may be employed. On the third and fourth days give the whole orange or grapefruit and on the fifth day other foods may be added. Large meals should not be attempted in less than a week. These instructions are for the long fast. A short fast requires less care in breaking. In breaking a short fast I commonly give a whole glass of juice every two hours the first day and three fruit meals the second day. I would emphasize that the routines I employ are not sacred. Other routines will prove equally satisfactory. Dr. Lindlahr used to break fasts with a handful of popcorn.

Almost any food may be employed in breaking a fast, although greater care must be exercised if the concentrated types of food are employed for this purpose. There are individual factors that must receive attention. Sinclair tells of breaking a fast on a large, thoroughly ripe Japanese persimmon, and says that "it doubled me up with the most alarming cramps." A friend of his had the same experience from the juice of an orange; "but he was a man with whom acid fruits had always disagreed." The tendency of the long fast is to remove these digestive shortcomings, but it is not always completely successful, and this is especially so where the fast has not been carried to completion.

FALLACIES ABOUT BREAKING FASTS

A few fallacies about breaking a fast deserve attention. Dr. Kritzer says: "In breaking a long fast it is wise to consult the patient's wishes as to the particular food desired for the first meal. Any food wished for should be granted—even if it is meat, ice cream, chocolate or any other food outside of the fruit and vegetable kingdom.

"In this instance the patient's appetite is fully reliable and the food thus craved may supply an essential need. Should such a request be denied, the patient's improvement may be retarded."

It is true that a long fast tends to restore taste and food desires to a more healthful condition and render them more reliable; but many patients crave the foods they have previously been in the habit of consuming. These reversions to the old habit-cravings are distinctly not to be respected on any specious notion that the foods "craved" supply some essential need. It is a common experience to see a faster crave, at the end of a fast, the foods he has always eaten. Fed differently and given a second fast, he craves at the end of the second fast, the foods he had following the first fast.

There are no food elements in chocolate that cannot be supplied by other foods and one would be foolish to permit his patient to return to his disease building diet. I saw two fasts broken on chocolate and I don't care to see it done again; neither do I care to see a fast broken on ice cream.

If we assume that the "patient's appetite is fully reliable after a long fast," there is no reason why we should limit the satisfaction of his desires to the first meal. We may permit him to follow the lead of his appetite at every meal and have all the chocolate and ice cream he desires. Not only should we permit him to have the food his appetite calls for, but, we should also permit him to have as much as his appetite calls for. Yet we all know that this cannot be done. A man breaks a long fast on bread and meat sandwiches and is dead in twenty-four hours. His appetite simply was not reliable.

In breaking a fast it is always wiser to play safe and use tried and tested methods and follow this up wtih an adequate diet and not go off after wild theories and funny notions.

Dr. Kritzer also says: "It is best to break a fast at five o'clock in the afternoon, thus the patient has an opportunity of thoroughly digesting his meal before retiring. It also affords the digestive organs a considerable rest between the first and second meals."

There is no time of day that is best for breaking a fast. There is no reason why the meal should be thoroughly digested before retiring. If the fast is properly broken, there will be no need for twelve to fourteen hours of rest for the stomach, between the first meal and the second meal. The second glass of orange juice may be given one hour after the first, instead of a day later. I would not hesitates to break a fast at midnight or at any time upon the return of hunger. If the fast is broken before the return of hunger, it may be broken at any hour during the day. Ritualistic feeding following the fast, is no more necessary than at other times. Let us employ our intelligence.

HUNGER AFTER THE FAST

My experience agrees well with that of Carrington, who says that after a long fast the faster is ravenous and "eating must be kept under control at all costs for the few days during which it lasts." He adds that after the first few days, if controlled, "the extreme" voraciousness will disappear and "will not return." He refers to this period as the "danger period," and says that, once it has passed, there is no longer the *desire* "for the great *bulk* of food which previously existed." He points out that there is also the absence of the pre-fasting "craving" for "hot, or spicy, or stimulating viands."

This agrees well with my own experiences and observations. The period of hunger that follows a long fast lasts two weeks and more. The patient continually complains that he is not getting enough to eat. He will gain in strength and weight, he will feel good in general, but there will be that persistent demand for more food. It is not wise to try to satisfy this demand; to do so will invariably lead to overeating and often to trouble. The demand for food will be satisfied by moderate eating in two weeks or less in most cases, after which the patient will no longer be troubled by the persistent hunger. Patients who refuse to control their eating during this period, but who eat on the sly and fill up to their belly's content, commonly put on weight very rapidly, the face and other parts of the body becoming puffy, indicating a water-logged condition, and, in all cases, they undo much of the benefits they derived from the period of abstinence.

The secret of the past popularity of the milk diet seems to lie here. Patients were given a fast and then put on a milk diet. They were given milk at half hour intervals all through the day and, while this over-feeding on milk destroyed much of the benefits of the fast, it satisfied the hunger of the person who had just ended a long fast. The patients put on weight in a hurry, although it was more water than flesh they accumulated, and the weight would not hold up under working conditions. The diet was a psychological success and caused the doctors who employed it less trouble than they experienced in trying to feed their patients rationally.

Professor Russel H. Chittenden confirms the view that the fast destroys the "craving" for abnormal substances and large quantities of foods. He says: "In the latter part of September, 1903, Doctor Underhill attempted to return to his original mode of living, but found difficulty in consuming the daily quantities of food he had formerly been in the habit of eating."—*Physiological Economy in*

Nutrition, p. 78. Dr. Underhill had not been on a fast, but had been on a controlled diet for a prolonged period.

Dr. Chas. E. Page says: "Accustomed to distention from the bulky character of the old diet, if only a physiological ration of the pure and more nutritious food be swallowed, the stomach misses the stimulus of distention; time will be required (in some cases) for the stomach to remodel itself as regards size—unless a large proportion of fruit is used in conjunction with the cereals." After the preliminary period of persistent hunger has been successfully passed, the stomach seems to rest content with less food. If the patient will control himself during this period, all will be well thereafter.

OVEREATING AFTER THE FAST

The persistent and unusual hunger that immediately succeeds a fast of considerable duration often if not guarded against results in supplying a greater abundance of food than necessity requires. If the unself-disciplined individual is turned loose after a fast and not controlled, he is sure to undo much or all of the benefit he gained from the fast. At this stage he is in urgent need of firm supervision.

The most difficult patients to handle after the fast are those who are anxious to gain weight in a hurry. Gaining weight often becomes an obsession with these patients. They demand great quantities of food, worry because they are not gaining faster, rapidly develop into gluttons, and defeat their own ends by their over-eating, worry and tension. There is a tendency on the part of the faster to overeat, not alone because he is hungry, but also because he is desirous of regaining his weight. His friends also urge him to eat. Sinclair truly says: "A person at the end of a (long) fast is an agitating sight to his neighbors, and their one impulse is to get a 'square meal' into him as quickly as possible."

FOOD AFTER THE FAST

When the fast is broken and eating is resumed, there is not only the need to meet the daily needs for nutriment, but also the need to replenish the body's exhausted reserve stores. This is to say, in addition to meeting the daily expenditures consequent upon the daily activities of life, the body also seeks to set aside another reserve stock in anticipation of a subsequent period of nutritive stringency. For this reason, the demand for food is commonly greater than what may be regarded as normal, at least for a short period following the fast. This is a period when unusual care should be exercised in the choice of foods, as, in laying up new reserves stores, it is essential that they be adequate, not alone in quantity, but also in quality, to meet any subsequent period of abstinence with all flags flying. In spite of the faulty diet of the American people, our nutritive reserves are commonly much more adequate in quality than we should expect.

After a fast the diet should be of the very best from the standpoint of its nutritive qualities. No canned and bottled juices should be used in breaking the fast. Only fresh fruits and fresh vegetables should be used. If any dried foods are to be employed in the diet, only sun-dried foods should be used. Certainly every food employed should have its full content of vitamins and minerals. Canned foods, sulphured fruits, denatured foods of all kinds, over-cooked foods, and foods that have been hashed or mangled, so that they have sustained vital losses through oxidation, are not to be considered. The loss of minerals and vitamins cannot possibly be compensated by the use of vitamin pills of whatever nature nor by the use of mineral preparations from any source. These things must be obtained from natural foods.

There is greater need for protein after a long fast than for carbohydrates. As the fasting individual who has had a long fast will build tissue rapidly, he will require more protein than that contained in a maintenance diet. High grade proteins will be required and these should be as fresh and wholesome as the market affords. It should hardly be necessary to add that the full portion of protein daily cannot be started from the first day the fast is broken. Caution must be observed in breaking an extended fast and the patient brought gradually from the fast to full meals.

Gaining Weight After the Fast

CHAPTER XXXI

The gain in weight after a fast is usually very rapid. Often it is almost as rapid as the loss during the fast. People that were formerly always underweight and emaciated, due to impaired digestion and assimilation, will become normal in weight. Nervous patients and those who have long been emaciated often gain very slowly. As there are a number of factors which determine the rate of weight-loss so there are a number of factors which determine the rate of weight-gain. We cannot close our eyes to the complexity of the problem. The increased ability of the cells to take up and appropriate nutrient materials that is always seen to result from fasting is a factor in determining the gain in weight that follows the fast. More gain on less food is the rule.

Both Morgulis and von Seeland confirmed, experimentally, in their animals a fact that has been repeatedly emphasized by the advocates of fasting, that thin people, while they lose weight on a fast, tend to regain more weight after the fast than they lose during the fast, so that the ultimate result is a gain of weight. We note this in patients who previously were unable to gain on any type of diet. There are only occasional exceptions to this rule. It is as though the renovation which the fasting organism undergoes not only creates a food hunger, but also increases the ability to digest and assimilate food, for we often see gains, sometimes surprisingly rapid ones, on a diet that the average person would lose weight on. The ability to utilize food is certainly increased. It is certain that in the thin people we care for in this country, not one in a thousand of them is thin for lack of food; commonly they are "eating their heads off." They are underweight because they do not digest and assimilate what they eat. The organic corrections that occur during a fast change all this.

Studying the liver cells of a fasting salamander, Morgulis found that after four days of feeding, both cells and nuclei had gained 34 and 31 per cent respectively. In another four days, eight days in all, the cell body had increased 143 per cent. After only fourteen days of feeding, the liver nuclei had reached normal size although the cells were still under sized. The epithelial cells lining the duodenum increased even more rapidly than did the liver cells. Their bodies and nuclei increasing 45 and 24 per cent respectively in the first four days of feeding. He says "the same holds true for the regeneration of the pancreatic cells except for minor details of the process." These gains were seen after long months without food, during which time the body as a whole lost 50 per cent. The liver cells, being food reservoirs, lost 52 per cent the first month, 74 per cent in two months and 80 to 85 per cent in three months.

Morgulis says: "the recuperation of the cells is shown when the animals are nourished again after having fasted three and a half months. The regeneration of the cells is marvelously rapid, the original normal condition being practically restored after 14 days of feeding." Protozoa show an astounding capacity for recuperation when feeding is resumed after an enforced fast. Some of them regain normal size in only two days. Other forms require as much as fifteen days. Recovery "is the inverse of that during inanition." Cell-divisions begin three to five days after feeding is resumed.

Carlson and Kunde found that at the end of a fast, subjects are able to maintain themselves and even gain weight on much smaller amounts of food than they had formerly thought necessary to keep them going, thus corroborating in the laboratory, a fact of observation that every one experienced in conducting fasts has seen many times. Kunde says: "It seems that the merchanism by which the cells of an extremely emaciated body, rendered thus by starvation (fasting) but organically sound, utilizes food must be quite different from that which occurs after emaciation from sickness, when not only body substances must be built up, but functional disturbances as well. Certainly the body is not able to utilize food on such an economical basis under ordinary conditions of nutrition."

It is not necessary to assume that the "mechanism" of food utilization is different in emaciation produced by fasting from that produced by sickness. We need only to recognize that it is less efficient after sickness because of damages from toxins, drugs and from functional weaknesses. On the other hand, we need to know that rapid gains in weight do often follow sickness and this is especially so if the sickness was accompanied by fasting.

Carlson and Kunde give one case where a subject gained 17.38 lbs. in the first seven days after the completion of a fast, and the body weight came back to normal despite the fact that during the first five days after the fast only one meal a day was eaten, and that a very moderate one. But it would be impossible to gain so much weight in such a short time without consuming enough food to put on this much weight, unless excessive water drinking produced a water-logged state of the tissues. There was either over-eating or over-drinking or both, and thus, much of the benefits of the fast were destroyed. Another of Carlson and Kunde's fasters gained 17.2 lbs. during the first week after a fast. Such rapid gains are not desirable.

Mrs. Sinclair lost twelve pounds in ten days during her first fast, and then gained twenty-two pounds in seventeen days following the fast. Mr. Sinclair gained four and a half pounds on the third day after breaking his fast. In twenty-four days he gained a total of twenty-two pounds. This gain, be it noted, followed a twelve days fast, which occasioned a loss of seventeen pounds. He tells us: "I had always been lean and dyspeptic looking, with what my friends called a 'spiritual' expression. I now became as round as a butter-ball, and so brown and rosy in the face that I was a joke to all who saw me." A slow, steady growth of tissue following a fast is far more satisfactory than any rapid laying on of fat. This is the more sure method employed by nature; in contrast with the quick, temporary and "stimulating" gains that man seems to prefer. The stability of the slow growing oak is certainly preferable to the instability of the rapidly growing mushroom.

There is no reason why the emaciated person should not fast. Indeed, there is often every reason why he should. The fast is sometimes the only thing that will enable him to gain weight. Special weight gaining diets are not required. The milk diet is frequently employed after a fast to force a rapid gain in weight. This I consider not to be necessary, but as tending to actually undo some or all of the benefits derived from the fast.

Von Seeland, subjected chickens to intermittent short fasts, using mature birds for this purpose. These fasts lasted one to two days. His fasting birds, although getting less food than the control birds, became heavier than the latter. He states that the increase in weight was due to an increase in real flesh—protein material—and not to a mere increase in fat. He states that the periodic fasting makes the body heavier, stronger and more solid. Morgulis experimenting with salamanders secured opposite results. "Kagan found," says Morgulis, that "the power of resistance declines with each new experience of starvation. The organism which recovered from inanition through the consumption of a liberal quantity of food still shows the effects of the previous experience °°° and when the inanition is repeated dies sooner than the normal organism."

While Dr. Morgulis thinks that the results of his experiments and those of Kagan, contradict the results claimed by Von Seeland, he says, "they do not necessarily disprove his contention of the invigorating influence of brief fasts inasmuch as in our own experiments the duration of each fast was considerably greater." It should be quite obvious that a series of intermittent fasts must not be long ones. It is quite obvious that subsequent recovery will depend upon the character of the food eaten as well as upon other factors, such as sunshine, exercise, etc. Much depends, too, upon the length of the period between the fasts. We frequently put patients upon intermittent short fasts and secure just such results as Von Seeland reports in his chickens.

Morgulis says that his intermittently fasted salamanders—"with one-half the amount of food reached somewhat more than two-thirds of the body weight of the continually fed salamanders." This points to a remarkable improvement in nutritive power and function, but it is too much to ask one-half the amount of food to produce greater results. Von Seeland did not limit his fasting chickens to one-half the food eaten by the control chickens.

Fasting is not something to play with. It is only a part of the health program. Feeding after the fast and the general *Hygienic* care of the patient are even more important. Laboratory experimenters, with their antiquated and synthetic diets, certainly are not to be trusted in this matter of feeding after a fast.

I am convinced from my own experience with patients, that a too rapid gain in flesh following the fast does not build as solid and healthful flesh as a slow rate of gain. Milk diet enthusiasts produce a flesh-gain after a fast, by their over-feeding, which is almost as rapid as the loss during the fast. But such flesh is watery, flabby and soon lost when one becomes active and returns to other foods. I prefer to feed patients an abundance of fresh fruits and green vegetables and limited quantities of proteins, starches and fats. Flesh gained at a slower rate is more solid and stays with the patient. A too rapid growth in children is not productive of sound tissue. I am convinced that the same is true of a too rapid gain after a fast.

A few do not gain rapidly for more than a week or two weeks after breaking the fast. With many, a short fast does not suffice to occasion a gain in weight. Many factors are at work to prevent a gain in these cases and the short fast is not sufficient to restore the nutritive functions to a vigorous state.

The most rapid gains in weight are seen after a long fast. All cases, however, will gain at a fairly rapid rate if the underlying causes of defective nutrition are corrected. This depends on many factors other than fasting and the intelligent person, be he doctor or patient, will not fail to attend to all necessary factors and influences.

In those animals that periodically undergo protracted periods of fasting, a tendency to acquire, during the feeding season, large stores of fat, is seen. Among these animals, as the Russian bear and the Alaskan fur-seal bull, the period of abstinence from food is often of long duration, so that a large supply of nutriment is necessary. Frequent fasting in man may result in the same tendency although I have never seen a clear case of the development of such a tendency from repeated fasts.

Living After the Fast

"The fast is in vain," says Tilden, "if the patient returns to his old habits. This is true of convalescing in general." The results of the fast will be more or less temporary unless one lives properly thereafter. Fasting will not make one "disease" proof. Orthobionomic living is essential thereafter if one desires to remain in good health.

One woman who placed her whole family on a fast wrote Sinclair of the experience. "Mama had indigestion," she says. After her mother had protestingly fasted for some time, the lady described her mother's condition thus: "Mama is now comfortably eating boiled ham and stuffed peppers, and fruit cake and cherry pie and green olives and what not at the same meal. She is well, though. But of course she will get sick again."

Fasting is but a means to an end. It is a cleansing process and a physiological rest which prepares the body for future right living. It is, therefore, necessary that the work begun by the fast be continued and completed after the fast.

Most fasting advocates advise great care in breaking the fast and in subsequent feeding and then feed abominably. Dr. Eales, for example, followed his thirty days fast with an exceedingly bad diet. He broke his fast on Horlick's Malted Milk and was soon eating such meals as the following: "Glass of malted milk with raw egg, and ate one poached egg later." Dinner (6 P.M.) "two soft-boiled eggs, glass of milk, little rice and strawberries." He also mentions that he "had a cup of coffee" with some friends.

Dewey's personal diet consisted chiefly of meat, fish, eggs, milk, pastries and bread, with but few vegetables, these chiefly of the starchier varieties. He was opposed to acid fruits, declaring they all contain potash which decomposes the gastric juice and that "there is never any desire for acid fruits through real hunger, especially those of the hyperacid kinds: they are simply taken to gratify the lower sense—relish." Acid fruits can be "taken with apparent impunity" "only by the young and old who can generate gastric juice copiously."

The demoralizing influence of all acids, fruit acids included, exerted upon gastric secretion, is undoubted. But this does not necessitate abstaining from acid fruits and does not prove them to be harmful. It only calls for eating them alone. Dr. Dewey knew nothing of food combining. He referred to apple eating as converting the human stomach into a cider mill and declared that "by their ravishing flavor and apparent ease of digestion, apples still play an important part in the 'fall of man' from that higher state, the Eden without its dyspepsia." It was his notion that if we "eat from hunger" and not "from mere relish," we would eat right without much attention being given to what we eat. While there is perhaps more truth in this than is generally recognized, it is, unfortunately, not absolutely true.

Pearson lived for the first week after his fast was broken on about 2 oz. of sweet chocolate, 2 oz. of peanuts and 1 sometimes 2 chocolate malted milks, from the soda fountain, a day.

Tanner tells us of his own overeating, that after his fast (he was dyspeptic before going on the fast) he ate "sufficient food in the first twenty-four hours after breaking the fast to gain nine pounds, and thirty-six pounds in eight days, all that I had lost." If I can judge by the results of over-feeding that I have observed after a fast, Tanner's gain in weight was a puffy, water-logged mass of material that cannot by any stretch of the imagination be called healthy or desirable. His uncontrolled eating was a dangerous procedure and he was in luck to escape with his life. It would not be wise for others to attempt this foolish stuffing. The inability of the undisciplined individuals of our country and age to control themselves means that they should not undertake to feed themselves at all after a fast. They should be controlled by a man of experience.

It will be quite obvious to the student of diet that the style of eating followed by these men must inevitably undo much of the benefits derived from the fast.

In many quarters it is the almost invariable practice to follow the fast with such a diet. The milk diet undoes much of the benefit derived from the period of abstinence. Dr. Hazzard also condemns the milk diet following the fast. Sinclair noted that very frequently the milk diet disagrees with people, and says: "Inasmuch as there is nothing that poisons me quite so quickly as milk, I had to look farther for my solution."

He further says concerning his experience with milk, "I was never able to take the milk diet for any length of time but once, and that after my first twelve-day fast. After my second fast it seemed to go wrong with me, and I think the reason was that I did not begin it until a week after breaking the fast, having got along on orange juice and figs in the meantime. Also I tried on many occasions to take the milk diet after a short fast of three or four days, and always the milk has disagreed with me and poisoned me. I take this to mean that, in my own case, at any rate, so much milk can only be absorbed when the tissues are greatly reduced; and I have known others who have had the same experience."

It is quite true that after a long fast one is capable of absorbing large quantities of milk, but there still remains the question of why one should do so. Why go on the fast in the first place if it is to be followed by worse gluttony than ever?

Dewey was opposed to special exercises. Ragabliati was of the opinion that exercises are not necessary to health and life, and that the ordinary movements supplied by the ordinary business of life are physiologically sufficient for this purpose. This is obviously not true in many occupations. Besides, exercise serves many purposes and few, if any, of the occupations of modern life supply all of the body's needs for exercise.

If we are to continue to enjoy good health after a fast, proper diet, adequate and fitting exercise, sunshine, fresh air, mental poise, rest and sleep and freedom from devitalizing habits are essential. The length of time through which the results of a fast will last depends upon how one lives after the fast.

"Diseases," when treated by drug and serum methods, frequently recur after they appear to be *cured*. I am frequently asked if this is true of fasting-*cured* cases. To answer this question correctly, it is necessary that the reader distinguish between "regular" methods of treating "disease" and fasting. Drugs and serums succeed only in suppressing the symptoms of "disease," so that an apparent *cure* often results. But suppression of symptoms does not constitute a real recovery. Fasting does remove the internal causes of "disease." If purifies the organism. Recovery by this means is genuine, and is not merely a forced suppression of symptoms.

But fasting cannot make one "disease"-proof. If a certain mode of eating and living makes a man sick once, it can do so a thousand times if he returns to it. When a man has recovered through fasting, if he resumes over-eating and wrong eating and sensuality and inebriety, excesses, dissipations and other forms of wrong living, he will again build "disease" in his body. It may be the same condition or some other, but he is certain to evolve some form of "disease" if he does not live rightly after his body has been cleansed. If, like the Biblical sow that was washed, he returns to his wallowing in the mire, he cannot help but become dirty again and will require another bath. But if he will live as he should live, he may be fully assured that he will not have a recurrence of his troubles. Once "disease" has been remedied by *Hygienic* methods, the person cannot again have the "disease" without building it all over again.

Sinclair likens a man who needs a fast "every now and then," to the man who spends his time sweeping rain water out of his house, instead of repairing the roof. If there is need for you to fast at frequent intervals, this is because your eating and living habits are wrong. If you give up drinking you will not need to be sobered up at frequent intervals.

Enervation, established as a chronic state following enervating habits, lowers and perverts functioning of the organs of the body, some functions being weakened more than others. If we do not build enervation and toxemia by taxing the organism to the very limit, no pathology will develop. Lighten the toxic over-load with which the organism has been burdened, cultivate conservative habits of living, guide the mind into new channels of thought, poise and control the emotions, and getting well and remaining well is no longer a game of chance.

Fasting in Health

CHAPTER XXXIII

Writing in *Physical Culture* (May, 1915), Mr. Carrington says: "If a well man starts going without food, he begins to starve (not fast). The nearer well you are the less you should fast." Mr. Macfadden takes a similar view, saying that fasting by healthy persons "represents more nearly cases of *starvation* than of *fasting*. A man can only fast with benefit when he is ill. If he is well, and goes without his food, he commences to starve at once; and the two processes are very different. Hence the physiological experts observed only cases of starvation, and not fasting cases at all. The therapeutic side of the question seems to have been missed by them entirely!" —*Encyclopedia of Physical Culture*, Vol. III.

Mr. Macfadden is discussing Prof. Gano Benedict's voluminous work. *The Influence of Inanition on Metabolism* (A Carnegie Institute Report), which is devoted entirely to observations of fasting in so-called normal or healthy individuals. Nowhere in the massive volume does Prof. Benedict consider the value of fasting in sickness. His experimental fasts were of two to seven days duration, the subjects being young men in good health. Strange, is it not, that studying Benedict's reports, and finding nothing in them to indicate that the young men suffered in any way from *starvation*, Mr. Macfadden should stress the alleged fact that when a healthy man misses a few meals he begins to starve.

Incorrect as this view is, it has been held by others. Jennings says: "Take a healthy child from food while its vital machinery is in full operation, and it will use up its own building material and fall to ruin in two or three weeks." He seems not to have been talking of the regular physical activities of the child when he said "with its vital machinery in full operation." He contrasts the activities of the healthy child with that of the sick one and speaks almost wholly of the activities of the internal organs. But he does give the healthy child two or three weeks of activity before it uses up all of its resources. It should be obvious that an adult would require a much longer period of abstinence to use up his resources.

In *Vitality, Fasting and Nutrition,* Mr. Carrington takes a similar view. He emphasizes the fact that his observations of fasting have been confined to sick fasters and have not been made upon healthy fasters. He asks the question: would the effects of fasting be the same in the case of a sick man as in that of a healthy man? He says: "My answer to this is a decided No! The effects of fasting in such cases are very different." Indeed, he says that we should expect this *a priori* "since the effects of anything would doubtless be different in healthy and in diseased bodies." "I have just drawn a picture of the effects of starvation in the case of a well person," he says. But this "picture" is one that he had conjured up in his own mind and not one that he had seen as he confesses. Let us look at his "picture." He says: "Were a really healthy person to commence going without food and continue this for a number of days, we can easily picture the result in our imaginations—a starved and shrunken body; hollow, staring eyes; parched and shrunken skin; perhaps a wandering mind; emaciation, weakness; and a ravenous, uncontrollable appetite—these are a few of the many symptoms we can imagine as following upon this outrage upon nature. What the exact symptoms would be; how long life could be sustained under the circumstances; these are questions I am totally unable to answer—since I have never had the opportunity of observing the effects of starvation upon the healthy body."

Note that this picture is a wholly imaginary one. Mr. Carrington could have known better at the time he wrote that pin-picture of starvation horror. He had just presented a short history of fasting through the ages in which he had recounted the long fasts undergone for religious purposes. He could have known that none of these symptoms were real. The fact is that the healthy man entombed in a mine by a cave-in or shipwrecked at sea, or a healthy animal forced by circumstances to do without food, goes without food as easily and with no more wandering of the mind, or parching and shrinking of the skin than occurs in the sick person abstaining from food. Prof. Levanzin's fast of 31 days undertaken at Carnegie Institute was taken while in good health. This fast was undergone after Mr. Carrington's book was written, but there were many long fasts prior to that date by healthy men and Mr. Carrington could have known of these.

Mr. Macfadden's statements about fasting by the healthy were published after the famous experiments in Madison Square Garden, in which several athletes took part. After watching a large group of healthy men and women fast and engage in severe athletic contests, with no signs of starvation resulting, how was it possible for him to take the view he did? With some of the fasters losing no weight and one or two of them registering gains, how can it be said that the fasting healthy man will waste rapidly? We know very well that such is not the case.

The healthy man, no more than the sick man, does not begin to starve as soon as he omits his first meal. He lives, as does the sick man, upon his stored reserves and begins to starve only after these are exhausted. Let us never forget that the body carries a store of food that may be called upon at any time that need arises.

Fasting in disease is very different in many particulars from fasting in health, but fundamentally, fasting under the two sets of circumstances is the same process. The view of fasting by the healthy taken by Mr. Macfadden and Mr. Carrington is a very superficial one. A perfectly healthy man may derive no benefit from a fast, but that he is starving so long as he is living on his reserves is no more true of the healthy man than of the sick man. We may add the obvious fact that there is no such thing known to us a perfectly healthy man, so that there may be no one who cannot derive benefit from a fast.

So far as experiments made upon healthy animals and men have shown, there is the same hoarding or conserving of reserves and the same rigid control of autolysis in healthy animals and men as in diseased ones, when these fast. Tissues are lost in the same order. Loss of tissue in the healthy faster is proportioned to his activity, whereas, in the sick man or woman, there may be a rapid loss of weight in the early part of the fast, due to the inferior quality of the tissues. Indeed, there is often much more rapid loss of weight in the fasting sick man than in the fasting well man. Let us grant, then, that there is a certain difference between fasting by the well and fasting by the sick—this difference is certainly not fundamental.

It will be recalled that there is great activity in those animals that fast during the mating season. Some of these fast for prolonged periods. Yet they know none of the signs of starvation that Mr. Carrington conjured up in his imagination as likely developments in the healthy faster. The fact is that his picture of "starvation" in the healthy faster is so like the picture presented by the regular physician in presenting his objections to fasting, as to arouse the suspicion that Mr. Carrington has subconsciously borrowed the description.

Fasting in Acute Disease

CHAPTER XXXIV

"Instead of using medicine, rather fast a day," wrote Plutarch, who was much closer to the primitive practices of mankind than we are today. By *medicine* he could only have meant drugs. Someone else has said: ""Wise people, falling into ailment, take a bath, go to bed, and fast, leaving nature to do her own work of cure, and not hindering her beneficent operations." This is the rule of nature in acute disease: *Go to bed, keep warm, and abstain from all food until hunger returns.* Writing in Trall's *Journal,* Sept. 1857, S. M. Landis, M.D., says: "In acute and inflammatory diseases, no food should be used." Discussing rheumatic fever in his editorial in the *Journal,* March, 1857, Trall says: "No food should be taken until the fever has nearly subsided, and the coat on the tongue begins to clean off." Going without food in these cases not only relieves pain, but it rests the heart and relieves the kidneys. Fasting in fevers was commonly employed by Neapolitan physicians some hundred and fifty years ago. They frequently permitted their fever patients to go for as long as forty days without food. When in pneumonia and pleurisy, the patient is fed, not only is the toxic saturation kept up, but feeding retards resolution; that is, it prevents the inflamed lungs and pleura from returning to normal. This may result in abscess formation.

One of the first indications of illness is a failing appetite. Indeed the desire for food often fails a few days before any other symptoms appear. The common expression, applied alike to horse and man, "off his feed," describes the instinctive abstinence from food that nature enforces when the power to digest food is low or absent. The loss of digestive power and digestive conditions is proportioned to the severity of the remedial action. If the illness begins "suddenly" while the stomach is filled with food or if there is a serious accident or shock to the nervous system, vomiting immediately empties the stomach. Thus does nature indicate, both in animals and man, that in acute disease, no food should be taken.

Writing of the vomiting that occurs in sea-sickness, Dr. Shew asserted that "almost all persons are benefited by it" (sea sickness), and explained the benefit thus: "It is by the beneficial power of fasting that the benefit of sea sickness is caused." Only false teachings can induce people to go on eating regularly in the face of the fact that the food is vomited as promptly as it is ingested. For this false teaching we have the medical profession to thank.

FALSE TEACHINGS OF MEDICAL "SCIENCE"

Physicians have taught the people that there are specific diseases requiring specific causes and that the sick must be fed "to keep up their strength," while being "cured" of their diseases. So long as we believe that the "cure" of a common "disease" depends upon the accidental or providentially ordained discovery of some mysterious compound, we are likely to continue overlooking the plainest indications of nature and go on killing the sick in the time-honored way.

Not merely in low chronic conditions, but in acute conditions, with high temperature as well, overfeeding is prescribed and enforced. Indeed, a high calorie diet is now the rule in fevers. Dr. Kellogg insists on sugar in some form, even in the most violent stages of acute "disease.' This insistence is not based on physiology, but on his fear of bacteria. He says that bacteria "will not grow or at least are not virulent and active in producing toxins, in the presence of sugar." Fear and false theories lead men away from nature and physiology and cause them to do many absurd and damaging things. With all due respect to Dr. Kellogg, his influence in this matter is highly pernicious and prejudicial to the health and recovery of the sick. The indications of nature are the true guide in a search for health. Ephemeral theories of mis-called science often do much harm.

INSTINCTIVE REPUGNANCE TO FOOD IN ACUTE ILLNESS

Animals will not eat when sick. It has long been known that when animals are severely injured they refuse food. Shock, severe injury of any kind, fever, pain, inflammation, poisoning, reduce or suspend digestive power and reduce the nutritive functions throughout the body. The human animal has no desire for food when ill; in fact, there is a positive repugnance to food, coupled with an inability to digest and utilize it. But, all too often, the human animal disregards his repugnance to food and the discomforts that follow eating in spite of this, and eats because he has become convinced that he will die if he does not eat.

When animals, young or old, become sick they instinctively re-frain from eating. *Warmth, Quiet and Fasting,* with a little water, are all they want. When they take nourishment, it is a sure sign that they are recovering. They eat but little at first and gradually eat more as they grow better. They never worry about calories or protein requirements either. *Warmth, Quiet* (rest) and *Fasting,* with a little water, as demanded by thirst, are the needs of a sick man or woman. A sick animal cannot be made to eat; but sick men, women and children can be induced to eat to "keep up their strength." Feeding, with relapses galore, until death ends the various tragedies, is common on both sides of the Atlantic. Every year the loss of life among useful men is appalling. They develop a "spring cold," then eat to keep up their strength; but the eating strengthens the toxins and weakens the body, until friends are shocked by their death.

Dr. Hazzard claims, and I believe rightly, that while appetite may be and often is present in "disease," true hunger never is. I believe that, with a few possible exceptions, this is as true of chronic as of acute "disease." Liek says that objection to fasting on the part of adults, is usually due not to the working of the instinct but to that of a faulty working intelligence." He illustrates this with a story about a fat woman doctor upon whom he performed an abdominal operation, which was followed by septic developments. Although she admitted she did not have the slightest desire for food and that even the thought of food produced nausea, she thought "she ought to eat something to keep up her strength" and "was worrying for days because she had the idea that she ought to be given strengthening food." He very appropriately remarks that "her stomach possessed more sense than her brain." His remark would have been nearer the mark, had he said that her organic instincts possessed more intelligence than her medical instructors who educated her into the false belief that "the sick must eat to keep up their strength."

Dr. Densmore says: "Quite generally, in severe attacks, the patient has no appetite—food is positively repulsive; but when there seems to be craving for food, it will be found to be a fictitious longing caused by inflammation and not from need of nourishment.

This fictitious appetite usually disappears with the first twenty-four hours of the fast. The effort of the true physician must be to assist Nature, and to be guided by her. If there should still be found longing for food at the expiration of forty-eight hours fasting, it will be evidence that food is needed. °°° The more serious the attack of illness, the longer duration of fast needed. From three to six days will be found advisable in extreme cases. Let nature be absolutely trusted; when the patient has been denied food long enough to overcome the inflammation which is liable to be mistaken for appetite, then give nourishment as soon and no sooner than the patient craves food."—
How Nature Cures, p. 23.

I do not agree that in cases of severe acute illness where the fictitious desire for food persists beyond forty-eight hours of fasting, it indicates a real need for food. There can be no digestion of food in these cases and there is no urgent need for food so long as the patient's reserves are not exhausted. The reappearance of a keen appetite in the sick is a sure indication of returning health and strength. The absence of desire for food, whether caused by illness, grief, anger, excitement, fatigue, or other cause, is nature's way of saying that the digestive organs are, for the time being, incapable of digesting food.

FEEDING TO KEEP UP STRENGTH

The idea that dominates the physician, the nurses and the relatives of the sick person is that the vital power or strength "must be supported with food" while the "conflict with disease" rages. This supposed need for food to support life, great in proportion to the apparent gravity of the patient's condition, would seem to make the natural or instinctive aversion to food a serious mistake of nature. "The force of custom," wrote Dr. Densmore, "is one of the strongest powers, and doctors and nurses for generations have been in the habit of urging invalids to partake of food, not infrequently to their serious injury." Because we believe that recovery from illness depends on nourishment "our unreasoning sympathy and solicitude prompt us to urge our invalid friends to partake of food. Whatever the origin of the custom, it is one universally to be condemned; when one is seriously ill a fast is indicated."—*How Nature Cures*, p. 21.

One thing is certain; either nature or the physician is mistaken. The furred tongue and loss of relish for food, the absence of "hunger contractions," the mental depression; in short, the entire absence of every physiological requirement for digestion, with, in many conditions, the presence of inflammation and even ulceration in the digestive tract, makes it impossible to sustain the patient's strength by feeding.

Enforced feeding of the sick is a war againt nature, dangerous in proportion to the gravity of the patient's condition. The poisonous products of undigested or imperfectly digested food must handicap the patient who is fed during an acute illness. The stuff-to-kill doctor who feeds milk, eggs, meat broths, etc., were he not so blind, should be able to see that he is killing his patient.

NO POWER TO DIGEST IN ACUTE SICKNESS

Beaumont showed that there is no digestion in serious acute illness. He says of one of his experiments, that, this "experiment has considerable pathological importance. In febrile diathesis, very little or no gastric juice is secreted. Hence the importance of withholding food from the stomach in febrile complaints. It can afford no nourishment; but is actually a source of irritation to that organ, and, consequently, to the whole system. No solvent can be secreted under these circumstances; and food is as insoluble in the stomach, as lead would be under ordinary circumstances." *Certainly no food should be eaten until normal secretions have been restored.*

A few years ago Prof. Carlson confirmed the findings of Beaumont and several of his successors. He showed that gastric secretion is absent during gastritis and fevers. The absence of hunger in fever has been shown to be associated with absence of the "hunger contractions" of the stomach. "Hunger contractions" have been shown to be absent in nausea, gastritis, tonsilitis, influenza and colds. In dogs these "hunger contractions" have been shown to be absent in infection and pneumonia. The absence of hunger is a concomitant of the absence of gastric and salivary secretions and the absence of the "hunger contractions." It is, in other words, an evidence of a suspension of the digestive process.

It is unfortunate that few, save *Natural Hygienists,* have ever based their care of the acutely ill upon the fact that there is no power to digest food when there is fever, pain, inflammation and severe poisoning. The practitioners of all schools have continued to urge food upon their acutely ill patients in spite of the protests of nature and in the face of the mounting physiological knowledge of the lack of power to digest food under such circumstances.

Pain, inflammation, fever, headaches, mental disturbances, etc., take away the appetite, inhibit secretion and excretion, impair digestion and render it injurious to eat under such conditions. Pain, inflammation and fever in all forms of *acute "disease"* inhibit the secretion of digestive juices, "take away the appetite" and render digestion practically impossible. The dryness of the mouth in fevers is matched by a similar dryness all along the digestive tract. It can be of no advantage to urge food upon a patient suffering with an *acute "disease,"* for there is then no digestive power to work it up. There is an almost total absence of the digestive juices. The little of these present, are of such poor quality that they could not properly digest even small amounts of food. Along with the absence of the power to digest and the absence of the digestive juices, there is lacking the keen relish for food which is so essential to normal digestion. Pain inhibits digestion and secretion. Fever inhibits these. So does inflammation. Food taken under such conditions is not digested. Nature has temporarily suspended the digestive functions. This is necessary in order that her undivided attention can be given to the task of recovery. Energy that is ordinarily consumed in the work of digesting, absorbing and assimilating food is now being used to carry on the restorative processes. The muscles of the stomach and intestine are in about the same condition as the muscles of the arm.

In acute disease the digestive system is as little fit to digest food as the limbs are for locomotion—both require rest. What is to be gained by eating when there is no ability to digest food? Why should physicians insist upon the patient eating when there is no desire for food, or when there is an actual aversion to food? Dr. Emmett Densmore laid down as the first rule to be followed when illness develops: "Partake of no food during forty-eight hours; after that time continue an absolute fast from food until the patient has pronounced natural hunger." He says that "at all such times (when there is fever and inflammation) all food must absolutely be withheld from the patient. This may be only for a day, or for many days; no food is to be taken until all symptoms of fever have entirely abated, and none then until the patient has a decided appetite and relish for it."

Jennings says: "It is of no advantage to urge food upon the stomach when there is no digestive power to work it up. There is never any danger of starvation so long as there are reserve forces sufficient to hold the citadel of life and start anew its mainsprings. For when sustenance becomes a prime necessity, the digestive apparatus will be clothed with power enough to work up some new material, and a call made for it proportioned to the ability to use it. And if there is not power within the domain of life to save the organism, it must perish."

Trall declared that when the body is struggling to throw off the toxins of "*disease*," the patient "has no ability, until the struggle is decided, to digest food; and to cram his stomach with it, or to irritate the digestive organs with tonics and stimulants, is merely adding fuel to the fire." The stuff-to-kill doctor shuts his eyes to this important fact and, ignoring all the instinctive indications that food is not desirable and all the physiological evidences that food cannot be digested if consumed, insists that "the sick must eat to keep up their strength."

NO NOURISHMENT WITHOUT DIGESTION

In all types of acute disease the whole organism is engaged in the work of eliminating toxins, not in that of assimilating food, hence, it is perfectly natural that the body should rebel against food. Anorexia, foul breath, coated tongue, nausea, vomiting, fetid discharges, the excretion of much mucus, constipation alternating with diarrhea, etc., all indicate that the organs are engaged in the work of vicarious or compensatory elimination, and are not able to digest food. It is not possible to nourish the body by feeding under such circumstances.

"Science and physiology teach," says Dr. Densmore, "that digestion of food can only be performed satisfactorily when there is secretion of the digestive juices; and also that there can be no adequate secretion of the digestive juices, where there is inflammation, or from any cause an absence of appetite. ° ° ° If, as physiologists teach, there can be no effective digestion except from the secretion of digestive juices, and if there is almost no secretion of digestive juices where there is high temperature, we ought to expect that there would be as much emaciation of the fever patient while partaking of food as while fasting; and this is precisely what will be seen to be the result by any physician who will make the experiment. Common sense teaches that if food is taken and not digested, such food does not help nourish the system. If no food at all be taken the processes of life are carried on by consuming the tissues; and if food be taken and not digested the processes of life must be supported by the same consumption of tissues, with the further result that the undigested food must be excreted from the body, which at a glance will be seen to be a strain upon the vital powers, calling for an additional consumption of tissue, and inevitably delaying the restoration of the patient."—*How Nature Cures*, p.p. 21-22.

RECTAL AND SKIN FEEDING

It may be objected to all of this that the patient should be fed so-called pre-digested foods. Our reply is that there are no pre-digested foods and little ability to absorb them if there were. Efforts to feed so-called pre-digested foods have proved failures, even when the foods were not vomited. Well did Dr. Dewey say: "Pre-digested foods! If they nourish the sick, why not feed the well? Why not abolish our kitchens at an immense saving in the time, expense and worry of cooking and live on them at an immense saving of the tax of digestion and the digestive juices? Brethren of the Medical Profession, make haste to let the world know when you have found a case in which you have made use of the lower bowel so to nourish the sick body that it didn't waste while the cure was going on."

Rectal feeding is absurd. It feeds nothing. The colon is busy excreting, not absorbing, and the so-called food injected into the colon, not being digested, could not be used if it were absorbed. The least it can do is ferment and putrify and add to the discomforts and expenditures of the patient. Lavage or stomach tube or duodenal feeding are delusions. When such large quantities of fluid are being poured out, there is no absorption from the stomach and intestine. To feed under such conditions, when there is no absorption, and also no digestion, is not to nourish the body. Food adds to the putrescence and to the danger.

The body never performs any of what Dr. Tilden calls "Hindu tricks," in this matter of taking nourishment. It does not digest and absorb food when digestion is suspended and the membranes of the stomach and intestine are exuding matter instead of absorbing it. It is exuding fluid to aid in expelling the mass of putrescence in the food tube, and to protect the walls of the tube and any irritated surface. Sometimes nature even rejects water, expelling it by vomiting as often as it is forced down. How foolish in such cases to continue to force food and drugs on the patient and water into his stomach. Nature is trying to protect herself by this vomiting. She even guards against water by creating a bad taste in the mouth that causes the patient to refuse water. Dr. Lindlahr likened the process to a sponge. During health, the sponge (intestine) is busy absorbing, during a fast or in *acute "disease"* the sponge is being squeezed.

Skin feeding is another absurdity. The skin will not absorb food, and it would not be prepared for use by the organism, if it did do so, as was shown in our study of digestion in a previous volume. I have heard physicians tell of feeding patients through the skin. Milk baths, olive oil rubs and other unphysiological procedures are employed, and then, if the patient does not die, the physician tells us how long he kept his patient alive by such absurd practices. Had the physician not been ignorant of the internal resources of the body he would have known that the patient would have lived just as long without such mis-called feeding. Skin foods are delusions. Intravenous feeding is also a delusion.

GASTRO-INTESTINAL DECOMPOSITION

If bacteriologists desire to make cultures of "pathogenic" organism, they use meat broths, meat jellies and boiled milk. These substances provide equally as good culture media for microbes in the digestive tract, when fed to patients who are acutely ill, as when used in the laboratory, and generate just as much putrescence. The physician who would not feed a putrid culture medium to a patient, will blindly feed the patient the culture medium and see it become putrid in the digestive tract. Dr. Josian Oldfield says, in *Fasting for Health and Life*: "If friends were only present at the post mortem and could see and smell for themselves the foul and filthy contents of the stomach and intestines of those nurse-bullied dying patients, they would pray, as I pray, that when their last days are come they may be allowed to die in quietude and cleanliness, taking only sips of pure water, and such fruit juices as their thirsty cells crave for, until peaceful dissolution takes place."

What Dr. Oldfield overlooks is that the members of his own profession, who are present at the post mortems and are allowed to see and smell the putrescence in the digestive tract, prescribed the foods the nurse or fond relative forced upon the patient and that these same medical men trained the nurse and taught the relatives. Food that is not digested undergoes decomposition, forming a mass of toxins more or less of which are absorbed to further poison and sicken the patient. A veritable cess pool is formed under the diaphragm that is much more dangerous to the individual than any cess pool that may be in the neighborhood. To get rid of this rotting, fermenting mass of food and the toxins it has formed requires a needless expenditure of energy. Nature is trying to conserve energy. This is precisely the reason she has temporarily suspended the digestive functions. It is little less than criminal to force the organism to divide its energies and attentions between the work of healing and the added task of eliminating a rotting septic mass from the digestive tract. The only sensible thing to do is to keep the digestive tract free of all such matter. Nature herself indicates this in the strongest possible manner, for not only is all desire for food cut off, but the most tempting dishes are not relished by the sick person. There is a positive disinclination to take food.

Bear in mind that the food decomposed and poisoned the patient because his digestive power had been greatly impaired, and that to give more food, under such conditions, is only to add to the poisoning. The "disease" will last until the poisons have been eliminated and the decomposing food has been voided. Fever, vomiting and purging are nature's methods of getting rid of the poison, and when these cases are fasted and not fed, such troubles soon end. There is no danger in them. Feeding and drugging are the elements of danger. Never permit a patient to be drugged, and never permit the physician to reduce (suppress) his fever.

One of our rules for caring for the sick is to stop the absorption of all toxins from the outside. Feeding during *acute "disease"* does just the opposite. It keeps the digestive tract full of decaying animal and vegetable matter, which the body must void or absorb. Putrescence arising from gastro-intestinal decomposition, grafted onto the pre-existing enervation, toxemia and dyscrasia, forms the cause of practically all the so-called "diseases" from which man suffers.

In health the body is "potentized with immunizing power" and can to a large extent, render innocuous the toxic substances arising from decomposition. The secretions of the stomach and intestine take care of such substances for us every day of our lives. When wrong eating and poor hygiene have broken down the body's resistance and deranged digestion, so that decomposition produces toxins in excess of the immunizing power of these secretions, trouble begins;

the body must defend itself against these toxins, and this defense we call "disease."

When the decomposition overwhelms the immunizing power of the digestive secretions, vomiting and purging, so commonly regarded as evil, are the conservative and defensive measures which nature employs in expelling the putrescence. To absorb the fermenting and putrefying contents of the digestive tract into the bloodstream would mean death. This does not occur. The absorbents reverse their ordinary activities and, instead of taking up the fluid contents of the digestive tract, pour a large amount of fluid (blood-serum), into the stomach and intestine to dilute and neutralize the decomposing matter and wash it away. The great quantity of fluid flushes the entire alimentary canal and the vomiting and purging complete the work of carrying the toxic matter from the body's cavities.

THE STOMACH AND INTESTINES IN ACUTE ILLNESS

A standard medical author thus describes the stomach in acute gastritis: "The gastric mucous membrane of such a stomach is red and swollen, it secretes little gastric juice, and this contains very little acid but much mucus. The patient has uncomfortable feelings in his abdomen, with headache, lassitude, some nausea, often vomiting. The vomiting relieves him considerably, for it removes the irritating substance. The tongue is coated, and the flow of saliva is increased. If this decomposing, fermenting, irritating mass is not vomited, but reaches the bowel, colic and diarrhea are the result. As a rule the patient is well in about one day, although he may not have much appetite for the next two or three days."

With the stomach in this condition, with appetite lacking, and with no digestive juice secreted, eating would be worse than folly. It would seem criminal to add more food to the "decomposing, fermenting, irritating mass" in the stomach. Fasting in such a condition is the only rational procedure. Yet in typhoid fever, with the stomach in an even worse condition, with the intestines in a much worse state and with temperature high, most medical men insist upon heavy feeding; a high calorie diet being generally recommended and employed. Not in acute gastritis and typhoid only, but in cholera and other intestinal ills, it is the custom to insist upon plenty of good nourishing food. Indeed, food is literally forced upon the sick. Part of the recognized formula of nursing invalids is to tickle their palates with food dainties. Food is urged upon their unwilling stomach in spite of strong protests.

NAUSEA AND VOMITING

Nausea and vomiting are common symptoms in acute disease of all forms. If food is taken it is commonly vomited. Where vomiting does not take place, the food is likely to be thrown out by means of a diarrhea. What can be more ill-advised than to persuade a patient to take food, knowing that it will be vomited immediately? By rejecting food, does the body not indicate in the strongest possible manner, that food is not needed and cannot be used? Yet food is literally forced upon the sick patient, "by order of the physician," in spite of the fact that his whole system rebels against it, and in spite of the nausea and vomiting that follow taking it. Physicians resort to *sedatives, anti-emetics* and *tonics* in their efforts to force the rebellious digestive system into submission.

FEEDING INCREASES SUFFERING

To feed under such conditions causes the temperature to rise and the pains and general discomfort of the patient to increase. Much of the restlessness and uneasiness usually observed in fever patients of all kinds is due to feeding and drugging. The fasting patient is comparatively comfortable and rests well, and makes a more rapid and satisfactory recovery. Dr. Jennings says: "The more you feed a sick man, the sicker you make him." Again, "Don't aggravate the troubles of a sick fellowman by forcing him to swallow food against the protest of his stomach."

Let us see what happens if we feed in acute "disease." The first thing the patient and physician note is an increase in symptoms. The fever goes up, the pulse increases, pain and other symptoms become more intense; the patient is caused much unnecessary suffering, and the patient's relatives are caused much needless anxiety. Graham declared that "the more they nourish (feed) a body while diseased action is kept up in it, the more they increase the disease." Again "when the body is seriously diseased °°° entire and protracted fasting would be the very best means in many cases of removing disease and restoring health. I have seen wonderful effects result from experiments of this kind."—*Science of Human Life.* He also called attention to the fact that eating increases the pain, inflammation, discomfort, fever and irritableness of the sick and that it does so in proportion to the amount of food eaten and in direct ratio to its supposed nutritive qualities, while fasting reduces the "violence" of the "disease" and renders recovery more certain. All forms of acute disease are cut short and made comfortable by fasting. Fever rapidly abates and inflammation quickly subsides.

COMPENSATION

Disease is labor, action, struggle—it is often violent action. Rapid heart action, rapid breathing, vomiting, diarrhea, etc., etc., represent increased effort. This uses up energy. It often leaves the patient exhausted at the end of his strenuous effort. It may so completely exhaust him as to end his life. Disease frequently means a greater expenditure of energy than the normal activities of health require, hence the urgent need for conservation of energy in every possible way. So great is the intensity of the effort, so fully are the powers of life concentrated upon the work in hand, there is no energy available with which to carry on the work of digestion. The suspension of digestive secretions, cessation of the rhythmic contractions of the stomach and intestines and the withdrawal of the desire for food are, therefore, compensatory measures, equally with the prostration of the patient, designed to conserve energy on the one hand that it may be available for use on the other.

Dr. Jennings wrote of this conservative measure seen in all acute disease: "The great, extensive, and complicated nutritive apparatus, that requires a large amount of force to convert raw material into living structure, is put at rest, that the forces saved thereby may be transferred to the recuperative machinery within their respective limits, so that there is no call for food,and none should be offered until the crisis is passed, or a point is reached where some nutritive labor can be performed, and there is a natural call for nutriment. ***
And food has no more to do with the production of vitality, than the timber, planks, bolts and canvas for the ship have in supplying ship-carpenters and sailors. In the mass of diseases—such as simple, continued, or remittent fever, scarlet fever, measles, mild bilious fevers—and most of the disorders that are termed febrile, that require a few days to do up their recuperative work in, the proper course of treatment to be pursued, is exceedingly plain and simple. So long as there is no call for nutriment, a cup of cool water is all that is needed for the inner man."—*Tree of Life*, pp. 186-187.

The urgent demand for increased effort which the presence of toxins occasions is the reason for the increased, even violent effort. But violent effort in one direction requires reduced effort, by way of compensation, in other directions. Fasting by the acutely ill is definitely a compensatory measure and its urgency is in direct proportion to the severity of the symptoms. There remains digestive power in a cold, in pneumonia there is none. By this is meant that the more ill is the patient the greater is the need to refrain from eating. Curious as it may appear at first thought, health and hunger come together.

PHYSIOLOGICAL REST
"Nothing is remedial," wrote Trall, "except conditions which economize the vital expenditures." The amount of work done by the heart, liver, lungs, kidneys, glands, etc., is largely determined by the amount of food eaten. Why should these organs and the stomach and intestines be given more work to do by eating? Haven't they enough work to perform under the circumstances? Nature demands physiological rest, not physiological over-work. Her call for rest comes in unmistakable terms. Why, then, shall the organs be forced to do extra work by the use of stimulants or by feeding? To stop the use of food for a time affords the most complete rest to the whole vital economy.

Fasting, or physiological rest is the surest way of economizing vital expenditures. Walter pointed out that "the patient often grows stronger through the process of fasting and always better." It should be understood that when food is eaten by the sick man or woman, much of the vital energies must be diverted from the work of purification to that of ridding the body of the unwanted and unusable food. Even in those mild acute diseases, such as the cold, in which but part of the body's energies have been mobilized for the work of disease, and in which considerable digestive power remains, with, perhaps, some desire for food, fasting often means the difference between a mild illness with quick recovery of physiological equilibrium and a severe illness that is long drawn out, or that may end in death.

PREVENTION
Tilden says: "All acute disease could be prevented if anticipated by a fast of sufficient duration to lower the accumulated toxins

below the toleration point. An anticipatory fast establishes a dependable immunization to any so-called disease. If started too late, it will eliminate or render very mild the worst types of epidemics. If this were generally known and acted upon by towns and cities in ordering the people to fast for a few days, and to follow the fast by light eating, epidemics would be shorn of their virulence, and in time rendered impotent or prevented entirely. Only the vulnerable— those pronouncedly toxemic—are attacked (?) by epidemics."

Fasting does not remove the cause of "disease"—*toxemia*. It merely allows the body to do its work of elimination more efficiently by not putting any hindrances in the way. Fasting does not stop the processes commonly called "disease"—nor does it shorten their duration—feeding and treatment do often suppress these processes, always impede them, and almost always lengthen their duration. The lengths of time the courses of self-limited "diseases" are said to run are times they run under the feeding and treating plans. Under fasting and resting they never run so long.

Nature indicates in the strongest possible manner her desire to fast in acute "disease." In proportion to its severity, so-called "disease" means a loss of digestive conditions and digestive power. Anorexia, nausea, vomiting and the absence of all relish for food should convince anyone, who is not a convert to the doctrine of "total depravity," that no food should be given. Due to our distrust of our natural instincts, we all too often disregard the patent demands of Nature and eat in spite of the closed-for-repairs sign she has hung out—an action invariably pursued by Nature.

If fasting were instituted at the first sign of trouble, few acute diseases would ever become very severe and many of them would be so mild as to lead to the thought that the patient would not have been very sick any way. Unfortunately, it is the custom to continue eating when symptoms appear. As Dr. Page ably put it, *Natural Cure*, p. 146: "Nearly all patients continue eating regularly, until food becomes actually disagreeable, even loathsome, often; and after this every effort is exhausted to produce some toothsome compound to 'tempt the appetite.' Furthermore, and often worst of all, after the entire failure of this program, the patient can, and usually does, take to gruel or some sort of 'extract' which he can drink by holding his breath. All this tends to aggravate the acute symptoms, and to fasten the disease in a chronic form upon the rheumatic patient, or to insure rheumatic fever; and the same principle holds in nearly all acute disorders, it is well to remember."

Page also says: "There is neither pleasure nor nourishment in forced feeding—only pain, poisoning and starving. The fasting cure universally and rationally applied, would save thousands of lives every year. For example, there would be practically no 'typhoid fever,' as all fevers would be aborted in a few days of stomach rest; and never a death or prolonged illness from whooping-cough, which is always a stomach cough from inflammation of that organ. In my busy practice of forty years, no fever has developed into 'typhoid;' nor has there been any whooping beyond a few days, and never a death."

NO DANGER OF STARVATION

There is no danger of the patient dying of starvation in the process of getting well. Let us bear in mind that the body is possessed of reserve food stores which will meet its needs for nutriment for a prolonged period. In acute "disease" the body can supply its nutritive needs from these food reserves with less effort and with less waste of energy and substance than is required to supply them from raw materials. We believe that man requires food all the time because we have learned to think of him as an engine or a machine that can run only so long as he is supplied with fuel. This absurd mechanistic view of life insists upon ignoring every prompting of instinct and treating man as an inanimate machine is treated.

Let the sick eat only when Nature calls for food. A large number of cases will recover, whether they feed or fast, but there is also a very large number of cases who will die, if they are fed, who would otherwise recover. To fast or to feed—this is often the issue of to live or to die.

PAIN

Pains that seem unbearable without the use of *narcotics* and *anodynes* rapidly lessen while one fasts, so that within a short time to a few days the patient is comfortable. Repeatedly have I watched the almost unbearable pains of acute articular rheumatism subside and the patient become comfortable after three or four days of fasting. In the last stages of cancer, when nothing is done for the patient except to dose him with opium, and when pains induced by opium are as great (or greater) as those resulting from the cancer, a fast will restore comfort and permit the patient to die in peace.

TORTURE OF HOPELESS CASES

"Feed the patient anything his fancy may desire; he is going to die anyway," is the advice frequently given by physicians when the patient has been brought so low that death seems inevitable. This is shameful cruelty and often results in death in cases that would otherwise recover. Why make the dying man more miserable? Why increase his suffering? "Do take a little more, dear, just to please me," coaxes the misguided wife or mother. Or a dominating, but ignorant nurse uses all of her mental power and masterful force to get the weak, perhaps, dying patient, to swallow more boiled milk, more meat broth or more egg custard, which decomposes rather than digests in the patient's digestive tract.

FASTING IN FEVERS

Trall insisted that "strictly speaking, fever and food are antagonistic ideas. No simple fever, if well-managed, requires dieting in any way, save the negative one of starvation, until its violence is abated."—*Hydropathic Encyclopedia*, Vol. I, p. 447. Again he says: "If you give food in the early stage of a fever, you do not feed the system, you only aggravate the fever. Why? Because the vital powers are so occupied in the remedial effort that they cannot digest or assimilate. That is why so many fever patients are *fed to death* by the nurses and doctors *** In fever it (the living system) cannot digest food."—*Jennings-Trall Debate*.

Fever indicates poisoning, usually decomposition in the intestines. It means that there is a mass of rotting food in the food tube poisoning the body. It means something else—namely: *nutrition is suspended until the poisoning is overcome.* It means that no food should be given to the patient until all fever and other symptoms are gone. It means that nothing but water, as demanded by thirst, should be given to the patient. So long as there is fever and diarrhea, no food, of whatever character, can be of any use to the body. If the patient appears to be hungry, it is thirst. Give him water, for food will not relieve the thirst.

The following quotation from Trall is to the point in this connection: "Food should not be taken at all until the violence of the fever is materially abated, and then very small quantities of the simplest food only should be permitted, as gruel, with a little toasted bread or cracker, boiled rice, mealy potatoes, baked apples, etc. There is not a more mischievous or more irrational error abroad in relation to the treatment of fever than the almost universal practice of stuffing the patient continually with stimulating slops, under the name of mild nourishing diet, beef tea, mutton broth, chicken soup, panada, etc. The fever will always starve out before the patient is injured by abstinence, at least under hydropathic treatment, and the appetite will always return when the system is capable of assimilating food."—*Hydropathic Encyclopedia*, Vol. II, p. 84

In speaking of the treatment of smallpox, Dr. Shew declared, *Hydropathic Family Physician*, p. 249: "Most fever patients are allowed to eat too much. Some may be allowed too little; but this must be the exception to the rule. In all severe fevers, the system absolutely refuses nourishment; that is, it is not digested or made into blood. Hence all nutriment in such cases is worse than useless, since if it does not go to nourish the system, it must only prove a source of irritation and harm. If the disease is severe, then it would be best as long as the fever lasts, to give no nourishment whatever. In mild cases it would of course be otherwise, although it would harm no one to fast a few days, but would, on the contrary, do them good. When nourishment is given, it should be some bland and anti-feverish kind. Good and well-ripened fruit in its season would be especially useful, taken always at the time of a regular meal."

TYPHOID

Typhoid fever patients become comfortable in three to four days if the fast is instituted at the outset of the "disease," and in from seven to ten days are convalescing. The patient will have such a comfortable sickness and recover so speedily that friends and relatives will declare he was not sick. And, indeed, he will not be very sick. It requires feeding and drugging to convert those simple natural processes we call acute *"diseases"* into serious and complicated troubles. It is not possible to have a typical case of typhoid fever, as described in allopathic text-books, without typical text-book treatment. Unthwarted nature never builds such complications and such serious "disease" as are described in allopathic works. All this mass of pathology is built by drugging, serum squirting and feeding.

In a voluminous work on diet, contributed to by a number of medical authorities in dietetics and edited by G. A. Sutherland, M.D., F.R.C.E., and entitled *A System of Diet and Dietetics* (published by the Physicians and Surgeons Book Co., of New York) I find a few interesting paragraphs in the chapter on *Diet In Fever and Acute Infectious Disease*, contributed by Claude E. Ker, M.D., F.R.C.P., Ed., which are worth quoting. He says, in discussing the "starvation treatment" in enteric fever (typhoid fever):

"The same idea which underlies the empty bowel theory is no doubt responsible for the attempts made to treat enteric fever with either no food by the mouth at all, or at the most with very little quantities. Thus Queirolo has recommended that feeding should be entirely rectal, a lemonade made up with a little hydrochloric acid being the only drink allowed, provided that the bowel of a patient so treated was first emptied by a dose of calomel, or other suitable purgative. Such method of dieting should secure complete rest for the affected parts and absolutely exclude the possibility of fermenting masses of partially digested material lying in the gut. The nutritive value, however, of rectal feeding in a prolonged disease is so limited that this method may be fairly regarded as a treatment by starvation.

"Similar in its objects and effects is the method suggested by Williams, who, believing that the exhausting diarrhea of the fever is due to improper feeding, endeavors to secure that the bowels shall, as far as possible, remain empty. Only water is allowed in severe cases, sometimes for days at a time, and he regards half a pint of milk in twenty-four hours as a liberal diet, seldom apparently exceeding this amount until the temperature is normal. The method seems drastic, but I have reason to know that the cases do remarkably well. I have often marvelled at the amount of starvation which a typhoid case can safely tolerate after a hemorrhage, and it is only rational to suppose that the patient would support starvation even better before such a depressing complication had occurred. Under such a regime Williams probably more nearly attains the ideal of the 'empty bowel' than any other observer. It seems almost incredible that patients so treated should occasionally gain weight and that they do not in any case waste more than patients more liberally fed; but it is, after all, obvious that, if food is not assimilated there is no benefit to be derived from it, and in many cases of enteric fever assimilation is undoubtedly extremely poor.

"The theoretical objection to both these methods of treatment is that, if ulceration has once started such a remarkably low diet would apparently give the intestinal lesions only a poor chance of repair. On the other hand, it is possible that the absence of irritation would go far to counterbalance this defect, apparently as the patient seems to stand the starvation so well. If plenty of water was supplied this would be more easily understood, but some of Williams' patients were limited, for a time at least, to one pint of water per diem, which seems to be a most inadequate amount."

Ker is unwilling to recommend what he mistakenly calls the "starvation treatment," but thinks there is much to be learned from such things and adds: "It encourages us to starve for two or three days, if necessary, severe cases with marked gastric and intestinal disturbances, probably very much to their advantage. It is, however, unnecessarily severe for the average patient, even while we admit that in enteric fever there is no certainty as to what may happen from day to day."

We have it stated that the exhausting diarrhea of typhoid is probably due to improper feeding.

We have it admitted that a "starvation treatment" seems complete rest for the affected parts of the intestine.

We have it admitted that typhoid patients may "starve" for days and make remarkable improvement during this time.

We have it admitted that they may do this even after a hemorrhage.

We also have it admitted that in this "disease" "assimilation is undoubtedly extremely poor." (It is so poor that there is none).

We have it admitted that "starvation" leaves no rotting food in the intestines to irritate and poison the inflamed and ulcerated intestinal wall.

Every one of these things, *Hygienists* have been pointing out for over a hundred years. We have been denounced as "quacks" and "ignorant pretenders" for so doing and our methods have been rejected by the medical profession as a whole, and, even now, the authorities, in adopting our methods in part, and in reporting favorably upon them, neglect to give credit where credit is plainly due. But Ker overlooks the important fact that where typhoid patients are not fed, ulceration is not likely to occur, and that hemorrhages are extremely rare, while he seems to be wholly unaware of the body's ability to heal wounds, broken bones, open sores, ulcers, etc., while fasting.

The theoretical objection offered to fasting, in enteric fever, is based on ignorance. It completely ignores the preceding statement that "assimilation is undoubtedly extremely poor," and it appears to be made in utter ignorance of the body's own internal resources. The author does not seem to be cognizant of the fact that repair of tissues does go on during a fast. What is more, he overlooks the fact that if feeding is stopped at the "onset" of the "*disease*" there is not likely to be any ulceration or any hemorrhage. Besides this, the patient is more comfortable and the "disease" of shorter duration—providing no drugging is resorted to. It is encouraging to note that he does not offer, as an objection, the old notion that fasting lowers one's resistance to germs.

The fault I find with the method of Queirolo is that he does not stop feeding at the *outset* instead of waiting until the "*disease*" becomes well developed and not that it is "too severe for the average patient." On the contrary, it is the easiest, safest and best plan. The feeding and drugging plan is the drastic plan; the plan that intensifies and prolongs the patient's suffering. It is no ordeal to do without food in acute illness. The ordeal consists in eating at such times. All we ask when acutely sick is to be let alone and to be free of worry of any kind.

PNEUMONIA

If fasting is instituted at the very outset in pneumonia, the patient will not be very sick, the exudate into the lungs will not be great and resolution will be hastened. Death in pneumonia will be very rare.

APPENDICITIS

All medical authorities admit the great value of fasting in appendicitis and recommend its employment, if the patient refuses an operation or, if for some other reason an operation is considered inadvisable. The pains of appendicitis practically cease after about three days of fasting.

RHEUMATISM

Page quotes Casey A. Wood, M.D., Professor of Chemistry in the Medical Department of Bishop's College, Montreal, in an article in the *Canada Medical Record*, entitled "Starvation in the treatment of Acute Articular Rheumatism," as giving the "history of seven cases where the patients were speedily restored to health by simply abstaining from food from four to eight days, and he says he could have given the history of forty more from his own practice." No drugs were used.

"In no case did this treatment fail." The cases reported "included men and women of different ages, temperaments, occupations, and social positions." Dr. Wood says: "From the quick and almost invariably good results to be obtained by simple abstinence from food, I am inclined to the idea that rheumatism is, after all, only a phase of indigestion." Dr. Page adds: "In chronic rheumatism he obtained less positive results, but did not venture to try fasts of longer duration." Dr. Wood concludes by saying that "this treatment, obviating as it does, almost entirely, danger of cardiac complications, will be bound to realize all that has been claimed for it—a simple, reliable remedy for a disease that has long baffled the physician's skill."

COUGHS

Most coughs can be stopped by a twenty-four to seventy-two hours fast; then, if the errors in eating are corrected, the cough is gone forever. Relief comes in the very worst cases of bronchial asthma in from twenty-four to seventy-two hours of fasting so that the sufferer can lie down and sleep in comfort.

DIARRHEA — DYSENTERY

Vomiting, restlessness, diarrhea and gross fatness are some of the symptoms of the *surfeit disease* and its proper care is, not soothing syrups, but fasting. Imagine feeding a patient who is having twenty to thirty bowel movements in twenty-four hours; or one that is vomiting frequently! Dysentery *medicines* may be entirely dispensed with if the sufferer will resort to fasting. Fasting in diarrhea is certainly better than the employment of *astringents* and *narcotics*, such as opium.

Oswald says: "For the incipient stages of the disorder the great specific is *fasting*. Denutrition or the temporary deprivation of food, exercises an astringent influence, as part of its general constructive effect. The organism, stinted in the supply of its vital resources, soon begins to curtail its current expenditure. The movements of the respiratory process decrease; the temperature of the body sinks, the secretion of bile and uric acid is diminished, and before long the retrenchments of the assimilative process react on the functions of the intestinal organs; the colon contracts, and the smaller intestines retain all but the most irritating ingesta."

WASTING BY THE ACUTELY ILL DESPITE FEEDING

Dewey emphasized the fact that the body of the acutely ill always wastes, no matter what he is fed nor how much. Indeed, he insisted that in typhoid and other severe fevers, the patient that is fed wastes most. This fact that in acute disease wasting goes on whether food is eaten or not, and that in fact, it is frequently true that the more the patient is fed, the greater the wasting, shows unmistakably that no food is absorbed and used during acute illness. Certainly, if it cannot be digested, it will not be absorbed and if it is not absorbed, it will not be assimilated, and if it is not assimilated, it can do the patient no good.

Ker believes in feeding to "keep up the strength of the patient," as do all "orthodox" medical men. Feeding in acute "disease" does not keep up strength and does not prevent the wasting of the patient. "In all acute diseases," says Dr. Dewey, "in which there is a high pulse and temperature, pain or discomfort, aversion to food, a foul, dry mouth and tongue, thirst, etc., wasting of the body goes on no matter what the feeding, until a clear, moist tongue and mouth and hunger mark the close of the disease, when food can be taken with relish and digested. This makes it clearly evident that we cannot save the muscles and fat by feeding under these adverse conditions."

The wasted bodies of patients who have been fed through acute illness is the strongest kind of evidence, to those who are capable of seeing, that the food they were fed was not digested and assimilated, and that their own tissues were drawn upon to provide the materials necessary to carry on the processes of life. We may go a step further and say that in practically every instance the wasting will be greater and the *"disease"* will be of longer duration if the patient is fed than if he is fasted. Liek says: "From my observations on children and animals, I have come to the conclusion that, particularly in acute diseases, fasting greatly favors the process of healing."

If the food eaten is not digested, of what value can it be to the sick man or woman? A two hundred pound man may become sick with typhoid fever. He will loose weight no matter how much he is fed, until, when he is well, he is but a shadow of his former self. In fact, the more he is fed the sicker he becomes, the more prolonged his illness, and the more he will lose in weight. What more conclusive evidence is needed to prove that the food eaten does harm and not good? What is true of typhoid is also true of other "diseases."

WEAKNESS

Weakness in *acute "disease"* is not properly attributed to the fast. Indeed, the fasting patient will not become as weak as the eating patient. He is more likely to grow stronger as the fast progresses. I am pleased to present the following *orthodox* testimony, on this point, by Dr. Liek, who says: "Those who are sick feel weak. Those who have been operated upon and who wake up from the narcosis are greatly enfeebled. According to the text books, we can overcome that weakness with strengthening food. Nothing is more obvious. Hence, we inquire for the most nourishing and strengthening foods and give them to patients. That idea is, of course, completely mistaken. The patient has been weakened not by a short fast, but by the disease, by the after-effects of the narcosis, the shock of the operation, etc." It should be obvious that the weaker the patient is, the less able is he to take and digest nourishment. The weaker he is the greater is the need for rest.

Fasting in Chronic Disease

CHAPTER XXXV

Nobody who thoroughly understands fasting, harbors any doubts about its possibilities and limitations. Most people who have voluntarily resorted to fasting for recovery from chronic illness, have done so as a last resort. They are usually in a very bad condition before they consent to fast. That the results have been so great, when we consider the type of patients that fast, is remarkable. That there are those who fast with only meager results must be expected, from the fact that so many of those who consent to fast are nearing death at the time. Fasting does not enable the body to accomplish miracles. But ninety-five per cent of chronic sufferers may undergo a properly supervised fast wtih every hope of good results.

DIETING VERSUS FASTING

A light diet, such as the eliminating diet, is offered as a substitute for fasting, particularly in chronic *"disease."* While we employ such diets quite often and recognize their value and utility, they are not the equal of the fast. One difficulty with them lies in the fact that the patient eats just enough food to keep his appetite alive, but not enough to satisfy it. My experience with fasting and light eating, and so-called "fruit fasts" has been the same as that of Sinclair's; namely, that the light eating is just enough to keep one ravenous, whereas on the fast all desire for food soon ceases. He also says that on the "fruit fasts" he would get so weak he could not stand up— "far weaker than I ever became on an out-and-out fast." In many cases, a fruit diet following a short fast, causes the patient to feel weaker than during the fast.

Many of those who freely employ fasting in *acute "disease,"* when there is no power to digest food, and no demand for food, object to fasting in *chronic "disease,"* where there still exists more or less digestive power and an appetite, even though morbid. For example, Dr. Kritzer cautions against fasting where there is a strong abnormal craving for food, due to gastric disorder. He thinks the mental process involved in the suppression of such a strong craving is unwholesome, that it produces a general tension which is not conducive to elimination. It may even contribute to the manufacture of new toxins, for, at best, there is an increase of acids in the system during the fast with corresponding lessening in the alkalinity of the blood which normally bathes the tissues."

Continuing, he says, "Fasting is not indicated in the treatment of chronic diseases. On the contrary, such patients should be dieted on foods rich in organic salts until their semi-starved tissues become revitalized and capable of promoting better tissue changes—metabolism." I need hardly discuss these statements at this place as they are sufficiently answered in preceding pages. They are based on mistaken notions about chemistry changes in the body during the fast and on psychological half-truths that are the present vogue. The value of fasting is too well-established to be overthrown by these fallacies.

Dr. Kellogg says: "It is true, as above admitted, that during a prolonged fast, any surplus of protein which may be present, may be used up and accumulated tissue wastes may be lessened in amount. But the amount of such accumulation is too small to justify the expensive method adopted by the faster for their elimination. The faster, in order to free himself of three pounds of waste or undesirable material, sacrifices an amount of healthy and useful tissue ten times as great. Why should one throw away thirty pounds of good muscle, brain, nerve, heart and other useful, vital machinery, in order to get rid of three pounds of waste material, which can be easily gotten rid of by simply restricting the diet and increasing the intake of water?" If restricted eating and water gluttony could do what fasting does, perhaps there would be no need for a fast in chronic cases. But the restricted eating seldom accomplishes these—perhaps never produces all of the benefits of fasting. Fasting accomplishes more than the mere removal of a possible three pounds of excess protein.

LOST APPETITE

A horse does not have to be acutely ill to be "off his feed." A cow does not have to be acutely sick to refuse food. I have watched sick cows straggling along in the rear of the herd, not sick enough to stay off their feet, but refusing food. A dog or a cat may refuse food because of a slight indisposition. In man we frequently observe a lack of desire for food when there is discomfort and distress in the abdomen or when there is a headache, even though there is no suggestion of acute illness. Indeed, one of the most common complaints of the chronic sufferer is this: "I have lost my appetite." Frequently the complaint takes this form: "I eat, but I do not enjoy my food." Another very common complaint is: "'Everything I eat turns to gas." Others complain of suffering after every meal. As often as not the chronic sufferer is more interested in regaining his appetite than in getting well of his relatively mild symptoms.

Physicians commonly prescribe *tonics* and *digestants* for these patients and urge them to "eat plenty of good nourishing food." They prescribe their drugs with the deliberate intention of whipping up a jaded appetite into renewed vigor, foolishly calling this *curing* the patient of lost appetite. When a patient is heard to complain that "nothing tastes good," we may be sure that he is in need of a fast. He will usually attempt, by the employment of seasonings, condiments, sweetenings, etc., which he adds to his foods, to make them taste good to him, but he also fails in this attempt. Nothing will as surely and as speedily restore the desire for food and the pleasures of eating as a fast. Just as sexual abstinence is the surest and best *aphrodisiac,* so abstinence from food is the best *appetizer.*

PLENTY OF GOOD NOURISHING FOOD

" 'Nourishment!' " is the prevailing cry of those who would cure us," says Adolph Just in his *Return to Nature;* " 'you need more nourishment!' But how can a body be nourished when it is incapable of absorbing, and especially incapable of expelling, that which has already been stuffed into it? The fact is that in nearly every instance the sufferer to whom more nourishment is recommended is one who is already brought low by excessive nourishment—he is actually pining through over plus!" These patients are not only incapable of absorbing, but, also, of digesting food. How foolish, to give more food when it cannot be digested, absorbed and assimilated! Not more food, but more ability to assimilate and excrete, is needed and this must be first provided through rest, fasting and hygiene before food is to be thought of.

How foolish to insist on feeding under conditions of an already existing plethora! Why insist on "plenty of good nourishing food" under conditions in which food cannot be digested and assimilated? Nature knows full well how to guard and protect and this is the meaning of the lack of desire for food, nausea, vomiting, distress after eating and other symptoms of protest. When digestion has been pushed and "stimulants" and drugs have been given for the purpose of forcing a reluctant appetite, we only add more burden to an already overtaxed organism. Fasting may here be used to best advantage. If the feeding person finds himself growing sicker, with frequent diarrhea and vomiting, with occasional nausea and constipation, and loss of appetite, with, perhaps, headache, coated tongue, foul taste and breath, he certainly needs a fast and if he had not lost his ability to interpret the language of his senses, he would need no urging to get him to fast. Why must man eat "from obvious necessity" when food is repugnant? How disgusting to persuade one to eat food knowing that it will be vomited immediately!

FEAR OF FASTING UNFOUNDED

The thin and weak individual, knowing little or nothing of fasting, may be excused for his fear of fasting, but the plethoric and overweight individual certainly cannot be excused. The bear eats heartily of nuts, honey, fruits, flesh, etc., while these are plentiful, and puts on a great store of fat with which to sustain his body during the winter season. The frog also stores up considerable fat for this occasion. There are hundreds of thousands of men and women who carry greater stores of fat than the bear or frog, who imagine that if they miss so much as a single meal they will begin to grow weak. They carry sufficient fat and other food reserves to last them for weeks and even months. They could fast for prolonged periods, not only without harm to themselves, but with positive benefit. Thin people also carry a reserve supply and may safely fast for considerable periods if they are properly supervised.

STARVATION FROM OVER-FEEDING

Great numbers of the chronic sufferers who habitually over-eat are very thin and grow progressively thinner with the passage of time. Indeed, one frequently hears them remark: "the more I eat the thinner I get." How true it is that they are slowly starving from over-consumption of food which they cannot digest. Dr. Dewey frequently speaks of the "starvation of over-feeding." Dr. King-Chambers spoke of the "starvation of over-repletion." Drs. Page and Rabagliati use similar expressions. Fasting literature is full of records of cases that had been suffering while surfeiting and who recovered health through fasting, regaining their normal weight when eating was resumed.

FICTIONAL DESIRE FOR FOOD

Many chronic sufferers think they are ravenous. They feel that their supposed desire for food should be satisfied. There is a great mass of chronic sufferers who eat three square meals and two lunches a day and are "always hungry." They say that they become "very weak" if they miss a meal. Others eat all through the day and several times at night. They are never satisfied. These people, over-looking or never having known that bad habits will in the end dominate and pervert our instincts, believe that their fictional demands for food are valid and should be gratified. These people are never actually hungry. They are food drunkards. They suffer from neuroses. Their troubles have grown out of habitual over-eating. Dr. Page says of such patients: "So inveterate is this mania for eating, even when to continue is like turning coals upon the dead ashes and clinkers of an expired fire, that, in ordinary practice, it is well nigh impossible to induce any class of patients to abstain from food at the beginning of an attack or to give the fasting cure a fair trial at any stage of the disease."

UNDIGESTED FOOD IN THE STOMACH

It is not unusual, in certain cases of indigestion, to have food remain in the stomach two or three days. Beaumont found that food taken in certain morbid states "remains undigested for twenty-four or forty-eight hours, or even more, increasing the derangement of the whole alimentary canal, and aggravating the general symptoms of the disease." He points out that all of this prolonged retention of undigested food in the stomach is often without discomfort or pain of some sort and without the patient's knowledge that it is present. Many *Hygienists* have observed this same phenomenon. For example, Carrington says that he has seen cases where food was ejected from the stomach three days after it was eaten. The food was thus lying in the stomach for seventy-two hours without being digested. He says of one of these cases that the man was not conscious that there was anything wrong with his stomach. An amazing amount of pathology often exists in the stomach of those who regard themselves as healthy and as possessing good digestion. These patients habitually mistake the morbid sensations of their stomach for hunger.

Carrington says that "the fact that food frequently remains in the stomach of quite light eaters when they are indisposed, and 'out of condition,' is certain." It should also be noted that emotional upsets will suspend the process of digestion and cause food to be retained for prolonged periods in the stomach. Rabagliati says: "Indeed, food is occasionally, or even not infrequently, still in the stomach twenty-four, thirty-six, and even forty-eight hours after it has been taken." Carrington tells us that he has known of cases in which large quantities of food were vomited at the end of three days of fasting. I have seen a number of such cases in my own practice. I think that it must be admitted, to use Carrington's words, that it "would be a common sense procedure to wait until this mass of rubbish was removed before again adding food." It is quite obvious that stomach digestion is not going on in these instances and that the food is rotting rather than digesting.

A young man once visited me who complained of headaches, catarrh of the stomach and nose and throat, hyperacidity of the stomach, constipation and nervousness. He was extremely ravenous, but could digest nothing he ate. A few days before coming to see me he had arrived home from work with an almost irresistible desire for food. He ate a hearty supper and started for the Y.M.C.A., where he was to play in a basketball game. About six blocks from his home he suddenly became dizzy; everything became black and he fainted. This was followed by vomiting, which brought up not only his supper, but food he had consumed at noon the day before. It had not been digested. I placed this man on a short fast, then taught him how to live, with the result that his catarrh, hyperacidity, indigestion, constipation, headache, nervousness and morbid appetite all ended.

Physiologists say that an ordinary meal is digested (in the stomach) in from two to five hours. That this is the normal digestion time may be nearly true, but it is no unusual thing for food to remain in the stomach for a much longer period. This is especially true if there is some slight indisposition. Physiologists have assumed that if the food has passed out of the stomach into the intestine it has been digested—that is, it is assumed that gastric digestion is completed. That this is often not true is shown by the great amounts of undigested food that are found in the stools of thousands of patients. The stomach may empty itself of undigested and unwanted food, either by vomiting or by passing it on to the intestine. I wish here to revert to the contention of Dr. Hazzard that while "appetite" may be present in disease, genuine hunger never is. While such patients often insist that they are ravenous, it seems more likely that in every instance, they have mistaken their morbid symptoms for a demand for food.

INSTINCTIVE EATING

There have been men who approved of fasting in acute disease, but not in chronic disease, on the ground that so long as nature demands food, food should be taken. They have insisted upon being guided by instinct in this matter of eating or fasting. The demand for instinctive eating, instinctive fasting and instinctive living is quite fundamentally sound, but we must learn to discriminate between instinctive demands and morbid cravings. Morbid cravings are strengthened, not overcome, by appeasing them. Take the case of the patient previously mentioned, who was ravenous, ate a meal and shortly thereafter, vomited this along with food that had been consumed at noon the day before; how can we think of his supposed desire for food as an instinctive demand? It seems the height of absurdity to contend that appetite, such as he had before he ate supper that evening, should be satisfied. To me such contentions are on a par with the claim that the craving for opium, alcohol, tobacco, arsenic, etc., should be satisfied.

NATURE ACCEPTS THE FAST

In *chronic "disease"* digestion is not suspended. In many cases it seems not to be impaired. Appetite may and may not be present. There is not, therefore, the same necessity for fasting in *chronic "disease"* as in *acute "disease."* Yet, if the fast is entered into, nature usually signifies her willingness to undergo a long deferred fast, which she has probably repeatedly asked for but did not receive, by cutting off the appetite on the second or third day and perhaps by developing nausea, vomiting and repugnance to food, and by instituting the usual processes of elimination. As this course of action is invariably pursued by nature, we are forced to conclude that she welcomes the proffered opportunity for house cleaning.

ELIMINATION

Due to many causes waste accumulates during the entire life period of the body. The older the body and the more gluttony and sensuality have been indulged in, the greater the toxin saturation. These toxins are lost to the body during a fast. It is largely for this reason that fasting proves to be so valuable in *chronic "disease."*

The purification of the organism and the regeneration of its tissues restore the youthfulness of the body.

Dr. Lindlahr likened the digestive tract to a sponge. In health it absorbs the elements of nutrition; but in acute disease the process is reversed; the sponge is being squeezed and it throws off toxins. When the sponge is being squeezed the processes of digestion and absorption are at a standstill. In fact, as he said, the entire organism, in acute disease, is in a state of weakness, prostration and inactivity. The vital energies are concentrated upon the work of cleansing the body of its accumulated toxins. I need only to add that in chronic disease, when the patient fasts, the whole digestive tract enters upon the work of elimination and assists in freeing the body of its accumulated toxins.

PHYSIOLOGICAL REST

"Rest and fasting constitute the *proper treatment* of those suffering from overwork, overeating and sexual excesses." It should be obvious that when energy is low and functions are inefficient, a period of physiological rest will be beneficial. When the digestive function is so badly impaired that every meal is followed with gas or with nausea or when undigested food remains in the stomach for prolonged periods, a rest of the digestive system is imperative. Mr. Carrington, who insists upon the necessity of resting in disease, places greatest stress upon rest of the digestive system.

After pointing out that loss of appetite, seen in all acute diseases and common in chronic disease, is "the voice of nature forbidding us to eat," and lamenting the fact that physicians and nurses disregard this "voice of nature" and force food down the throats of "disgusted patients," Dr. T. L. Nichols says, "rest for the stomach, liver, all the organs of the nutritive system, may be the one thing needful. It is the only rest we will not permit. – In certain states of disease, where the organs of digestion are weakened and disordered, the best beginning of a cure may be total abstinence for a time from all kinds of food. There is no cure like it. If the stomach cannot digest, the best way is to give it a rest. It is the one thing which it needs." He also says, "for every disease of every organ of the body, the first condition is rest—rest for stomach, rest for brain. Broken bones and cut or torn muscles, must have rest, or there can be no cure. For the vital organs there must be, at least, diminished labor—intervals of rest—all the repose that is consistent with the necessary operations of life. In disease of the heart, we must diminish the amount of the circulating fluid, and remove all stimulants and excitements to action. It is chiefly through the stomach and nutritive system that we can act on the heart and brain, the more rest we can give to the stomach, the more chance."

When organs have been lashed into impotency by overwork and over-stimulation, rest alone can save, it alone can restore power. Dewey referred to fasting as the "rest cure," and emphasized the urgent necessity of rest in all acute and chronic diseases. Rest, he said, "is not to do any of the curing (healing) any more than it heals the broken bone or the wound; it is only going to furnish the condition for cure." By rest in this statement, he is referring to physiological rest. Using up nerve energy in business and the general affairs of life to the extent of having too little to take care of the food we eat is common in present-day society and is commonly met with increased food consumption, rather than by the physical and physiological rest the condition demands. If we are sick we "need plenty of good nourishing food"; if we are weak we need "more food." If we are tired and "out of sorts," we need "more food."

Sinclair went upon his first fast when, "after another spell of hard work I found myself unable to digest corn-meal mush and milk." He took a fast when nature compelled him to do so. The common mode of caring for the body in health and *"disease"* is a tragedy. It consists of eating food several times a day, of employing *stimulants* to whip up fatigued organs until they are exhausted, of yielding to indulgencies, and dissipations that waste the energies and substances of the body; of whipping into submission any and all organs and functions which attempt to correct matters; of cutting out offended organs and structures which are the seat of discomfort; and of neglecting any and all rational and radically remedial measures until some parts of the organism have become so badly damaged and the organic destruction is so great that recovery is all but impossible.

RELIEF OF PAIN

Fasting not only brings absolute comfort to those who have a fatal "disease," but it brings comfort in every other "disease," cuts all "diseases" short, and gives the sick man or woman the very best opportunity and the surest road out of suffering into health. Dr. Shew wrote: "Very seldom will toothache withstand twenty-four hours of entire abstinence from all food."—*Water cure in Pregnancy and Childbirth*, p. 63. Again, he wrote: "If a person has a toothache—no matter how bad—provided there is not swelling and ague in the face, it is cured with certainty within twenty-four hours by abstaining from all food and from all drinks, except water. At any rate, I have known no case where such treatment has failed of complete success." —*Family Physician*, p. 796.

PLEASURES OF THE PRACTITIONER

Dr. Arthur Vos grows poetic in his praise of the benefits of fasting in *chronic "disease."* He says : "I can conceive of no greater pleasure in the pursuit of my profession; than to witness a patient suffering from a chronic disease, gradually regaining his health under the administration of a fast and the application of proper dietetic and hygienic procedures. Though some patients have considerable distress during the first few days of a fast, the later feelings of buoyance and freedom of pain, both mentally and physically, make them willing to continue a method against which their prejudices at first strongly rebelled. To see the clouded eye clear up and regain its igneous brightness, to see the zanthically discolored parchment-like skin clear itself and become normally peaches and cream, to perceive the breath, at first heavily laden with unmentionable impurities, gradually lose its nauseous odor and become attar of roses, to experience the joys of fellowship that come back again with the correct mental attitude and a sane view of life, displacing the old, intoxicated, perverted and disjointed attitude toward the world and one's fellowmen, from the enjoyment of witnessing which neither struggle nor effort ought to deter. These devoutly-to-be-wished-for benefits and consummations and a thousand other patronymics come as the effects of a fast performed and properly conducted, provided, of course, subsequent treatment is carried on in a manner to continue the benefits received. This can be done by correcting the life through the application of the principles of hygiene and natural living."—*Fasting*, June, 1923.

SOME "ORTHODOX" TESTIMONY

Asclepiades used fasting 2,000 years ago, as did Thessalus of Tralles; Celsus employed fasting in jaundice and epilepsy; Avicenna used to fast his patients four or five weeks. Even Paracelsus declared, "Fasting is the greatest remedy." In the 17th Century, Dr. Hoffman wrote a treatise on fasting entitled *"Description of the Magnificent*

Results Obtained Through Fasting in All Diseases." In the 18th century, Dr. Anton Nikolai asked: "What is more sense, to feed the patient and give him medicine and keep him sick for the rest of his life, or make him thin for a while and make him absolutely well?"

Dr. Von Seeland, a Russian physician, says: "As a result of experiments, I have come to the conclusion that fasting is not only a therapeutic agent of the highest degree possible but also deserves consideration educationally." Dr. Adolph Mayer, a prominent German physician, says, in a book entitled *Fast Cures–Wondercures*: "I assert that fasting is the most efficient means for correcting any disease." He also asserts that "Fasting and surgery is all that is of any value in the professional armamentarium." Dr. Moeller, head of the sanatorium "Closchwitz," says, "fasting is the only natural evolutionary method whereby through a systemic cleansing you can restore yourself by degrees to physiologic normality." Dr. Osbeck, of Upsala, Professor of Surgery, was so successful with fasting treatments that the government ordered them investigated, and upon receipt of a favorable report from the committee, gave him a bonus of $5,000 and a yearly pension of $500. Fasting is now employed in several European sanatoriums, both in England and on the continent.

A FEW DISEASES CONSIDERED
When we see the eyes become brighter, the skin fairer and the breath sweeter from fasting, when we see pimples on the face clear up and not recur thereafter, when we observe all the other evidences of benefit to be derived from a period of abstinence, we are naturally encouraged to go on with our work in the more complicated states of the organism. It is a great mistake to expect one long fast to always be sufficient to enable the body to free itself of all of its accumulated debris. When we spend a lifetime piling up injuries in the body and storing up toxin, we cannot expect to always repair all of these injuries and excrete all of the retained waste in the short space of a few weeks, but we can repeat the fast where this is needed. It is not intended here to do more than consider a few so-called diseases, as object lessons in the use of the fast, as these are covered in greater number in Vol. VII of this series.

Denutrition or temporary abstinence from food, is the most effective, and, at the same time, the safest method for eliminating morbid elements from the system. Any flux, issue, diarrhea, bronchorrhea, dropsy, flow of fluid into the pleura (sac around the lungs), pericardium (sac around the heart), peritoneum (lining of the abdominal cavity) water on the brain, flow of pus from any chronic suppuration, polyuria, and others—any disturbance of the fluids of the body—is favorably influenced by total abstinence from food and water. All catarrhal conditions—rhinitis, ozena, bronchitis, colitis, metritis, cystitis, hay fever, asthma, and other catarrhal conditions—quickly cease to exist under a fast. When the abnormal flow of fluid is controlled, a proper dietary can be fitted to the body; and when impaired nerve-energy—enervation—is brought back to normal, health is restored.

Every meal eaten, every glass of milk or fluid drunk, raises blood-pressure. Every transfusion of blood raises blood-pressure. When people are sick with catarrh and nose bleeding, or tuberculosis and bleeding from the lungs, or tuberculosis of the bowels with diarrhea, etc., they should stop the intake of water and food, and the hemorrhage will surely cease within twenty-four hours. Then restricted eating should be practiced until hyperemia from plethory is overcome, after which, proper eating and respecting food limitations will bring dependable health.

The editor of an osteopathic journal, an ex-druggist, who still believes in drugs and particularly believes in their use in so-called syphilis, wrote Dr. Alvin N. Davis, of Pa., that Dr. Weger rejects fasting in the conditions labeled syphilis. In reply to a letter to him about the matter, Dr. Weger wrote to me, saying, "I certainly do fast syphilitics." The authenticated long fast of Ulrich Von Hutten, which was followed by an absolute and openly attested *cure* of "syphilis," is known to all students of medical history. This treatment of so-called "syphilis" found many zealous champions later on. The value of fasting in the conditions labeled "syphilis is beyond dispute. Nothing is more effective in the so-called primary and secondary stages. It is valuable also in the tertiary stage; but as this stage is due to drugs, its value is often less apparent. The truth of these things is not impaired by the failure of some individual to employ fasting in such conditions.

Tilden says: "Something more is necessary, however, than simply fasting to overcome and bring about absorption of a fibroid tumor. The proper local treatments for correcting uterine derangement and establishing proper nutrition are absolutely necessary in all cases, if dependable health is to be hoped for." This has not been our experience and we do not approve of the *scarification* and other local treatment employed by him. The wen is a cyst. Graham mentions seeing wens remedied by fasting. I have no desire to dispute this observation, for I have myself seen a very few such pathologies remedied by fasting. What I do want to point out, however, is that this is a rare occurrence. Commonly wens and other cysts are not much affected by the fast. Tilden was of this same opinion, saying that there is but one treatment for wens and this is surgical removal. Dr. Weger's observations led him to the same conclusion.

Dewey, Hazzard, Carrington, Macfadden and others record cases of recoveries from diabetes through fasting, before Allen made his experiments and gave the "Allen treatment" to the medical world.

All observers, who have had wide experience with fasting, record cases of improvement of eyesight while fasting, even an occasional case of blindness in which sight is restored. Often, hearing that has been faint for years, is brought up to the acuteness of childhood. In other cases complete deafness is remedied. I had one case of complete blindness in one eye that had existed for several years, in which complete and permanent recovery occurred during a fast undertaken to reduce weight. Another case was one of total deafness in one ear that had existed for twenty-five years. Perfect hearing in this ear was restored during a fast of more than thirty days, undertaken to remedy other troubles. So many pathological changes in the eyes and ears and their associated nerve and brain structures may result in blindness and deafness, it would be folly to expect vision and hearing to be restored in all cases of blindness and deafness. Such recoveries are not to be expected as a regular occurrence.

Carrington says: "lung tissue seems to possess the inherent power of healing itself in a far shorter time, and more effectually, than any other organ which may be diseased. I have repeatedly observed that, in all cases where a fast has been undertaken, in order to cure lung troubles of any description, such fasts have always terminated more speedily and more satisfactorily than in other cases; and such fasts are also undertaken far more easily, and the deprivation and lack of food noticed even less, in such cases, than in any other cases whatever."

He adds that cases of tuberculosis of the lungs are likely to collapse more or less frequently, when they fast, an extreme degree of debility being noted. This, he thinks is due to three chief factors:

The real condition of the tubercular is one of debility, but the condition is not apparent, due to the pressure of tonics and stimulants and to the over-feeding to which they are regularly subjected—over-feeding on meats, eggs, milk, and other stimulating foods. The real condition of the patient becomes apparent when the stimulants and the foods are withdrawn, the reaction being severe in proportion to the degree of debility. "The great sense of freedom which is experienced in the lungs, and the ability to talk and sing with greater clearness and facility, and with greater range and depth of tone, than has been experienced, perhaps, in months and years, will amply testify that the lungs are far sounder and more normal than they have been—perhaps ever!"—*Vitality, Fasting and Nutrition*, p. 497.

Short fasts are commonly employed in tuberculosis. It should be noted, however, that an amazing number of people are constantly under treatment for tuberculosis who do not have the disease. I once had a case of what I shall call "pseudo-tuberculosis" of the lungs to get well in a week. This case presented the following symptoms upon which the diagnosis had been made—weakness, loss of weight, habitual cough, night sweats, afternoon temperature, "positive" sputum and "spots" on the lungs, as revealed by x-ray. Several physicians had concurred in the diagnosis. Another similar case, which had been under treatment for tuberculosis for four years, growing steadily worse, completely recovered in six weeks.

Some of the most remarkable recoveries it has been my privilege to witness have been in cases of "incurable" heart disease. There are irremediable damages to the heart, but it does not always follow, because some physician has pronounced a given case of heart disease "incurable," that it is really irremediable. Fasting in heart disease is a sure means of giving the heart a rest. Eating places a load upon the heart. Overeating needlessly increases this burden. Fasting relieves the heart of the excess load it is carrying and provides an opportunity for rest.

Every day people die of "heart attack" or "heart failure" who are eating three square meals a day with extra food between meals. Often these deaths follow immediately upon the heels of a hearty meal, or occur while the sufferer is eating. If "plenty of good nourishing food" will prevent heart collapse, or will assist in the "cure" of heart disease, these patients should not die so regularly. The simple truth is that very few sufferers from heart disease, be they doctor or layman, fail to note from experience that their comforts depend to a great extent upon what and how much they eat. Heart "attacks," from simple acceleration and palpitation to the severe anginas, are in the great majority of instances, due to over-loading, fermentation, distention of stomach, and indigestion.

FASTING IN NERVOUS DISEASES

In many quarters there exists a strange prejudice against the employment of the fast in what are called "nervous diseases." It is customary to recommend a "full diet" in both nervous and mental diseases. This plan of care is far from satisfactory, but it is persisted in with a slavish adherence that would do justice to a better cause. This practice grows in great measure, out of the tendency to set the brain and nervous system apart from the remainder of the body and to think of it as not physical. There is the classification of diseases into "mental" and "physical" which grows out of this effort to think of the brain and nervous system as separate and distinct from the organism as a whole. But a moment's reflection should be sufficient to reveal the error of this view.

The human body is one vastly complex organism, the many parts of which are intimately connected and correlated in their functions and interdependencies. It is essential that we fully grasp the intricate interrelations of all parts of the organism before we can make any real progress in the science and art of caring for the well and the sick. The organs of the body are not isolated isonomies. Due to the close unity of the body it is utterly impossible for any one part of the body to become impaired without involving the whole organism in the consequences and impossible for any part to be impaired (except by violence) so long as it receives adequate support from its physiological partners. Parts of the body become impaired only after there is more or less general impairment. Organs do not become "diseased" independently of the rest of the organism.

In what way do "nervous" diseases differ from "physical" diseases? The nerves are also physical. They are parts of the body. They are not so completely removed from the physical as popular expressions seem to imply. They are neither ethereal, nor mental, nor spiritual in essence, and they do not call for non-physical means of care. They are organs and should be looked at from the organic point of view. Basically, nerve fibers are not greatly different from muscle fibers. Nerves are supplied with blood, they must have oxygen, food, and water; they are capable of being cut and torn by violence, or poisoned by toxins of various kinds.

The brain and nervous system are subject to the same laws of organization as is the rest of the body, are subject to the same nutritive requirements and are subject to poisoning, as well as are the muscles and glands. The nervous tissue may become inflamed, it may undergo atrophy. Its condition, strength, power and functioning ability depend wholly upon the composition, purity and quality of the blood with which it is supplied.

Another reason that we tend to think of and treat the nerves and brain as though they are separate and distinct from the general organism is the almost universal error of the medical profession, an error in which they have fully indoctrinated the lay public, of trying to treat one part of the body without reference to all other parts— an error that has given rise to all the evils of specialism. A full recognition of the unity of the body should cause this error to be rejected. The effects of over-eating upon nervous diseases are readily apparent to all who will take the trouble to observe them. Likewise, the benefits that flow from fasting in nervous and mental diseases have only to be observed to be appreciated. "The extreme rapid and invariably successful results at once prove the correctness of the contention," says Carrington.

It is usual for an increased nervous irritability to manifest when the mental and nervous patient is not fed, hence the advice to "feed him up." But this stuffing treatment only serves to smother symptoms, not to remove their causes. It is significant that when food is withheld for a few days, the nervous storm that ensues upon discontinuance of food, subsides and the patient progresses healthward. The remarkable manner in which attention, memory, association and the ability to reason with more than ordinary brilliance are acutened during a fast indicates as nothing else can, the benfits the brain derives from a period of physiological rest. Recoveries from insanity while fasting are equally dramatic evidence of this benefit.

Macfadden and Carrington relate the case of a man who had a paralyzed throat who fasted for ten days when "signs of life" appeared in the throat. He found he could again swallow and within a few days, the full power of his throat was restored. "Though in some cases," they say, "through the influence of fasting the blind have literally been made to see, the lame to walk, I feel that this case was perhaps one of the most remarkable of all with which I have come in contact." Fasting and prayer were prominent among the remedies employed by the ancients in epilepsy. Dr. Rabagliati says that the best remedy for epilepsy "consists of a careful restriction of the diet. *** I have for many years now advised restriction of the diet in epilepsy to two meals daily, and sometimes to one; and in acute cases have recommended further and great restriction to a pint or a pint and a half of milk daily for a considerable period of time. *** Fasting, in fact, seems to be of very great efficacy in the treatment of epilepsy."

The length of the fast in any condition will have to be determined by each individual case. In most cases, except tuberculosis, there can be no sound objection to a fast to completion, although this will seldom be necessary, and many patients will not want to fast so long, unless they must. The case should be carefully watched and the judgement of the experienced practitioner followed.

Fasting in Drug Addiction

CHAPTER XXXVI

Any form of drug addiction is an unintelligent seeking for "relief." Those who are comfortable seek no *soothing* poisons. Restless bodies and irritable nerves are *soothed*, often with the very occasion for the restlessness and irritability. The coffee user "relieves" her headache with more of the coffee that induced her headache in the first place. The morphine addict *soothes* his damaged nerves with more of the morphine that is responsible for their damage. There is no drug-hunger, no craving for a poison of any kind, as is popularly supposed to exist in the victims of drug habits. The supposed craving for poison of any kind is a peculiar and unbearable *nervousness* arising out of exhaustion and injury. It is not a loud call for more stimulation (irritation) or more narcotization (depression)—nor yet a call for more poisoning, more injury, greater exhaustion—but a cry of distress. The real need is rest and a cessation of abuse. The "relief" that follows the repetition of the poison-dose is fictional and unreal.

Addicts take their beer and tobacco to *soothe* their distressed nerves. They feel weak and faint without them. They are just as weak and faint with them, but they are unconscious of the fact. The drug merely temporarily wipes out their awareness of their true condition. A man becomes irritable and cranky when denied his tobacco. The irritableness and crankiness are merely part of his general uneasiness—an uneasiness that has grown out of and is perpetuated by his habitual poisoning of himself. That temporary respite from a sense of weakness and uneasiness, that temporary "relief" from misery and pain may be had from a re-narcotization of the nerves that are suffering from prior narcotization, leads the poor victim of the poison-vice to believe that his misery is a *craving* for his accustomed poison. This all adds up to the fact that the drug habit is the "relief" habit. Many drugs are said to be habit-forming. It is not the drug, but man that forms the habit. Man is, indeed, a habit-forming animal. For whatever reason he first takes the poison, he later takes it habitually as a means of escape from his intolerable suffering.

Nothing enables the alcoholic, the drug fiend, the tobacco addict, to overcome his "desire" for his accustomed poison and to return to a state of good health, as does fasting. To fully realize the truth of this statement, one needs merely to view the whiskey-sodden body of the drunkard before fasting and the fresh renewed body of the same person after a fast. In his whole countenance, from the sparkle in his eyes and the ruddiness of his cheeks to the pink glow of his renewed skin, and his whole demeanor, from the buoyant step to the gay spirits, the man has undergone a complete and thorough renovation and regeneration. Few drunkards have sufficient will power and physical stamina to abandon drink without help and nothing affords them greater and more certain assistance than the fast.

Dewey seems to have been the first to call attention to the great value of fasting in alcoholism. His book, *Chronic Alcoholism*, first published in 1899, is devoted to this subject, although he emphasized the value of fasting in this abnormality in his other and earlier works. Subsequent writers have also stressed the value of fasting in alcoholism. In his *Vitality, Fasting and Nutrition* Carrington says: "a fast is one of the easiest methods for the cure of alcoholism." I do not subscribe to the explanation he gives of how and why fasting puts an end to alcoholism, but I am satisfied with the foregoing statement as it stands. In his *Encyclopedia of Physical Culture,* Macfadden says: "There is no better method of giving a victim of this disease (alcoholism) an opportunity to again secure control of himself, at least in the beginning of the treatment, than can be suggested by a complete fast."

ALCOHOLISM

Since, apparently, fasting was first used in alcoholism and later employed in other drug addictions, it may be well to begin with a brief study of this addiction. It is now everywhere recognized that the alcoholic is a sick man (or woman), but nowhere, it would seem, is the true nature of the illness recognized. The development of the illness called alcoholism is so insidious that even the most thoughtful become enslaved to a remorseless habit, almost before they are aware of it. Starting the use of alcohol, usually in youth, when the energy reserves of the body are so great that almost any amount of indulgence seems perfectly safe, the habit progresses to a chronic illness that seems hopeless to the helpless inebriate. Fettered by chains of his own forging, weakened in body, mind and will by the very indulgence that he would discontinue, suffering unutterably when he does not take his alcohol, he will often commit crime to get the "relief" he seeks.

The suffering of the alcoholic is so much greater than that which his drinking causes the members of his family that he does not hesitate to spend all his money for more alcohol and let the family suffer for want of food or other necessities. He finds temporary "relief" from his suffering by re-narcotizing himself with alcohol. He may have started drinking to *drown* sorrows that refused to stay *drowned;* he now drinks because he is miserable—a misery induced by his prior drinking—and he finds a fictional surcease from his unutterable misery in more of the narcotic that induced his misery. He is a sick man. He is profoundly enervated. His injured nerves will give him no peace.

When it is recognized that alcoholism is a chronic illness, it will be easy to understand how and why fasting may be of service in the condition. It is a period of rest during which the much abused organism undergoes much-needed adjustments and repairs and recuperates its wasted energies. When the fast is ended and the system has been freed of its accumulated toxins, and what is even more important, the nervous system has been restored to health, the supposed craving for alcohol is no more.

Alcoholism is an illness involving structural abnormalities. The thickening and toughening of the membranes of the mouth, throat and stomach are necessary defensive expediences. Fatty degeneration of the liver or sclerosis of the liver are, of course, later developments. When the alcoholic fasts the thickened membranes are removed and new membranes are formed. The new membrane of the mouth, tongue, throat and stomach will not be a thickened, seared one, impervious alike to foods and poisons, but a thin, delicate and sensitive one that permits full appreciation of the fine delicate flavors of foods.

Glands and nerves that have been lashed into impotency by overstimulation, rest into full functional power when given an opportunity. Renewal of their power can come in no other way. Will nerve energy be restored through rest? Just as certainly as a night of sleep will permit recuperation from the expenditures of the day. The abused organism will heal itself through rest as the broken bone will knit through rest. Do we deny rest to a broken bone, a wound, an ulcer? Do these need other means of healing? Can we deny that restorative cell-action resides within and that it operates best while the body is at rest?

Dewey said that the only remedy for alcoholism is "through a rest from all irritation from other alcoholics or food." He says of fasting in alcoholism: "the fast cure is one of the very easiest after the first three or four days, and even the most desperate old chronics can fast on for two, three or even more weeks with only an increasing sense of comfort, and with no loss except disease and pounds. Was ever a cure for the alcholic disease more rational, more in line with the very laws of nature?" He declared that there are only the fewest cases of chronic alcoholism so desperate, so long continued that a fast will not result in a new stomach, a repaired and renewed nervous system and a new outlook upon life.

Of this new outlook upon life, resulting from the emancipation of the man from his slavery to alcohol and of his renewed health, it may be well to take a brief glance. Dewey said to the alcoholic: "let me presume that for a whole month you have been absent from your homes undergoing the rest (fasting) cure, aided by my encouragement, your homes the while having the 'peace be still' comfort you have not permitted for years. You will return to those homes saner men, and because of your clearer vision and soul power in reserve you will see far more in the countenance of that long suffering wife to love, honor and respect than you really were able to see in your days of food gluttony even before the alcoholic disease.

"And those children, as soon as they find that it is safe to be in the same house with you, will respond to your soul, born again, as the rose unfolds under the favoring conditions of June. It will take them a little time to overcome fear of your attacks of emotional insanity, but in time they will get accustomed to the dazzling light where they have only found darkness and violence. As certainly will this be the result as you comply with the conditions."

Secret *cures* for alcoholism involve the expenditure of hundreds of dollars, weeks of absence from home and work, the introduction into the body of poisons (dangerous drugs) which are often worse than alcohol, and, usually, if not always, failure. The folly of trying to *cure* one poison addiction by resort to another poison should be apparent to all who read these lines. Occasionally the medical profession announces the discovery of a drug that will *cure* alcoholism or other drug addiction. As often as these poison-*cures* for poison-addiction are announced, they fail. Still the merry search for such a magic drug continues.

To the question: How long must I fast for alcoholism, Dewey replies: "Until you get into such comfort of body and mind that fasting will be a luxury. You will fast until there is a perfectly clean tongue and you feel capable of fasting unlimited. You will fast until there is a slight hint that some food of the nourishing kind is craved. Some of you will not get this felicity in less than a month others sooner, and others will require even more time. The time is of no special account when cure is so certain and for such diseases as yours." When the alcoholic has fully recovered from his illness and hunger has returned, no form of alcoholic drink will tempt him and should he attempt to drink some form, he will discover that he no longer "likes" it. It will *bite* and *sting* as it did when he first took it as a youth. He will be a free man again—no longer a slave to King Alcohol.

NICOTINISM

Let us look at tobacco next. Nicotinism, like alcoholism, is a chronic illness that is more or less willfully, although largely ignorantly cultivated. Young people usually begin the use of tobacco because it is "being done." It is the "proper thing." They must be in style, they must conform to the approved usages of the society in which they live and of which they are a part. Being in Rome, they must "do as the Romans do." Poor purblind fools! They know not what chains they are forging for themselves.

All that has been previously said about the use of alcohol, opium, etc., as a means of securing "relief" from uneasiness and distress, applies with full force to the use of tobacco. To chew or snuff, to smoke a pipe, cigar or cigarette, is to "relieve" distress—the distress of profound enervation. It is to re-narcotize the outraged nerves of the user of tobacco, to again cover up or hide from consciousness the true condition of the slave of Lady Nicotine.

Many tobacco-slaves try repeatedly to discontinue the use of the poison, but fail to succeed. They return to the poison-vice rather than endure the irritableness, grouchiness, "nervousness," and uneasiness that the prior use of tobacco has induced. They lack the determination to "tough it out," until the nerves have repaired themselves; they lack the will power to carry through; they are unwilling to bear the suffering, but return again and again to the fictional "relief" offered by another dose of their accustomed poison.

To such as these fasting is a God-send. It makes discontinuing the tobacco-vice easy, almost pleasant. Indeed, in but a few days the very taste of the weed becomes obnoxious. It is no uncommon complaint of the old smoker, after a thorough overhauling, that he cannot get a cigar of the right brand, or that he cannot find a cigarette that he *likes*. The difficulty is not, however, as he thinks, in the tobacco, but in his improved nervous system, and in the regenerated membranes of his mouth and nose. I have seen heavy smokers, who smoked half a life-time, after a fast, become so "sensitive" to the obnoxious fumes of tobacco that the odor of a cigar wafted to their nostrils from a block away was objectionable to them.

COFFEE, TEA, COCOA

It should not be necessary to devote space to coffee, tea, chocolate and cocoa addiction. These poisonous substances (caffeine-containing drugs) are used by many millions of people for the same reasons that tobacco and alcohol are employed—to "relieve" distress. Caffeine is classed as a stimulant and is commonly employed by the enervated and weak to "sustain" them in their work or to keep them awake at night. Stimulation is wasteful of the energy of life, producing enervation. The headache, nervousness, unease, and suffering of the caffeine addict drives him, or her, to more of the same poison that produced his, or her, enervation in the first place.

OTHER POISON HABITS

Other drug habits, such as the opium and morphine habit, the cocaine habit, the chloral habit, etc., are developed in much the same manner and follow much the same course in their development as the tobacco and alcohol habits. First resorted to in our search for "relief" from strain and tension, or from pain, or sleeplessness, or because of our mad search for thrills, the use of these drugs becomes a habit. This damages and enervates the nervous system to such an extent that the user is uneasy, uncomfortable, in pain and distress. He returns to his narcotic as a means of escaping from his intolerable suffering. Drug addiction is a phase of man's *incurable* escapism.

The drug addict uses no more intelligence in his search for "relief" from his exhaustion, unease and actual pain than does the sufferer with the jumping ache of a diseased tooth. His groaning nerves will not permit him to sleep and his distress cries out for "relief."

"Relief" he will have if he has to die to get it. His resort to alcohol or morphine or cocaine or other "relieving" poison is no more a matter of morals than the forceps of the dentist.

OPIUM ADDICTION

The opium and morphine habits are often the result of the use of these drugs by the physician in the treatment of some disease that can be more readily, and certainly more rationally cared for by *Hygienic* measures. The medical profession stands convicted of the crime of producing thousands of drug-addicts. As it pleads guilty to the charge, there seems to be no reason to labor the point. Cocaine using often becomes habitual as a result of using proprietary catarrh "remedies." Chloral and barbiturate addiction is a common result of the use of these drugs for purposes of inducing "sleep" in insomnia. Had the medical profession not taught mankind for ages that poisons are beneficent, these forms of poison addiction would be unknown.

Macfadden's *Encyclopedia of Physical Culture* says: "Fasting is the most valuable of all forms of treatment for overcoming the pathologic condition of the body brought about by the habitual use of poison. Fasting gives the body an opportunity to readjust itself in a normal way and also hastens the elimination of any poison remaining in the system. The drug-fiend has lost his appetite anyway, and by means of a fast will regain a normal condition of the alimentary canal in a fraction of the time that would otherwise be consumed in the process. Especially the mind will clear and gain strength, and he will much sooner find himself in possession of the moral impulse and the will to fight his habit."

The digestive system and the nervous system of the dope addict are somewhat the same as those of the alcohol addict and from the same cause—habitual lashing with poisons. Rest—physical, mental and physiological—is the great need. In a remarkably short time, the fasting patient finds his supposed "craving" for morphine or other poisons, has disappeared. It is, of course, necessary to discontinue the use of the drug. Experience has shown just what we should expect on a priori grounds to be true, namely, that the abrupt withdrawal of all drugs at the very outset is far more satisfactory in the long run than any effort to gradually withdraw it. The "tapering off" process continues the injury and keeps alive the suffering that causes resort to the drug.

Violent *reactions* often follow the withdrawal of the drug. For this reason, it is essential to take great care of the patient. Mania following the withdrawal of morphine or opium, or delirium tremens following the withdrawal of alcohol are similar developments. They indicate the gravity of the injury to the nervous system and reveal how important and urgent is the need to get away from the use of the poison. It is much better, in cases of mania, to completely emerse the body of the patient in warm water for two to three hours, even if he has to be strapped in the tub, until his nerves become quiet, than to resort to even a small dose of the drug. A cold cloth or a cold pack should be placed on the head while the patient is thus emersed in the hot bath.

Bear in mind that these violent *reactions* soon cease as the patient fasts. With the gradual recovery of energy, repair of his damaged nervous system and regeneration of his membranes, the "call" for the "soothing" morphine, chlorate, cocaine, etc., grows so faint that it is easy to discontinue its use. Of the cases of morphinism I have assisted in caring for in this manner, not one, so far as I have learned, has ever returned to its use.

AFTER-CARE OF THE ADDICT

It seems necessary to point out that any return to the prior mode of living, after the fast, will reproduce a state of enervation and toxemia, thus giving rise to more suffering, which may tempt the "relief" seeker to again resort to the old "relief" measure. If he does this, he may again find himself in the grip of addiction. Only by first-class habits of living can any man guarantee himself against evils of all kinds. The eating habits of the former addict are of special importance.

The medical profession now says that drunkenness is a disease. They have not considered it so for any great length of time. On the other hand, the fact that it is a disease has long been recognized in *Hygienic* circles. I take the following statement from A *History of the Vegetarian Movement* by Charles W. Forward, published in London in 1878: "A remarkable instance of success in the treatment of intemperance by means of a vegetarian diet was that of Dr. James C. Jackson, of Dansville, N. Y. Writing in 'The Laws of Life,' Dr. Jackson stated that "it is now twenty-five years since I took the position that drunkenness is a disease arising out of waste of the nerve tissue, oftentimes finding the center of its expression in the solar plexus or network of nerves that lies behind the stomach, and reflecting itself to the brain and spinal column by means of the great sympathetic. Since that time there have been under my care not less than a hundred habitual drunkards, some of them with such a desire for liquor that if they could get it they would keep drunk all the time; others having periodic turns of drunkenness, during the paroxysms of which they would remain drunk for a week or a fortnight at a time. Everyone of these persons was so far gone as to have lost all self-respect, character, and position, and many of them fine estates. In only two instances have I failed to give back good health and sobriety where these individuals have been under my personal management and direction; and of all the agencies that have been brought to bear upon them, save the psychological, none have proved themselves so effective as those of diet and bathing. It is morally and physically impossible for any man to remain a drunkard who can be induced to forego the use of tobacco, tea, coffee, spicy condiments, common salt, flesh meats, and medical drugs. If his diet consists of grains, fruits and vegetables, simply cooked, and he keeps his skin clean, he cannot, for any length of time, retain an appetite for strong drink. The desire dies out of him, and in its stead cooks up a disgust. This disgust is as decidedly moral as it is physical. His better nature revolts at the thought of drinking, and the power in him to resist is strengthened thereby. The proof of this can be seen at any time in our institution, where we have always persons under treatment for inebriety. The testimony is simple, is uniform, is incontrovertible.' And further on, Dr. Jackson declared, 'I have found it impossible to cure drunkards while I allowed them the use of flesh-meats. I regard animal flesh as lying right across the way of restoration. Aside from its nutrition, it contains some element or substance which so excites the nervous system as in the long run to exhaust it, to wear out its tissues, and to render it incapable of normal action.'"

Note that he taught that both flesh and alcohol and other "stimulants" produce enervation—"waste of nervous tissue." Enervation is the basic fact in all addiction and to avoid re-cultivation of a drug addiction, it is essential that the individual so live that he does not enervate himself. While Dr. Jackson, in the foregoing, emphasizes addiction to alcohol, what he says is applicable to any drug addiction. It should also be stated that flesh eating is far from being the only or the greatest enervating factor in the lives of our people.

All sources of enervation should be studiously avoided. A well-nourished body, the energies of which are conserved by first-class habits, will not feel the "need" for stimulants and will not "need" to be "relieved" of discomforts and pains.

Fasting Versus Eliminating Diets

CHAPTER XXXVII

Writing in the *Critique* (Dec. 1931, p. 646-7) Tilden says: "The foregoing may lead to the belief that I am in the habit of advising patients through long periods of fasting. This is not true. I do not believe in the need of long fasts. In years gone by I required of my patients more fasting than I do now. Since having had the opportunity of watching patients individually from the beginning to the end of one or more month's stay with me, I have proved to my entire satisfaction that long fasts are neither necessary nor beneficial, but often do harm." He adds that "very light eating, instead of fasting over a long period of time, brings much better results—with proper nursing, it should be understood."

A statement of this nature, coming from a man of the vast experience of Tilden, is not to be lightly brushed aside. It should reveal to my readers the importance of competent supervision of a fast and the folly of attempting long fasts out of enthusiasm and half-information. That a long fast may prove harmful in some cases is certain and to undertake such a fast without supervision is unwise. I have cared for numerous cases that a long fast was the only thing that brought any genuine improvement; I have seen many more where a long fast would have been dangerous. I have had two patients to die and another to sustain considerable temporary injury because they refused to break their fasts when I advised and persisted in fasting for days after I wanted it broken. A patient who takes the bit in his teeth and runs away with the apple cart in this manner is also almost certain to run into trouble. The practitioner supervising a fast is justified in refusing further responsibility in a case when the patient refuses to follow instructions.

Whoever arbitrarily rules out the long fast thereby cuts himself off from a remarkable means of enabling the body to renovate its tissues. There is also the time factor. It is possible for the body to do for itself in a few weeks of fasting what it will require months and even years to accomplish on limited diets. This is an important factor in the institutional care of a patient who has neither the time nor the money, nor the patience to get well by any long drawn-out process of dieting. The fast will also assure less suffering, more profound body changes and more certainty of success.

There is today much loose talking and writing about fasting by writers and lecturers and doctors who have never conducted and in the majority of instances, never even so much as observed a single fast. These people almost uniformly decry the long fast and advise, not fasting, but various kinds of diets and programs for "detoxication." Just why they insist on calling these programs and these diets, fasting, is difficult to determine.

The "detoxicating" program usually lasts from three days to seven days and consists of taking fruit juices or fruits and, sometimes, vegetable juices. With these go repeated enemas, large quantities of drinking water and purges or laxatives of various kinds. Their whole idea of "elimination" is that of emptying the digestive tract. They know nothing of fasting and its effects. How true are the words of Dr. Rabagliati that "the most popular criticisms of fasting are written by people who have never missed a meal in their lives." The periods of detoxication are arbitrarily limited and bear no necessary relation to the needs or condition of the patient, are seldom of sufficient duration to produce marked benefit, and are often accompanied with such drastic purging that the patient is weakened and made worse. Often the patients are sold machines to extract the juices from their fruits and vegetables and are urged to drink large quantities of juice to "alkalinize" their bodies. Greatly enervated and in need of rest, these patients spend so much time in their kitchens making juices that they wear themselves out and grow worse.

Few doctors of any school know enough about fasting to conduct a fast with confidence. They prefer the eliminating diet in all cases because their ignorance of the superior method is so great. A few of these men succeed in camouflaging their ignorance and inexperience behind the pretense that fasting is dangerous or that the eliminating diet is superior to the fast because it supplies the body with alkaline salts, while the fast depletes the supply of these. Their plausible arguments, based as they are, on half truths, deceive many who are not fully informed about fasting. Then, there are others, who, finding it much easier to get people to go on an eliminating diet than to get them to fast, prefer the eliminating diet.

Dr. T. L. Nichols, an outstanding *Hygienist* of the last century, laid great stress on the importance, in some cases, of what he called the "partial fast." He says: "I have known a case of serious organic disease, which I feared might prove speedily fatal, to be entirely cured by a seven-months fast on one very moderate and very pure meal a day." Following his lead, Dr. Rabagliati of England and Dr. Tilden of this country made frequent use of what Tilden often referred to as the "starvation diet." Indeed, Tilden said that the patient should be fed barely enough to sustain life. Macfadden and his staff also made frequent use of various "partial fasting" regimens. It will be readily recognized that limited feeding of this type constitutes a marked degree of physiological rest for the sick and enervated organism and constitutes a near approach to a complete fast. The student of the matter also knows that the originators of the "partial fasts" or "eliminating diets" did not regard them as *cures.* They knew what they were doing and were not fooled by the ideas that there are *curative* foods. I offer the following reasons why the eliminating diet is preferable to the fast in certain cases:

1. A few patients who know nothing of fasting, or who have been poisoned against it by someone else who knows nothing of fasting, are afraid of the fast. The eliminating diet should be employed in such cases. It frequently happens that after watching others fast and witnessing the results, these fearful ones ask to be permitted to fast but at the outset they refuse to fast.

2. Some patients are so greatly depleted in body that a fast of more than three or four days, or at most a few days, is inadvisable. Such a fast may profitably be followed by an eliminating diet. In such cases an eliminating diet may even include small quantities of proteins, carbohydrates and fats.

3. In mild, acute and in chronic "disease," in children who demand food and cannot be made to understand the reason for fasting and cannot be induced to cooperate with parent and doctor, the eliminating diet is usually very satisfactory.

The eliminating diet is of no value in acute "disease" and should not be employed in acute conditions. It proves to be of value in chronic conditions and following periods of indulgence in the healthy state. In the milder forms of acute "disease," such as the common cold, an eliminating diet may be used, although it is not as satisfactory as the fast. An eliminating diet (an orange or grapefruit diet) may also be used in boils and similar disturbances. Such a diet may also be employed in acute diarrhea, although the fast is far superior in such cases.

It sometimes happens that a patient is placed upon an eliminating diet and upon the second, third or fourth day, a crisis develops, just as occurs in many instances during the fast, and feeding must be discontinued. As in the fast, these crises are seen in toxic individuals. They are cleaning-out processes. In such cases the fast should have been instituted from the beginning. There are many cases of chronic "disease" in which the elminating diet proves to be of but little value. These patients make almost no improvement until they are placed upon a fast. I once cared for a lady, who, before coming to me, could not eat any food but meat, without great distress. Fruits and vegetables caused pain and distress and passed out in the stools as they were swallowed, having undergone no digestion. After a fast of eleven days, this patient could eat certain fruits and vegetables and juices, and digest them. Her progress, however, was very slow and at the time she passed from under my care she was able to take but a limited variety of foods. Her troubles had existed for over twenty years and there had been an abdominal operation and a permanent suppression of menstruation by means of the X-ray. We anticipate slow recoveries in such cases.

I see many cases of "nervous indigestion" of long standing, in which rational feeding and eliminating diets are not possible, until after a fast has prepared the way for these. The doctor who rejects fasting cuts himself off from a method that would spell certain success in many cases in which the eliminating diet means certain failure. The patient who rejects fasting often dooms himself to continued invalidism. I am proving these things every day by employing the fast, with the most happy results, in cases that several doctors have placed upon eliminating diets and failed to bring about even slight improvement.

John W. Armstrong, of England, after sixteen years of experience with fasting, says that "any attempt to tone down the principles of correct fasting, (by 'the attempts,' often successful, 'to cure disease by fasting' on the juices of fruits and water, or by vegetable juices and water) often disappoints both the faster and his advisers, and, those numerous 'failures,' merely illustrate the folly of raking ground that urgently requires not a stirring-up but a good downright prolonged system of digging." He adds that to anyone who has had opportunity to observe numerous cases on a fast and on light diets, it is very apparent that the patient progresses much better on the fast and that the body frequently protests vigorously against even the ingestion of fruit juices. He lists angina pectoris and other forms of heart trouble, most forms of rheumatism, influenza, phlebitis, dropsy, jaundice, eczema, psoriasis, and diabetes as among conditions in which this is especially noticeable. "The chronic, so-called incurable forms of disease," he says, "can—and mostly do—continue to flourish upon even so light a diet as fruit juice, not to mention whole fruits, milk, and fresh meat."

4. Some patients are compelled to continue with their work. While long fasts have been taken by both mental and physical workers who continued their activities during the fast, this is not advisable, particularly, if there is any strain connected with the mental work, or if the physical work is heavy. A short fast is easily possible for people who must continue their work. This may then be followed by an eliminating diet. Not everyone, however, can take a short fast and continue working. In such cases the eliminating diet is very convenient.

It is worthy of note that fasting is usually much easier than restricted diets. The fast produces less discomfort and the fasting patient is often the stronger of the two. Sinclair says that again and again he tried light fruit meals, "but with always the same result: the light meals are just enough to keep me ravenously hungry, and inevitably I found myself eating more and more." He also says that on the "fruit fasts" he found that he "could live on nothing but fruit for several days, but I would get so weak that I could not stand up—far weaker than I ever have become on an out-and-out fast." These experiences of Sinclair agree with my own. The fasting patient soon loses all desire for food—the patient eating an eliminating diet does not lose his appetite but does not eat enough to satisfy it; so, he is always hungry. I do not know how to explain why the patient on an eliminating diet is so often weaker than the fasting patient, but it is a fact I frequently observe.

During World War II, the Army Air Force conducted a series of experiments in the Gulf of Mexico, to aid them in solving problems connected with survival at sea. Men were put out in liferafts and permitted to remain on these for several days under all the weather conditions they were likely to encounter in the event they were forced down at sea. Each day they were taken aboard ship for examinations and tests. One 38-year old officer went without food and water for four days, also refraining from smoking during this period. He is said to have "felt no ill effects," while, the account adds, "Others on short rations, suffered more." The fact that the faster suffered less than those on short rations is no surprise to those of us who are experienced with fasting.

5. In many cases it is necessary to treat the family and friends more than the patient. In many cases where a fast is plainly needed and would be of the greatest good it is impossible to get the patient to fast, because of the unreasoning and uninformed opposition of the other members of the family and from the patient's immediate friends.

Even should the patient attempt to fast despite this opposition, those around him keep him so upset and disturbed that he is harmed more than helped. Unless this patient can be cared for away from the influence of family and friends, the eliminating diet will prove more practical, even if inferior. In institutional work, where patients often come long distances and can be away from their work or business for only a limited time, or have but limited funds, they must get results as speedily as possible. They cannot spend months or years at the institution.

Results may be achieved by fasting that can be achieved in no other way and results may be achieved in less time by fasting than by any other method. If only those who know nothing of fasting would let it alone! Was it not Ingersol who prayed to God to take care of his friends, saying he could take care of his enemies?

FOOD CURES

Diet *cures* are quite popular at this time and are now exploited from the housetops by all and sundry. There are "grape *cures*," "lemon *cures*," "orange *cures*," "onion *cures*," "garlic *cures*," and similar *cures*, galore. Juices of all kinds—vegetable juices and fruit juices—simple, mixed (compounded) in every conceivable manner, are urged upon the sick as *cures* for almost all the ills flesh is subject to. Food extracts, food concentrates, vitamin preparations, gland extracts, food pills, food powders, and other food-derived imitations of the products of the pharmaceutical houses are sold at big profits to a credulous and *cure*-deluded people.

Practically all parts and tissues of the body are bathed in a solution of food and oxygen constantly renewed—the blood and lymph—which yields to functioning organs and growing tissues the elements needed by them to sustain their special actions and support their growth. Every functional act and every process of repair and growth is a local demand on the whole resources of the system. The organ or tissue is local, the supply is general and mobile. The blood, if normal, contains ample resources to sustain alike all parts and all functions of the body. Healthy individuals find no difficulty in deriving nutritive support for all the organs and functions of their bodies from the same food. This means that ordinary natural foods contain ample diversity for all needs and that special foods are not required to support special functions or particular organs. If these foods are adequate for the healthy, they are equally adequate for the unhealthy and special foods to support weakened powers are of slight value. The present feeding plans seek specific foods for special organs or for "specific diseases" in the same way the old drugging plan sought specific drugs for special organs or for "specific diseases."

Food *cures* are based on two half-truths. Some of them are based on the notion that the sick body is full of acids and that alkaline foods must be supplied to neutralize the acids. Foods rich in bases are prescribed for this purpose and it is usual to urge their use in large quantities. Two fallacies are involved in this theory and practice. It is not true that the sick body is full of acids. It is true that the cell wastes are all acid and acid fermentation-products do get into the body from the digestive tract. But the body will not tolerate acids for a second. They are immediately "bound" with alkalies and neutralized. The other fallacy is the belief that the body utilizes food elements in proportion to the amount ingested. This is not true. Forcing large quantities of alkalies into the body does not assure their utilization. Indeed, one may be positive that the sick body will not be able to utilize them. Only a healthy body, possessed of full nerve force, is capable of properly digesting and assimilating foods. To overfeed the sick body on certain elements does not restore health.

DEFICIENCIES

The other half-truth upon which diet *cures* are based is that "diseases" are due to nutritive deficiencies, and *cure* follows an ade-

-469-

quate supply of the deficient element or elements. Efforts to meet this requirement may take the form of drinking large quantities of juices or of using food concentrates—substances rich in minerals or vitamins. All over America the gum-willis are talking "deficiency" to the people and all over America there are millions of people who are living testimonials to the failure of the theory and the practices built thereon. This is not to deny that deficiencies exist; rather, it is to point out that most deficiencies are due to failure of assimilation and can be corrected only by removing the causes that have impaired the nutritive processes. Enervation and toxemia and the mental and physical habits that are responsible for these are the chief causes of deficiency.

There are deficiencies, but they are almost never primary. Constitutional impairment—enervation and toxemia—is prior to the appearance of the nutritional imbalance. The toxic state is the large factor and the mineral and vitamin deficiencies are secondary to this. The truth of this is strikingly revealed in anemia, where the deficiency theory and the feeding practices based thereon are failures. Care that eliminates the toxemia is followed by immediate and marked improvement in the blood without any food at all, except water, being given. Goitre also presents a striking demonstration of this fact. Care based on the "deficiency" theory is a failure. Care based on the toxemia theory is a success.

The great object to be achieved is the elimination of toxins. Nothing more effectively promotes the elimination of toxins than a fast coupled with rest. No "eliminative" or "curative" diet can equal the fast for this purpose. Here is a true story of a woman who was cared for in the Health School. Among her troubles were brittle and corrugated finger nails. She had been assured that this trouble was due to calcium deficiency and for some time before coming to the Health School had been faithfully swallowing the calcium preparations that were prescribed for her. She was also using other food preparations that were prescribed for her. Nonetheless her nail condition grew worse instead of better. At the Health School she underwent a lengthy fast during which her nails completely recovered, so that when she left here all traces of the former difficulty had disappeared.

LESS FOOD BETTER
Writing in *Physical Culture*, May, 1915, Dortch Campbell says: "There is nothing that can be found as an actual substitute for fast-

ing, nothing which will give the full benefits of the fast." He is discussing various types of eliminating diets for those who "cannot fast." Among these diets, he mentions the grape diet, the apple diet, the tomato diet, the milk diet, etc. He says: "I am inclined to the opinion, however, that there are better fruits than grapes that may be used. An exclusive apple diet is superior, an exclusive orange diet more so because there is little nourishment in oranges. An exclusive tomato diet answers the same purpose."

The principle here expressed, that the diet gives better results as it approaches a fast, agrees perfectly with my experience in the matter. Not only is it true that the less "value" the food possesses, the more good the patient derives from its use, but it is also true that the less the patient takes of the food and the more nearly he fasts, the more rapidly he recovers. Tilden fed diluted fruit juices for an extended period and came to the same conclusion.

Fruit diets, vegetable diets, juice diets, mono-diets, etc., are valuable in the degree to which they reduce the amount of food daily ingested. Their value increases as the total amount of food eaten daily diminishes. The nearer one approaches a complete fast the more good one derives from his "curative" diet. In an article written a short time before his death and published posthumously in the October, 1940 *Review and Critique*, Dr. Tilden says: "How do fruits prevent clogging of the liver, kidney, and skin? By not causing clogging of these organs. Certainly not through eliminating properties—medicinal qualities. No! Nature eliminates, when given an opportunity. Clogging comes from ringing the changes on bread, meat, potatoes, puddings, pies, and coffee, until the body is burdened with waste. A fruit diet allows nature to work in an almost unobstructed manner. Every particle of fruit taken when the body is replete hinders elimination. This being true (and I have proved it daily for years in actual practice), then fruit does not assist elimination, except by its absence. When used, it has less influence than the other foods in preventing elimination." Consuming large quantities of juice water-logs the tissues and overworks the kidneys. The less juice ingested, the more rapidly the sick person improves.

A fast is more effective than any form of diet; not because fasting *cures* for it does nothing of the kind, but because it affords the body full opportunity for house-cleaning. The sick man is not so much in need of ingestion as he is of excretion. His body is already overloaded. More often than otherwise he is suffering from nutritive redundancy. Abstinence, or partial abstinence alone, can save him. In many cases of chronic illness it is not necessary to undergo a long fast, a short fast, or a series of short fasts to obtain the desired results. However, the most salutary effects of cutting down the food intake are best obtained by fasting. All that is needed in some cases is to cut down the total quantity of food consumed and of the proteins and starches in particular. But, even in these cases, the results obtained are never as far-reaching as those obtained while fasting. The reason for this will be evident to those who have mentally digested and assimilated the chapter on the rejuvenating effects of the fast.

That many do obtain relief from symptoms by the use of these various diets is not to be questioned. For, at their worst, they are usually better than the diet customarily eaten and their use usually means less gluttony, at least, for a while. But the man of experience is well aware that full health is almost never achieved, that the effects of the diets are never as profound and far-reaching as those of fasting and that the diets almost never achieve their results in as short space of time as does the fast. Using foods to *cure,* instead of removing the causes of disease and using foods to nourish the body, is fundamentally as unsound as using drugs to *cure.* Foods do not *cure.* Until we have discarded our faith in *cures,* there can be no intelligent approach to the problems presented by suffering and no proper use of foods by those who are ill.

I am not content with half-way measures. I have seen them fail too often, where a subsequent fast brought speedy results, to be fooled by the claims of the inexperienced and poorly informed. In many cases, failure has been so marked that the patient has been permanently soured upon the whole idea of fasting. In thus drawing a contrast between fasting and the eliminating diet, and pointing out the many limitations of the latter, I do not wish to appear to minimize its value. The eliminating diet is extremely important and no doctor, who does not fully understand the application of such a diet, is fully equipped to serve all patients who may consult him. He is seriously handicapped just as is the man who does not have a thorough working knowledge of fasting. The reader should refer to Volume II of this series for a full presentation of the eliminating diet.

CPSIA information can be obtained
at www.ICGtesting.com
Printed in the USA
BVHW082226130919
558287BV00001B/73/P